Cardiovascular System

Thomas F. Lüscher · Ulf Landmesser
(Editors)

Cardiovascular System

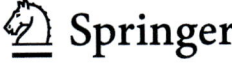

Editors
Thomas F. Lüscher
Center for Molecular Cardiology
University of Zurich
Schlieren - Zurich, Switzerland

Ulf Landmesser
Department of Cardiology
Charité – University Medicine Berlin
Berlin, Germany

ISBN 978-3-662-70151-5   ISBN 978-3-662-70152-2   (eBook)
https://doi.org/10.1007/978-3-662-70152-2

Translation from the German language edition: "Herz-Kreislauf" by Thomas F. Lüscher and Ulf Landmesser, © Der/die Herausgeber bzw. der/die Autor(en), exklusiv lizenziert an Springer-Verlag GmbH, DE, ein Teil von Springer Nature 2024. Published by Springer Berlin Heidelberg. All Rights Reserved.

This book is a translation of the original German edition "Herz-Kreislauf," 3rd edition, by Thomas F. Lüscher and Ulf Landmesser, published by Springer-Verlag GmbH, DE in 2024. The translation was done with the help of an artificial intelligence machine translation tool. A subsequent human revision was done primarily in terms of content, so that the book will read stylistically differently from a conventional translation. Springer Nature works continuously to further the development of tools for the production of books and on the related technologies to support the authors.

© The Editor(s) (if applicable) and The Author(s), under exclusive license to Springer-Verlag GmbH, DE, part of Springer Nature 2025.

This work is subject to copyright. All rights are solely and exclusively licensed by the Publisher, whether the whole or part of the material is concerned, specifically the rights of translation, reprinting, reuse of illustrations, recitation, broadcasting, reproduction on microfilms or in any other physical way, and transmission or information storage and retrieval, electronic adaptation, computer software, or by similar or dissimilar methodology now known or hereafter developed.
The use of general descriptive names, registered names, trademarks, service marks, etc. in this publication does not imply, even in the absence of a specific statement, that such names are exempt from the relevant protective laws and regulations and therefore free for general use.
The publisher, the authors and the editors are safe to assume that the advice and information in this book are believed to be true and accurate at the date of publication. Neither the publisher nor the authors or the editors give a warranty, expressed or implied, with respect to the material contained herein or for any errors or omissions that may have been made. The publisher remains neutral with regard to jurisdictional claims in published maps and institutional affiliations.

This Springer imprint is published by the registered company Springer-Verlag GmbH, DE, part of Springer Nature.
The registered company address is: Heidelberger Platz 3, 14197 Berlin, Germany

If disposing of this product, please recycle the paper.

Preface to the 3rd Edition

Cardiovascular diseases continue to be, especially in Western countries, the most common cause of illness and premature death. Accordingly, this group of diseases must receive significant attention at Medical School and during postgraduate training. In addition to their frequency, this group of diseases also plays an important role due to their variety and complexity and their severe complications and often fatal outcome. Therefore, students, senior house officers and fellows in training must understand the basic principles of their pathophysiology as well as recognize their typical symptoms and master the use of their diagnostics well as the major principles of their management. Due to their high incidence, such a basic knowledge is essentiel for all doctors and their patients, regardless of their later specialization.

The booklet aims to convey this basic knowledge to students, senior house officers and fellows in training in a concise and clear manner and indeed has enjoyed great popularity among readers with its first two editions. Now the module appears in a revised and expanded English edition ers to expand its reach worldwide. The booklet provides in a nutshell structured and richly illustrated figures of the disease phenotypes with tables, algorithms, and key points for the diagnosis and management of the most important cardiovascular conditions.

The current English edition includes all recent developments in the understanding, diagnosis and management of cardiovascular diseases. On the most common cardiovascular conditions. To that end, we have invited a number of highly experienced authors and experts for the respective conditions to assure that u the chapters are in line the latest findings. In doing so, we have focused the chapters on the essentials to provide students and trainees with the information they absolutely need for their exams and later for their clinical practice. Simple algorithms are intended to help in practice to easily diagnose the most important cardiovascular diseases and to memorize the most important diagnostic and therapeutic steps.

We sincerely hope that with the this booklet on Cardiovascular Diseasese, we can provide the students, Senior house officers and fellows in training , with the necessary knowledge they need for their studies in medicine and training in cardiology and their further professional development.

Thomas F.Lüscher
Ulf Landmesser
Zurich and Berlin
30 May 2023

Contents

1	**Anatomy and Physiology of the Cardiovascular System** .... 1 Thomas F. Lüscher and Ulf Landmesser	
2	**Cardiological Diagnostics** .... 11 Gerald Maurer and Christian Schmied	
3	**Epidemiology and Prevention** .... 33 Martin Halle and Thomas Münzel	
4	**Arterial Hypertension** .... 49 Felix Mahfoud, Roland Schmieder and Thomas F. Lüscher	
5	**Pulmonary Hypertension** .... 61 Irene M. Lang and Stephan Rosenkranz	
6	**Diabetes Mellitus** .... 77 Roger Lehmann and Nikolaus Marx	
7	**Atherosclerosis and Sequelae** .... 89 Andreas Zirlik and Ronald K. Binder	
8	**Myocardial Diseases** .... 121 Benjamin Meder and Urs Eriksson	
9	**Valvular Heart Diseases** .... 145 Christian Hengstenberg, Thomas Pilgrim, Philipp Bartko, Fabien Praz, Georg Goliasch and Stephan Windecker	
10	**Endocardial Diseases** .... 171 Alexander Lauten and Thomas F. Lüscher	
11	**Pericardial Diseases** .... 185 Thomas F. Lüscher, Matthias Greutmann and Jan Steffel	
12	**Conduction System Diseases—Cardiac Arrhythmias** .... 193 Jan Steffel and Thomas F. Lüscher	
13	**Heart Failure** .... 223 Bettina Heidecker and Otmar Pfister	
14	**Congenital Heart Defects** .... 241 Helmut Baumgartner and Gerhard-Paul Diller	

15 **Aortic Diseases** 255
    Martin Czerny and Christoph Nienaber

16 **Tumors of the Cardiovascular System** 265
    Tatiana Manuylova and Karin Klingel

17 **Diseases of the Venous System** 273
    Christine Espinola-Klein and Stavros Konstantinides

Editors and Contributors

About the Editors

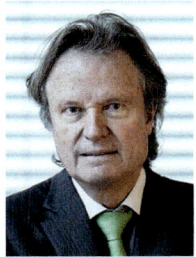

Prof. Dr. Thomas F. Lüscher MD, FRCP, FESC

Thomas F. Lüscher studied medicine at the University of Zurich and received his training as a specialist in internal medicine, clinical pharmacology, and cardiology at the University of Zurich, the Mayo Clinic in Rochester, Minnesota, USA, and the University of Basel.

From 1992 to 1994, he was a professor of pharmacotherapy at the University and University Hospitals of Basel, then for 4 years a professor and deputy clinical director of cardiology at the Inselspital and the University of Bern, and in 1996 he was appointed professor of cardiology and director of the department and later the clinic for cardiology at the University Hospital Zurich, as well as head of cardiovascular research at the Institute of Physiology of the University of Zurich.

Professor Lüscher founded and led the University Heart Center in Zurich until 2017 and then moved as Consultant and Director for Research, Education and Development to the Royal Brompton and Harefield Hospitals and to Imperial College and King's College in London in the United Kingdom. Professor Lüscher is active as a clinical and interventional cardiologist and as a researcher with a particular interest in endothelial function, lipids, hypertension, atherosclerosis, acute coronary syndrome, and heart failure. He is among the most cited scientists worldwide and has received numerous research awards. From 2009 to 2020, he was Editor-in-Chief of the *European Heart Journal* and continues to be the editor of the *ESC Textbook of Cardiovascular Medicine*. Additionally, he is President of the *European Society of Cardiology*.

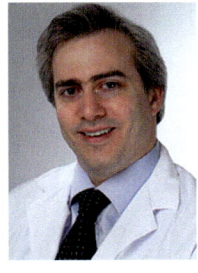

Univ.-Prof. Dr. med. Ulf Landmesser

*24 November 1970 in Dresden

Professor Ulf Landmesser has been the Director of the Clinic for Cardiology, Angiology, and Intensive Care Medicine, Campus Benjamin Franklin of the German Heart Center of the Charité (until 12/2022 Clinic for Cardiology at the Charité – Universitätsmedizin Berlin) since 2014 and since January 2023, he has been the Division Head of the German Heart Center of the Charité (DHZC).

After his medical studies at the Hannover Medical School, the University of Connecticut in Farmington (USA), and the National Heart & Lung Institute in London, he specialized in internal medicine and cardiology at the Hannover Medical School. In 2000/2001, he worked as a fellow of the Alexander von Humboldt Foundation at the Department of Cardiology of the Emory University School of Medicine, Atlanta (USA), and received the Outstanding Fellows in Cardiology Special Recognition

Award. In 2007, he was appointed as a senior cardiologist with a focus on acute and interventional cardiology and as the head of translational cardiovascular research at the Clinic for Cardiology of the University Hospital Zurich (Switzerland), where he later served as deputy director and professor at the Clinic for Cardiology. In 2012, he received the Götz Award, the official prize of the Medical Faculty of the University of Zurich in the field of cardiovascular prevention.

From 2009 to 2020, Professor Landmesser was Deputy Editor of the *European Heart Journal*, the leading cardiovascular journal in Europe. He has a particular research interest in the translational and clinical development of new personalized management and therapy strategies for cardiovascular diseases, with a focus on coronary heart disease. Furthermore, he is the scientific director of the Friede Springer-Cardiovascular Prevention Center @ Charité, founded in 2022.

About the Authors

Philipp Bartko Clinical Division of Cardiology, University Department of Internal Medicine II, Medical University Vienna, Vienna, Austria

Prof. Dr. med. Helmut Baumgartner Department of Cardiology III: Congenital and Valvular Heart Diseases, University Hospital, Munster, Germany

Primarius Priv.-Doz. Dr. Ronald K. Binder Department of Internal Medicine II, Cardiology and Intensive Care, Wels-Grieskirchen Hospital, Wels, Austria

Prof. Dr. Martin Czerny University Heart Center Freiburg • Bad Krozingen, Department of Cardiovascular Surgery, Albert-Ludwigs-University Freiburg, Freiburg im Breisgau, Germany

Prof. Dr. med. Gerhard-Paul Diller Department of Cardiology III: Congenital and Valvular Heart Diseases, University Hospital, Munster, Germany

Prof. Dr. med. Urs Eriksson MD, MSc ETH, FESC, FHFADepartement of Internal Medicine, Regional Hospital Wetzikon, Wetzikon, Switzerland

Univ.-Prof. Dr. Christine Espinola-Klein Department of Cardiology III-Angiology, Cardiology Center, University Medicine Mainz, Mainz, Germany

Georg Goliasch Clinical Division of Cardiology, Department on Internal Medicine III, University Hospital, Vienna, Austria

Prof. Dr. med. Matthias Greutmann Department of Cardiology and University Heart Center, University Hospital Zurich, Zurich, Switzerland

Editors and Contributors

Univ.-Prof. Dr. med. Martin Halle Preventive and Sports Medicine and Sports Cardiology, University Hospital rechts der Isar, Technical University Munich, Munich, Germany

PD Dr. Bettina Heidecker Department of Cardiology, German Heart Center Charité – University Medicine Berlin, Berlin, Germany

Prof. Dr. Christian Hengstenberg Division of Clinical Cardiology, Department of Internal Medicine II, University Hospital, Vienna, Austria

Prof. Dr. med. Karin Klingel Cardiopathology, Institute of Pathology and Neuropathology, University Hospital Tubingen, Tubingen, Germany

Univ.-Prof. Dr. Stavros Konstantinides Center for Thrombosis and Hemostasis, University Medicine Mainz, Mainz, Germany

Prof. Dr. med. Ulf Landmesser Department of Cardiology, Charité – University Medicine Berlin, Berlin, Germany

Prof. Dr. med. Irene M. Lang Clinical Division of Cardiology, Department of Internal Medicine II, Medical University Vienna, Vienna, Austria

Prof. Dr. Alexander Lauten Department for General and Interventional Cardiology and Rhythmology, Helios Klinikum, Erfurt, Germany

Prof. Dr. Roger Lehmann Department of Endokrinology, Diabetology and Clinical Nutrition, University Hospital, Switzerland, Zurich

Prof. Dr. med. Thomas F. Lüscher Heart Division, Royal Brompton and Harefield Hospitals GSTT, King's College and Imperial College, London, United Kingdom

Prof. Dr. med. Felix Mahfoud Department of Cardiology, University Heart Center Basel, University Hospital Basel, Basel, Switzerland

Dr. Tatiana Manuylova Cardiopathology, Institut for Pathology and Neuropathology, University Hospital, Tubingen, Germany

Univ.-Prof. Dr. med. Nikolaus Marx Department of Internal Medicine I – Cardiology, Angiology and Intensive Care, University Hospital Aachen, Aachen, Germany

Prof. Dr. med. Gerald Maurer Medical University Vienna, Vienna, Austria

Prof. Dr. med. Benjamin Meder FESC, RSMInstitut for Cardiomyopathies, Department of Cardiology, Angiology and Pneumology, Medical University Hospital, Heidelberg, Germany

Prof. Dr. Thomas Münzel Center for Cardiology, Cardiology I, University Medicine Mainz, Johannes Gutenberg-University, Mainz, Germany

Prof. Dr. med. Christoph Nienaber Heart Division, Royal Brompton Hospital, London, United Kingdom

Professor Otmar Pfister Department of Cardiology, University Heart Center Basel, University Hospital Basel, Basel, Switzerland

Thomas Pilgrim Deaprtment for Cardiology, University Hospital (Inselspital) Bern, Bern, Switzerland

Fabien Praz Department of Cardiology, University Hospital (Inselspital) Bern, Bern, Switzerland

Prof. Dr. med. Stephan Rosenkranz Department of Internal Medicine III Cardiology, Heart Center, University Hospital Cologne, Cologne, Germany

Prof. Dr. med. Christian Schmied Cardiology, Clinic Im Park, Zürich, Switzerland

Prof. Dr. med. Roland Schmieder Department of Nephrology and Hypertension, Friedrich-Alexander-University Erlangen-Nürnberg, Erlangen, Germany

Prof. Dr. med. Jan Steffel Elektrophysiology, Hirslanden Hospital and Klinik im Park, Zürich, Switzerland

Prof. Dr. Stephan Windecker Department of Cardiology, University Hospital (Inselspital) Bern, Bern, Switzerland

Univ. Prof. Dr. Andreas Zirlik University Heart Center Graz – Division of Cardiology, Medical University Graz and LKH-University Hospital Graz, Graz, Austria

Anatomy and Physiology of the Cardiovascular System

Thomas F. Lüscher and Ulf Landmesser

Contents

1.1 Anatomical Structure of the Heart – 3

1.2 Excitation Formation and Conduction – 4

1.3 Mechanics of the Heart Action and Hemodynamics – 4

1.4 Blood Supply of the Heart Muscle – 5

1.5 Peripheral Circulation and Blood Distribution – 8

Earlier versions were created with the collaboration of Jan Steffel and Christoph Wyss.

© The Author(s), under exclusive license to Springer-Verlag GmbH, DE, part of Springer Nature 2025
T. F. Lüscher and U. Landmesser (eds.), *Cardiovascular System*,
https://doi.org/10.1007/978-3-662-70152-2_1

The anatomy and physiology of the cardiovascular system are fundamentally covered in the preclinical studies and textbooks and are only briefly reviewed in this textbook. For more in depth studies, please refer to the textbooks of anatomy and physiology.

Humans have two circulatory systems, i.e. a high-pressure system (referred to as the arterial circulation) and a low-pressure system (referred to as the venous circulation), each with separate cardiac chambers or "pumps" (◘ Fig. 1.1). This include an atrium and a ventricle on the right side (low-pressure system with predominantly low oxygen content) and the left side (high-pressure system with high oxygen content), each separated by four heart valves that allow blood flow in only one direction.

The **right side of the heart** consists of the right atrium and right ventricle, which pumps blood with relatively low pressure (mean pressure: ~15 mmHg) through the **pulmonary circulation** to allow for gas exchange in the lungs, from where it flows to the left side of the heart, i.e. the left atrium.

The **left side of the heart** (consisting of the left atrium and left ventricle) pumps the now oxygen-rich blood through the **systemic circulation**, which supplies the individual organs with oxygen, requiring a significantly higher pressure (mean arterial pressure: ~85 mmHg). As the blood flows through the smaller arteries and arterioles, the pressure decreases due to the increasing distance from the heart and the increase in the total vascular diameter, so that in the capillaries of the organs, there is only a mean pressure of ~20 mmHg, which further drops to about 5 mmHg in the venules and veins (◘ Fig. 1.6).

The **high-pressure system** includes the left heart, the large arteries, and arterioles starting from the left ventricle. The **low-pressure system**, in which the blood

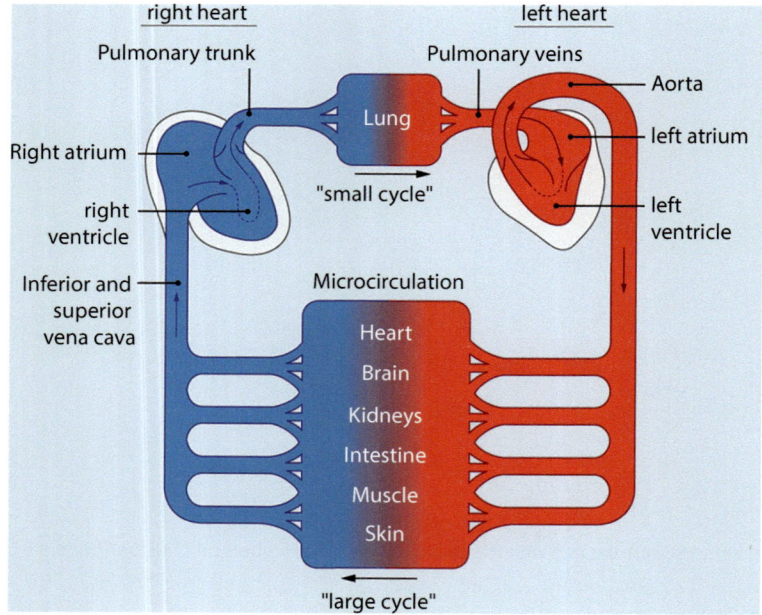

◘ **Fig. 1.1** Diagram of the arterial and venous circulatory system. (From Zilles/Tillmann, Anatomy, Springer 2010)

flows back to the right heart, consists of capillaries, venules, the right atrium and ventricle, as well as the pulmonary circulation and the left atrium.

> All blood vessels that lead blood away from the heart are called arteries, and all blood vessels that bring blood back from the organs to the heart are called veins. This nomenclature is independent of the respective oxygen content of the blood.

1.1 Anatomical Structure of the Heart

The heart is a hollow muscle (◘ Fig. 1.2) composed of various tissues: Inside, it is lined with endothelium (the so-called endocardium), in the middle, the actual heart muscle (myocardium) follows. On the outside, the heart is surrounded by nourishing connective tissue with fat pads and vessels (epicardium) as well as a serosa (pericardium). The entire organ is enclosed in a skin (pericardial sac), which is serous on the inside and contains connective tissue on the outside and normally contains no or only a small amount of fluid.

Each half of the heart is divided into an atrial chamber (atrium) and a ventricular chamber (ventricle): The human heart is thus a 4-chambered hollow organ. The heart has 4 heart valves that function and allow blood flow in only one direction. The atrioventricular valves are located between the atrium and ventricle (atrioventricular valves), the semilunar valves (semilunar valves) between the ventricle and the respective circulatory system.

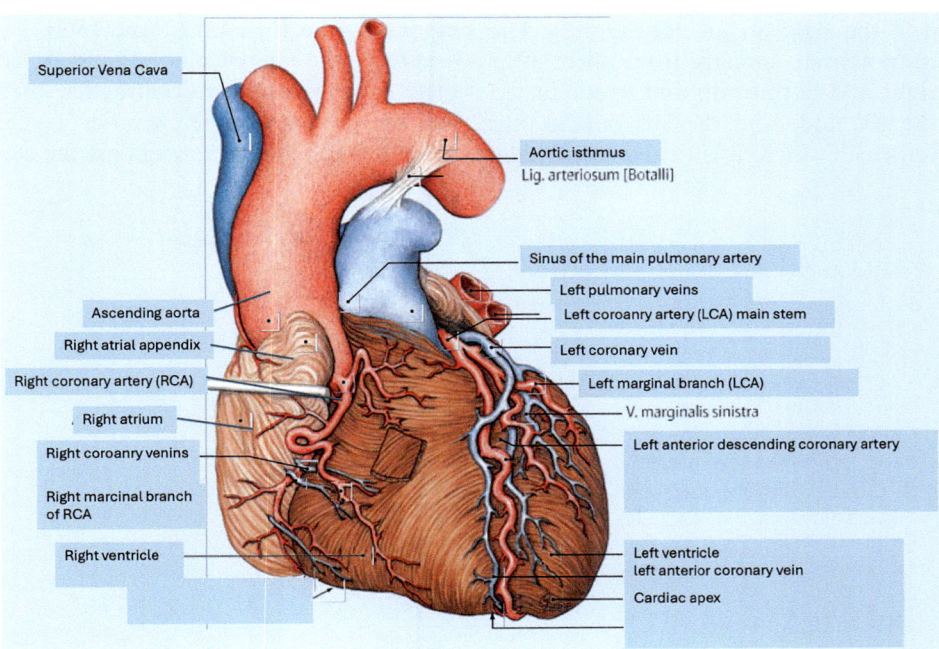

◘ Fig. 1.2 Structure and blood flow of the human heart and the major vessels. (From Zilles/Tillmann, Anatomy, Springer 2010)

- The atrioventricular valve of the left heart is bicuspid and is called the **mitral valve** (named after the liturgic headdress of bishops, the "mitra"; Sects. 9.3 and 9.4).
- The atrioventricular valve of the right heart is tricuspid and is accordingly called the **tricuspid valve** (▶ Sect. 9.5).
- The semilunar valves separating the ventricles from the major vessels are called the **aortic valve** (▶ Sect. 9.1 and 9.2) in the left heart and **pulmonary valve** in the right one, corresponding to the vessel into which they open.

1.2 Excitation Formation and Conduction

The heart contracts regularly with a basic frequency of 50–80 beats/min. Under physiological conditions, the action potential originates in the sinus node, which is located in the right atrium (◘ Fig. 1.3). The action potential spreads from there over the right and left atrium and is conducted via the AV node and the His bundle into the ventricles, where it is further conducted via the Tawara branches and Purkinje fibers into the working myocardium of the right and left ventricles. The repolarization of the myocardium occurs from the apex of the heart to the base and from epicardial to endocardial (▶ Sect. 12.1).

1.3 Mechanics of the Heart Action and Hemodynamics

The cardiac cycle is divided into several phases (◘ Fig. 1.4). The main part of the **filling of the ventricles** from the atria is achieved by the valve plane mechanism, i.e., the successive basal and apical displacement of the valve plane and the associated suction effect. Furthermore, towards the end of the electrical diastole, the atria contract (= atrial systole and ventricular diastole) and normally contribute to the filling of the ventricles (about 25–30% of the ventricular filling) (for changes in cardiac diseases see ▶ Sect. 12.4, 12.5 and 13.2).

Once the ventricular filling is complete, the **ventricular contraction** begins and the pressure in the chamber increases. Since this initially occurs against the closed

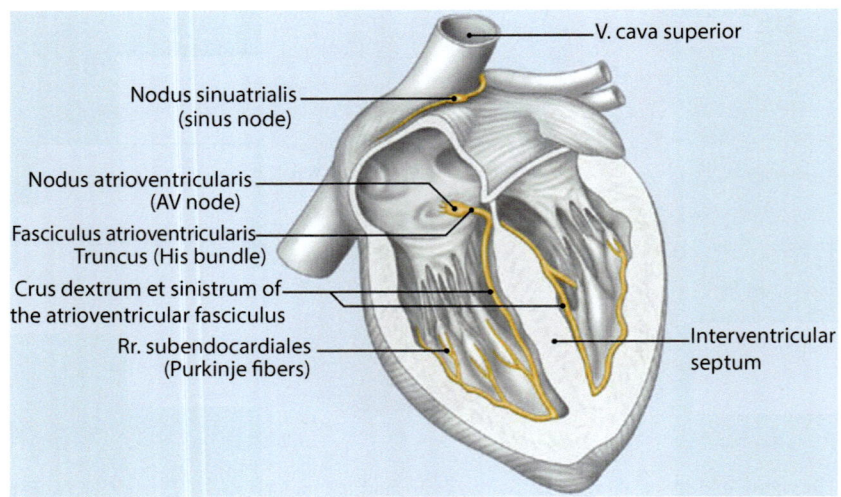

◘ **Fig. 1.3** Excitation formation and conduction system of the human heart. (From Zilles/Tillmann, Anatomy, Springer 2010)

semilunar valve, the first part of the contraction is also referred to as the **isovolumetric contraction phase**. If the pressure in the ventricle exceeds that of the subsequent large vessel, the semilunar valves open and the **ejection phase** begins. At the end of the ejection phase, the tension of the ventricular myocardium decreases again and the pressure in the ventricle drops. If the ventricular pressure falls below the pressure of the subsequent large vessel (aorta or pulmonary artery), the semilunar valves close. This is followed by the **isovolumetric relaxation phase**, which lasts until the ventricular pressure falls below the pressure of the respective atrium, causing the atrioventricular valves to open and the ventricles to fill again.

The pressure values of the left ventricle are several times higher than those of the right ventricle, corresponding to the higher resistance of the systemic circulation. The physiological hemodynamic normal values are given in ◘ Table 1.1. These change significantly in cardiovascular diseases such as arterial hypertension (see also ▶ Chap. 4 arterial), pulmonary hypertension (Sects. 5.1 and 5.2), cardiomyopathies (▶ Sect. 8.1) and heart failure (▶ Sect. 13.1).

The **cardiac output** (CO) is calculated from the product of stroke volume (SV) and heart rate and indicates the amount of blood that is pumped through the circulatory system per minute (normal: 4.5–5 L/min, and is reduced in heart failure (▶ Sect. 13.1) and increased in hyperthyroidism). The systemic blood pressure is calculated from CO and peripheral resistance, the pulmonary pressure analogously from CO and pulmonary resistance. Elevated pressure values in the pulmonary circulation are referred to as pulmonary hypertension (▶ Sect. 5.1), while elevated pressure values in the systemic circulation are referred to as (systemic) arterial hypertension (▶ Sect. 4.1).

The **peripheral resistance** is regulated predominantly in small arterioles by the activity of the sympathetic nervous system (◘ Fig. 1.5), the vagus nerve, and neurohumoral regulatory mechanisms (e.g., norepinephrine, renin-angiotensin-aldosterone system [RAAS], endothelin, vasopressin, natriuretic peptides) (▶ Sect. 13.1).

The **stroke volume** of the heart is predominantly regulated by the Frank-Starling mechanism (linking the initial length of myocardial fibres and the force generated) and inotropic hormones such as adrenaline (▶ Sect. 13.1).

1.4 Blood Supply of the Heart Muscle

The arteries that supply the myocardium are called **coronary arteries** (or **coronary arteries**, from Latin corona = crown) due to their crown-like course around the heart. The left and right coronary arteries originate from the left and right bulbus aortae, respectively.
- The left coronary artery (LCA) divides after a short main stem (LM) into the left circumflex (LCX) and the left anterior descending (LAD) coronary artery. Normally, the LAD supplies the left ventricle, the anterior wall of the right ventricle, and the majority of the interventricular septum, while in some the RCA or LCX maybe dominant (see below).
- The right coronary artery (RCA) divides into a main branch, the posterior descending (PDA) coronary artery, and (usually) a posterolateral branch (PLA). The RCA typically supplies the right atrium, the inferoposterior parts of the left ventricle and septum, as well as the right ventricle.
- If the RCA is dominant, it is referred to as the right-dominant type; if it is the LCA, it is referred to as the left-dominant type (▶ Sect. 7.2).

In the coronary circulation, especially in the left coronary system, blood flows—in

Table 1.1 Physiological hemodynamic values

Anatomical location	Hemodynamic parameter	Mean value (mmHg)	Range (mmHg)
Right atrium	A-wave	6	2–7
	V-wave	5	2–7
	Mean value	3	1–5
Right ventricle	Systolic pressure	25	15–30
	End-diastolic pressure	4	1–7
Pulmonary artery	Systolic pressure	25	15–30
	End-diastolic pressure	9	4–12
	Mean pressure	15	9–19
Capillary pressure	Mean value	9	4–12
Left atrium	A-wave	10	4–16
	V-wave	12	6–21
	Mean value	8	2–12
Left ventricle	Systolic pressure	130	90–140
	End-diastolic pressure	8	5–12
Central aorta	Systolic pressure	130	90–140
	End-diastolic pressure	70	60–90
	Mean pressure	85	70–105

contrast to other vascular areas—almost exclusively occurs during diastole due to the strong contraction of the left heart muscle. During systole the pressure in the myocardium compresses the arterioles and capillaries bringing coronary blood flow almost to a halt (◘ Fig. 1.6). Therefore, blood flow into the coronary system is determined by perfusion pressure, peripheral resistance, and heart rate, which dictates the duration of diastole. Since the electrical excitation of the ventricles always takes a certain minimum amount of time, the duration of systole is largely independent of heart rate. Consequently, with increasing heart rate, the duration of diastole and thus the perfusion time of the myocardium decreases. Conversely, the muscle of the right ventricle is much thinner, and the contraction is weaker, and the pressure conditions are much lower than in the left coronary, where arterial pressure values prevail; accordingly, the blood flow during systole in the branches of the RCA, which supply the right heart, hardly decreases.

1.5 Peripheral Circulation and Blood Distribution

In the peripheral circulation, the blood vessels branch out starting from the aorta or the main pulmonary artery. In doing so, the respective cross-section of the individual

Anatomy and Physiology of the Cardiovascular System

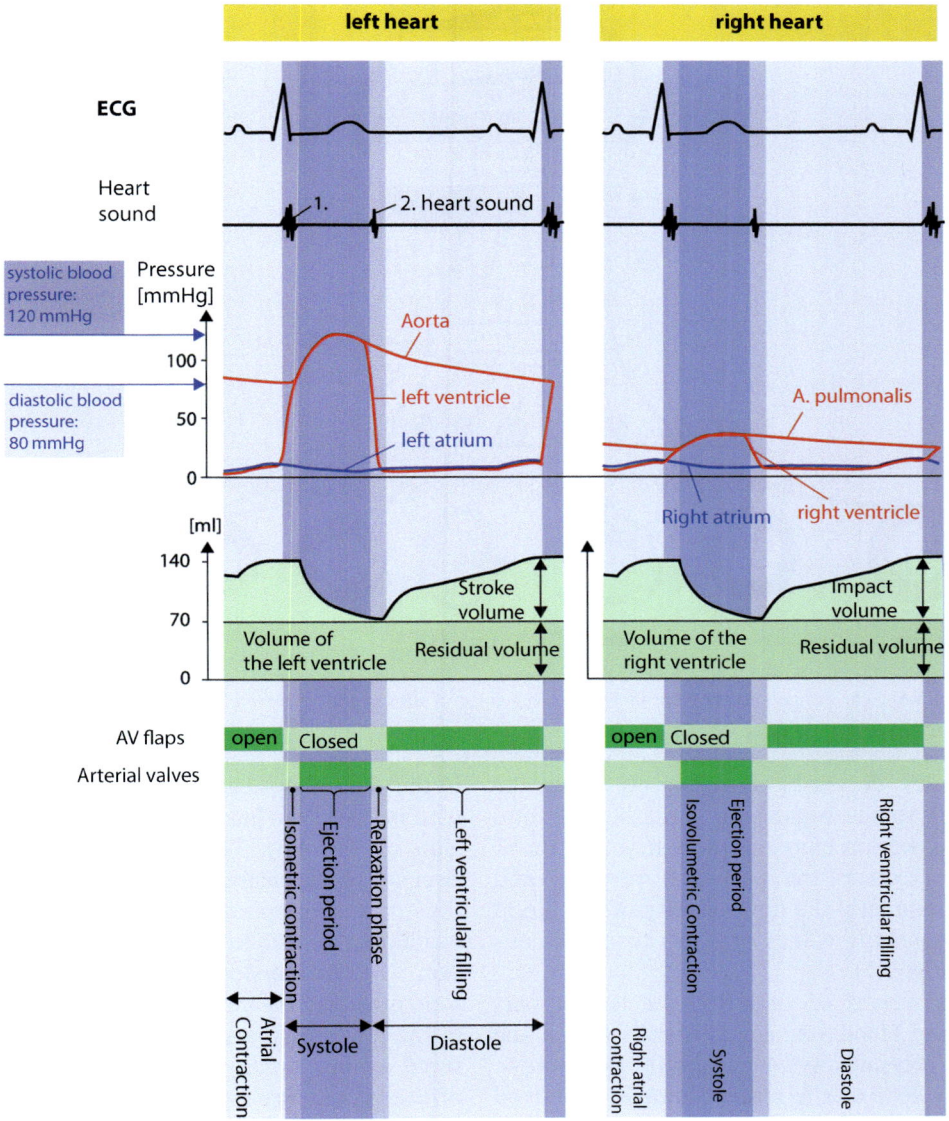

Fig. 1.4 Temporal relationship of ECG, valve opening and closing, and pressure-volume relationships in the right and left heart

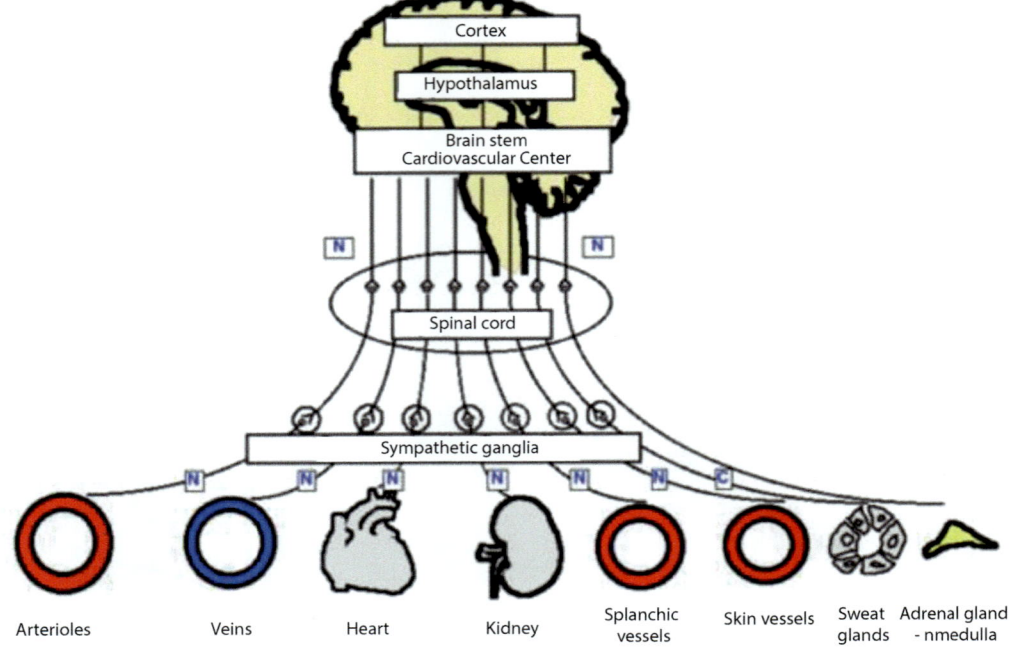

Fig. 1.5 The sympathetic nervous system as a regulator of the circulatory system and its organs

arteries decreases progressively from the heart to the organs. In contrast, the total cross-section increases more than 100 times. This reduces the perfusion pressure and consequently the flow velocity of the blood from resting values of 1 m/s to a few cm/s (◘ Fig. 1.7).

In terms of quantity, the largest part of the **blood volume**s is distributed in the low-pressure system (about two-thirds). Only 15% of the total volume is contained in the arterial system, with the rest distributed between the heart and the perfused organs (◘ Fig. 1.8). The venous part of the circulation, especially the large venae cavae, thus have an important reservoir function, which can be utilized during physical exertion. Due to the slow flow and low perfusion pressure, the return flow to the heart in the low-pressure system can only be ensured against gravity with the involvement of the venous valves and the muscle pump,

Anatomy and Physiology of the Cardiovascular System

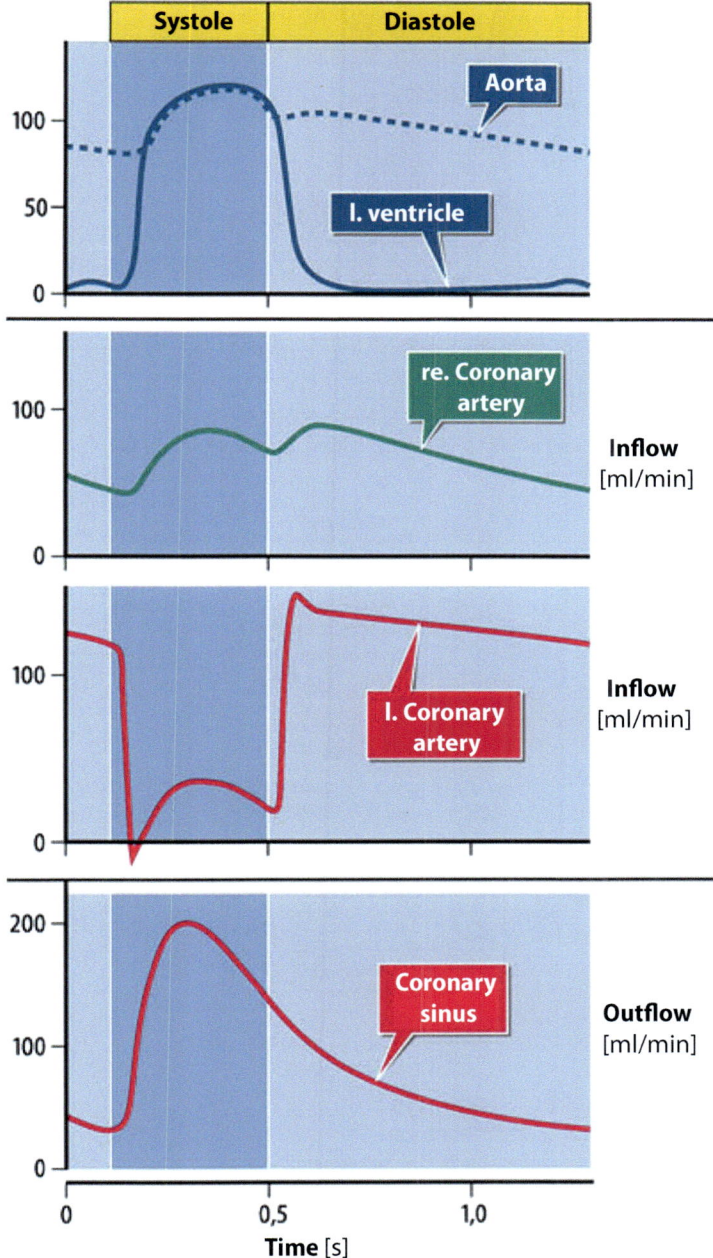

Fig. 1.6 Temporal relationship of pressure-volume ratios in the left ventricle and in the coronary arteries. Specifically, in the left coronary artery, blood flow occurs primarily during diastole. (From Schmidt/Lang/Heckmann, Physiology, Springer 2010)

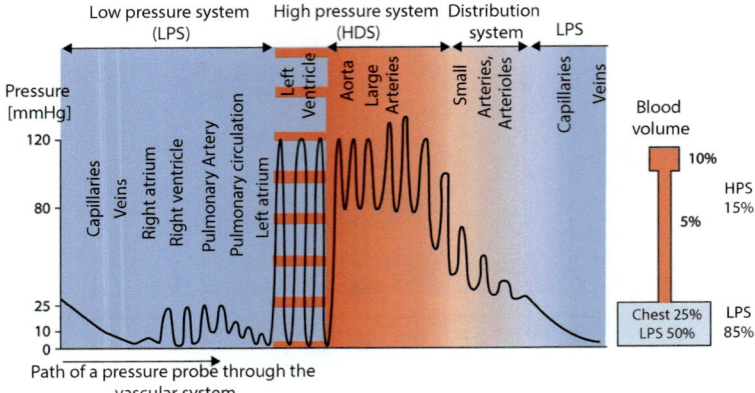

Fig. 1.7 Pressure conditions and blood volume distribution in the heart and vessels

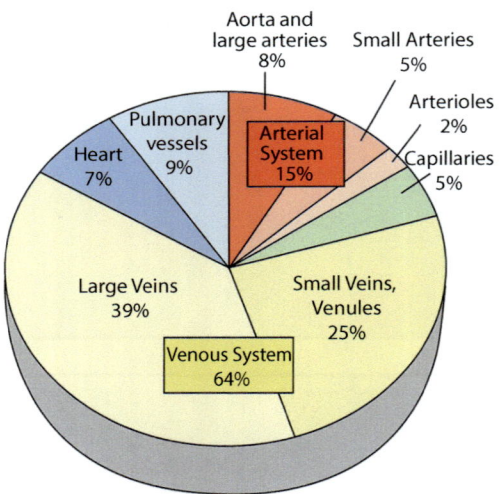

Fig. 1.8 Distribution of blood volume in the arterial and venous systems

as well as through the suction effect of the heart, which results from the displacement of the valve plane during systole.

Cardiological Diagnostics

Gerald Maurer and Christian Schmied

Contents

2.1 Medical History, Clinical Examination – 12

2.2 Electrocardiogram – 13
2.2.1 Resting ECG – 13
2.2.2 Exercise ECG – 13

2.3 Echocardiography – 15
2.3.1 Transthoracic Echocardiography (TTE) – 16
2.3.2 Transesophageal Echocardiography (TEE) – 18
2.3.3 Imaging Techniques – 19

2.4 Laboratory – 22

2.5 Non-invasive Imaging Techniques – 22
2.5.1 Conventional Radiology – 22
2.5.2 Computed Tomography (CT) – 24
2.5.3 Magnetic Resonance Imaging (MRI) – 24
2.5.4 Nuclear Medicine Procedures – 25

2.6 Coronary Angiography and Left Heart Catheterovation – 28

2.7 Right Heart Catheterization and Cardiac Output Determination – 31

Earlier versions were written in collaboration with, O. Gämperli, J. Steffel, and T. F. Lüscher.

© The Author(s), under exclusive license to Springer-Verlag GmbH, DE, part of Springer Nature 2025
T. F. Lüscher and U. Landmesser (eds.), *Cardiovascular System*,
https://doi.org/10.1007/978-3-662-70152-2_2

The cardiological examination of the patient begins, as in every specialty of medicine, with a detailed medical history and a physical examination. Depending on the question, diagnostic tests wills follow, including ECG, laboratory examinations, X-rays, echocardiography or other imaging modalities, and/or cardiac catheterization. For specific questions, computed tomography (CT), magnetic resonance imaging (MRI), and nuclear scans are also used.

2.1 Medical History, Clinical Examination

A carefully conducted medical history and a thorough physical examination are a central component of any cardiac evaluation. This provides the basis for further investigations , and not infrequently, a diagnosis can already be made without expensive and elaborate laboratory examinations and/or diagnosticsl tests. Furthermore, a number of diagnostic tests and procedures in cardiology are of great importance and an integral part of modern medicine.

The most important components of medical history and clinical examination are briefly repeated here but discussed in detail in the context of specific cardiovascular conditionss (e.g., myocardial infarction, valvular diseases, heart failure, etc.).

Cardiovascular Medical History
- Questions about cardiac symptoms such as reduced physical performance, palpitations, dyspnea, orthopnea (according to the NYHA classification), angina pectoris (according to the CCS classification, ▶ Sect. 7.2), edema/nycturia, claudication (according to Fontaine classification, ▶ Sect. 7.4), syncope or presyncope, dizziness, neurological symptoms, etc are essentiel in any cardiological work-up.
- Further, patients should be asked about cardiovascular lifestyle and risk factors (body weight/body mass index, weight development, diet, smoking, physical activity, home blood pressure measurements, diabetes mellitus, lipid metabolism disorders)
- Moreover previous illnesses and surgeries and allergies should be documented
- Family medical history should include hypertension, diabetes, coronary heart disease <60 years in parents/siblings)
- Medication history is also of great importance

Clinical Examination of the Cardiovascular System
- Inspection, including skin and mucous membrane color, skin turgor, habitus (including weight, weight distribution, and height), thorax shape, breathing pattern
- Palpation, including apex beat, thrills, collateral circulation
- Heart rate and blood pressure measurement (bilaterally, lying/sitting and standing after 3 minutes of rest, occlusion pressure measurement on legs, ankle-brachial index ▶ Sect. 7.4)
- Cardiac auscultation: 1st, 2nd heart sound, potential presence of a 3rd, 4th heart sound, systolic and diastolic murmurs, provocation maneuvers ("squatting")
- Auscultation of the carotid artery bilaterally, interscapular (▶ Sect. 7.7, renal arteries in the abdomen (▶ Sect. 4.3)
- Pulse status in extremities (regular/irregular, rapid/slow (▶ Sect. 12.4 and 12.5)
- Auscultation of the lungs (breathing rate, pattern, and lung sounds)
- Signs of congestion (lower leg edema, hepatosplenomegaly, jugular vein

distention, hepatojugular reflux; ▶ Sect. 13.3)
– Inspection, palpation, auscultation of the abdomen

2.2 Electrocardiogram

The electrocardiogram (ECG) is, alongside with blood pressure measurement, the most frequently used examination of the heart and is practically available in all hospitals and practices. The advantages of the ECG lie in its cost-effective acquisition and maintenance, its simple handling, and its high clinical significance.

2.2.1 Resting ECG

In the ECG (◘ Fig. 2.1), the sum of the electrical activity in the heart is represented over time using various leads. In the standard ECG, 12 leads are used. In the bipolar leads according to Einthoven, an electrode is placed on the right arm (red), one on the left arm (yellow), and one on the left leg (green), and these are then derived against each other (◘ Fig. 2.2). A grounding electrode is usually placed on the right leg (black). This results in lead I (right arm → left arm), lead II (right arm → left foot), and lead III (left arm → left foot). The connection of these 3 lead lines as a straight line forms the equilateral Einthoven triangle.

The bipolar Einthoven leads are supplemented by the leads according to Goldberger. Here, one of the aforementioned electrodes is derived against a composite electrode consisting of the other two electrodes. This results in the leads aVR (composite electrode between left arm and left foot → right arm), aVL (composite electrode between right arm and left foot → left arm), and aVF (composite electrode from both arms → left foot). If the limb leads according to Einthoven and Goldberger are represented as straight lines and these are shifted parallel so that they pass through a (fictitious) center of a circle, the so-called Cabrera circle is formed, from which the axis type of the QRS vector and the P wave can be determined (see also ▶ Chap. 12).

The limb leads according to Einthoven and Goldberger are supplemented in the standard 12-lead ECG by the chest wall leads according to Wilson. Unlike the former, which represent currents in the frontal plane very well, Wilson leads can represent potentials that run out of the frontal plane. For this purpose, all 3 limb leads are connected in the so-called Wilson composite electrode and 6 electrodes placed at standardized positions on the chest wall are derived against it. This results in the chest wall leads V_1–V_6. These can be supplemented beyond the standard 12-lead ECG by the so-called right precordial leads V_{1R}–V_{4R} (especially in case of suspected right heart infarction) as well as the posterior chest wall leads V_7–V_9 (posterior wall infarction with right heart involvement?).

Cardiovascular diseases are often associated with characteristic changes in individual or multiple ECG components (◘ Fig. 2.3).

> The ECG only measures the electrical activity of the heart's conduction system. Statements about structure and function can only be made indirectly.

For typical ECG changes and the interpretation of the resting ECG, see ▶ Sect. 7.2, 7.3 7.4 and 7.5 and ▶ Chap. 12.

2.2.2 Exercise ECG

Particularly in the context of a suspicion of coronary heart disease (CHD; ▶ Sect. 7.2)

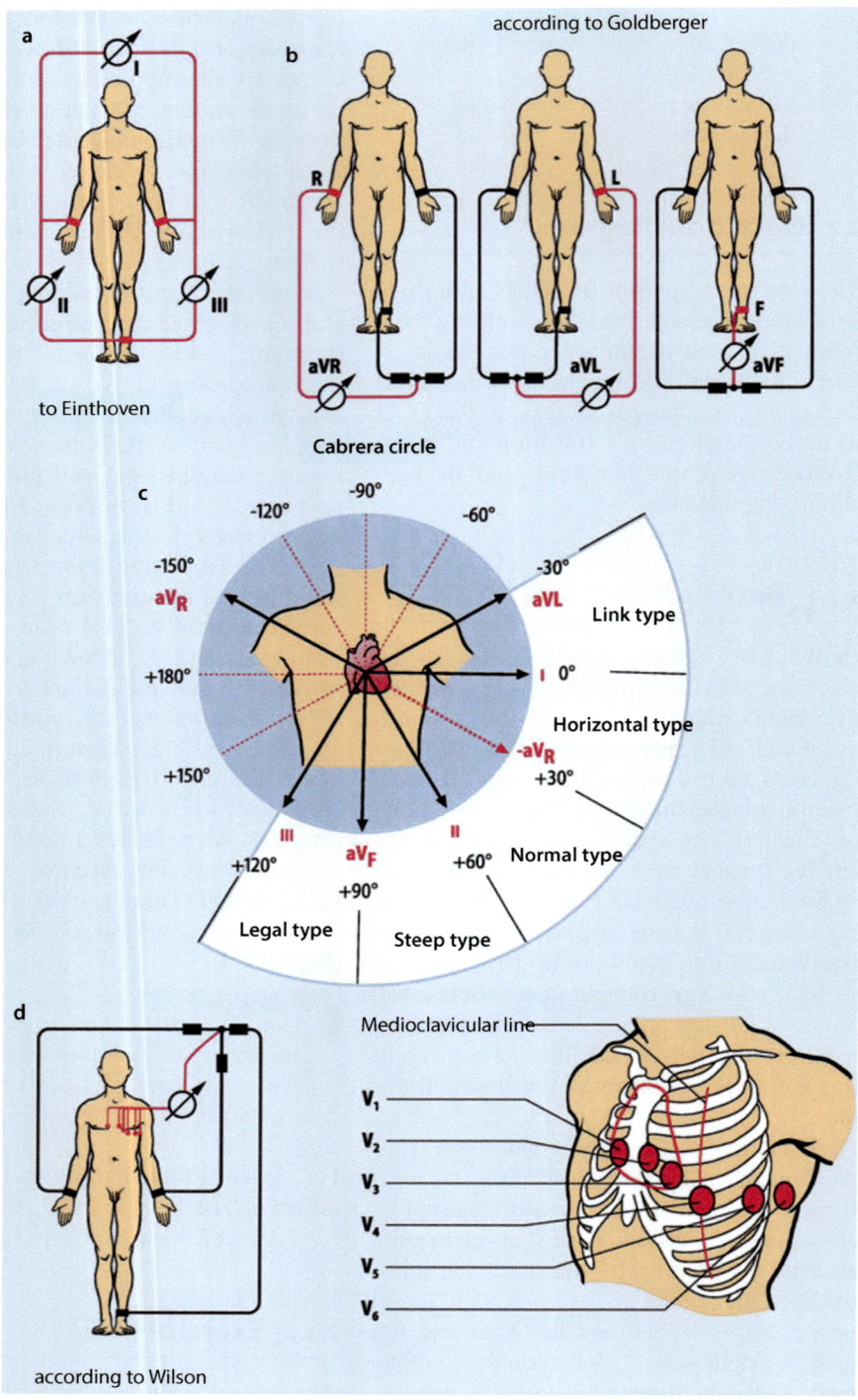

Fig. 2.1 a–d Placement of limb and chest wall electrodes and projection of the corresponding leads

Cardiological Diagnostics

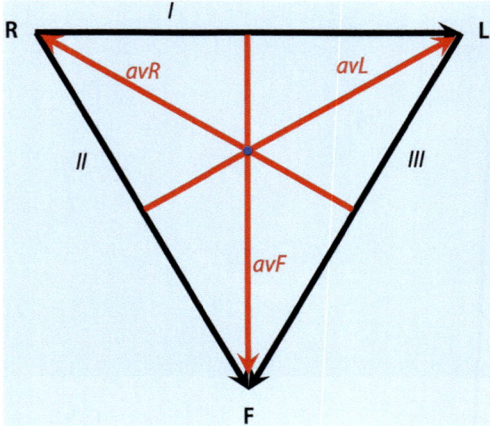

Fig. 2.2 Cabrera triangle: leads according to Einthoven (black) and Goldberger (red)

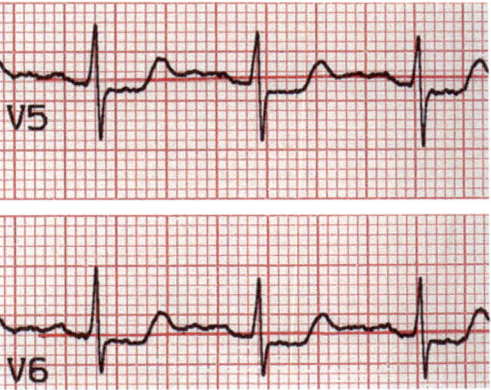

Fig. 2.3 Ischemia-suspect repolarization disorders (with typical ST-segement depression) during an exercise ergometry in V5 and V6

or exercise-induced symptoms, an ECG under physical stress can also be performed, usually on a bicycle or treadmill, in the form of an exercise ECG or an ergometry. In CHD, stress-induced ST-segment changes (Fig. 2.4) and anginal symptoms can be a reflection of myocardial ischemia. In addition, physical performance (according to age, gender, etc.), blood pressure progression (normal increase, blood pressure drop, lack of increase, hypertension), heart rate progression, and any rhythm disturbances can be assessed and used diagnostically.

However, the diagnostic accuracy of ergometry regarding possible myocardial ischemia is limited, especially in the case of a negative test result (sensitivity only 45–50%). In women, the diagnostic accuracy of ergometry is even worse than in men. The following overview shows clinical scenarios in which the significance of ergometry is also limited due to false positive results regarding ischemia. Caution is advised in cases of severe aortic stenosis, hypertrophic obstructive cardiomyopathy (HOCM), severe three-vessel or LM disease, active myccarditis, or immediately after a heart attack. The use of additional imaging techniques in conjunction with stress (echocardiography, cardiac magnetic resonance, nuclear scintigraphy) can significantly improve the sensitivity and specificity of the examination.

Frequently false positive test results in bicycle exercise test
- LBBB and other intraventricular conduction disorders
- Pacemaker rhythm (▶ Sect. 12.4)
- Wolff-Parkinson-White (WPW) syndrome (▶ Sect. 12.5)
- Pre-existing ST-T changes in the resting ECG
- Electrolyte disturbances
- Digoxin
- Left ventricular hypertrophy (Sects. 8.1 and 9.1)

2.3 Echocardiography

In echocardiography, an ultrasound examination of the heart is performed in real-time.

> In contrast to the ECG, echocardiography provides direct information about the anatomy and function of the heart.

Furthermore, with **Doppler sonography** (flow, color, and tissue Doppler), the flow

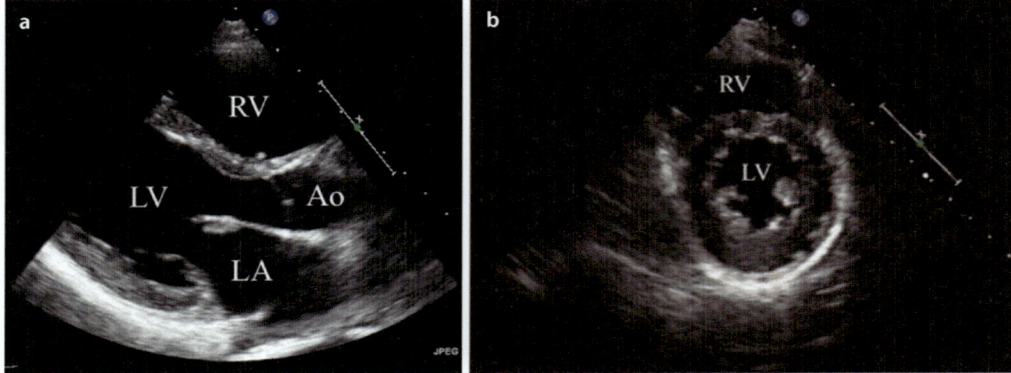

Fig. 2.4 Parasternal long axis view a, parasternal short axis view b. (*Ao*: Aorta, *LA*: left atrium, *LV*: left ventricle, *RV*: right ventricle)

conditions in the heart can be determined, which is particularly important for the diagnosis of valvUlan heart disease.

Echocardiography is technically demanding and requires some experience. Basically, various ultrasound techniques are used, the indication of which arises from the respective question or suspected diagnosis. The transducer is brought to the heart transthoracically or transesophageally.

2.3.1 Transthoracic Echocardiography (TTE)

In transthoracic echocardiography (TTE), there are various standard settings.

- **Parasternal Long Axis (◘ Fig. 2.4a)**
The transducer is placed in the 3rd–5th intercostal space, almost perpendicular, with a slight tilt towards the left shoulder.
The transducer should lie in the presumed long axis of the heart and anatomically displays the left ventricle with mitral valve, the left atrium, the left ventricular outflow tract (LVOT) with the aortic valve, and the proximal part of the ascending aorta as well as the right ventricle.

- **Parasternal Short Axis (◘ Fig. 2.4b):**
This is set by rotating the transducer from the parasternal long axis by 90° clockwise. In this way, depending on the question, any number of short-axis slices can be generated, and, among other things, the left ventricle from apical to basal, the valve planes, as well as the right-sided heart chambers and valves can be displayed.

- **Apical 4-Chamber View (◘ Fig. 2.5a)**
The transducer is placed in the area of the cardiac apex in the 5th–6th intercostal space, aimed towards the right shoulder. This apical plane provides an overview of all 4 heart chambers. By adjusting the transducer angle, the left ventricular outflow tract and the aortic valve can also be displayed with the 5-chamber view.

- **Apical 2-Chamber View (◘ Fig. 2.5b)**
Rotation from the 4-chamber view by about 80° counterclockwise provides the 2-chamber view, in which the left heart with atrium, ventricle, and mitral valve is displayed. Additionally, the left atrial appendage and the coronary sinus can usually also be visualized.

- **Apical 3-Chamber View (◘ Fig. 2.6a)**
Further rotation counterclockwise from the 2-chamber view results in the 3-chamber

Cardiological Diagnostics

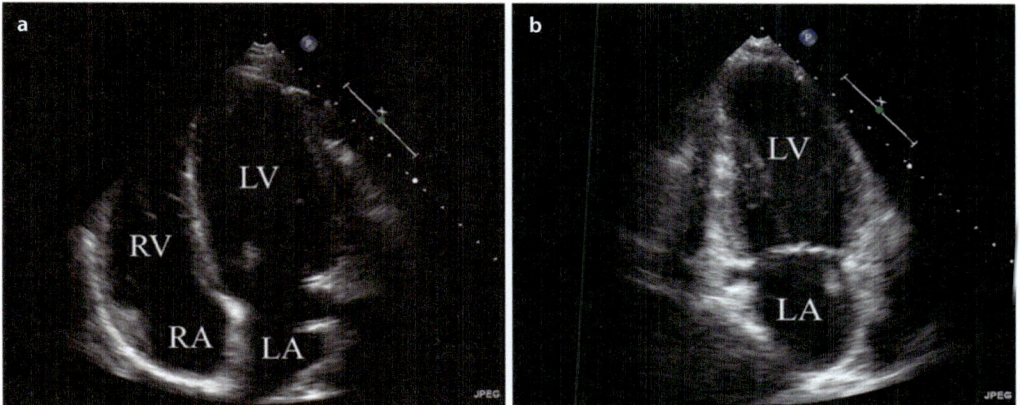

Fig. 2.5 Apical 4-chamber view a, apical 2-chamber view b. (*LV*: left ventricle; *RV*: right ventricle; *LA*: left atrium; *RA*: right atrium)

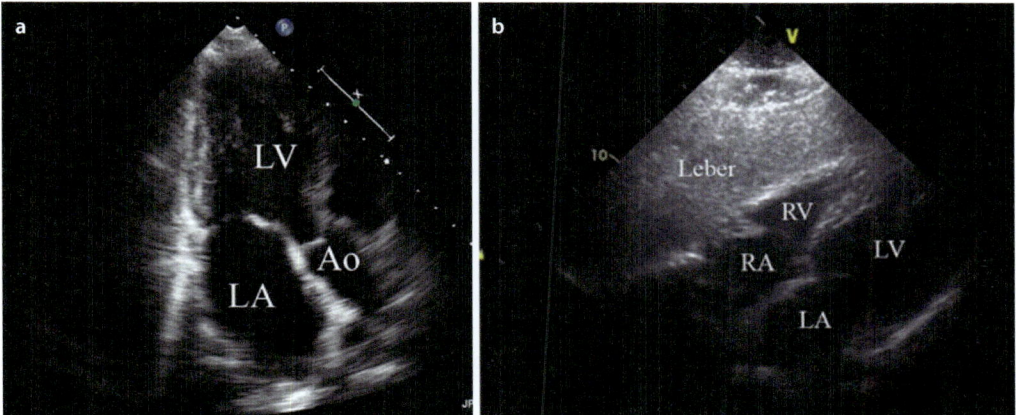

Fig. 2.6 Apical 3-chamber view a, subcostal plane b. (*Ao*: aorta, *LA*: left atrium, *LV*: left ventricle, *RA*: right atrium, *RV*: right ventricle)

view or the so-called RAO equivalent. The displayed structures correspond approximately to those of the parasternal long-axis slice.

Subcostal Plane (Fig. 2.6b)

The transducer is placed subxiphoidally with angulation towards the left shoulder. Through this technique, in addition to practically all cardiac structures that can be displayed transthoracically, the inferior vena cava or the hepatic veins and parts of the descending aorta can also be visualized. Additionally, the subcostal examination classically detects a pericardial effusion accurately. This view has proven particularly useful in patients who are difficult to image transthoracically.

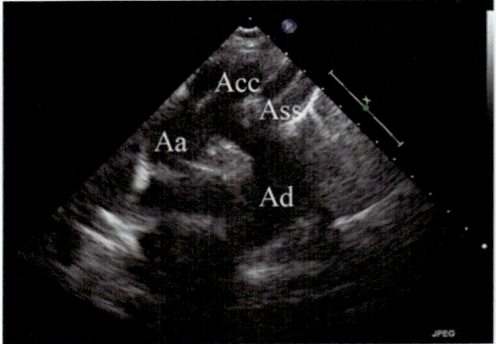

Fig. 2.7 Suprasternal acoustic window. (*aA:* ascending aorta, *aA:* descending aorta, *lccA:* left common carotid artery, *lsA:* left subclavian artery)

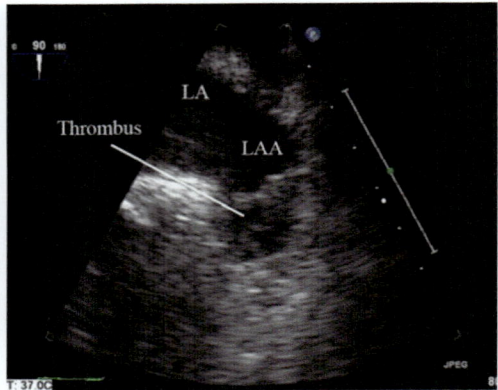

Fig. 2.8 Large thrombus in the left atrial appendage (*LAA*), visualized by transesophageal echocardiography. (*LA*: left atrium)

- **Suprasternal Acoustic Window (◘ Fig. 2.7)**

In the supine position and with the patient's head slightly reclined, the aortic arch and its adjacent structures can be visualized in this way.

A **right parasternal window** is sometimes used to evaluate aortic valve stenosis. For specific questions and in cases of difficult transthoracic examination conditions (such as in very obese patients, but also in patients with other extracardiac limitations like emphysema, chest deformities, or post-thoracotomy status), **transesophageal echocardiography** is used.

2.3.2 Transesophageal Echocardiography (TEE)

In TEE, the patient swallows a transducer, which is mounted on a modified gastroscope, after local pharyngeal anesthesia. Since this is uncomfortable and usually accompanied by a more or less pronounced gag reflex, TEE is generally performed under light sedation or short anesthesia. By positioning the probe in the esophagus, rotating the ultrasound probe (0°–180°), rotating the probe around its own axis, gentle angulation anteriorly and posteriorly, and tilting left or right, virtually all structures of the heart can be visualised. Due to the close anatomical proximity to the esophagus to the heart, TEE provides very good quality images, especially in the area of the atria. The risks of serious complications are minimal with proper technique and experience. However, dental injuries, bleeding, aspiration, and (in extreme cases) esophageal injuries up to perforation have been described and must be discussed accordingly in the informed consent conversation.

TEE is used, among other things, to assess valvular heart disease such as endocarditis or to rule out intracardiac thrombi (including in the left atrium and atrial appendage, which is well accessible to TEE due to its anatomy directly adjacent to the esophagus, ◘ Fig. 2.8). In addition, the thoracic aorta can be accurately examined for plaques or dissection. Finally, atrial shunt defects can be very well visualized using TEE (e.g. persistent foramen ovale [PFO]; atrial septal defect [ASD] or ventricular septal defect (VSD), ► Sect. 14.2, ◘ Fig. 14.2).

2.3.3 Imaging Techniques

Various imaging techniques are generally used in echocardiography:

- **B-Mode Technique**

In the B-mode technique (I.e. *brightness mode*), different echo amplitudes are displayed as grayscale of varying intensity. This results in a 2D cross-sectional image that allows morphological and functional assessment of the heart structures (◘ Fig. 2.9).

- **M-Mode Technique**

The M-mode method (i.e. *motion mode*, ◘ Fig. 2.9) allows the representation of dynamic structures, resulting in a temporally integrated image. The M-mode is primarily used for the quantification of cardiac dimensions or for structural functional analysis.

- **Doppler sonography**

Doppler sonography evaluates cardiovascular flow conditions either along a so-called sound beam (i.e. *continuous wave*, cw, ◘ Fig. 2.10) or at a specific, spatially assigned point (i.e. *pulsed wave*, pw).

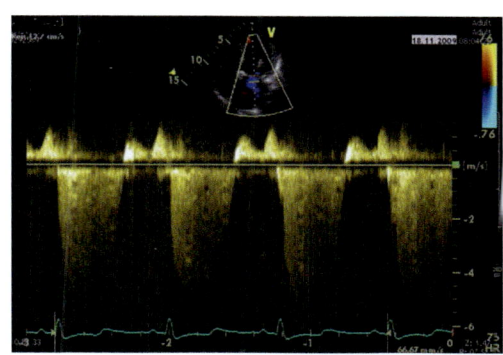

◘ **Fig. 2.10** Continuous-Wave Doppler (cw-Doppler) through the mitral valve in the apical 4-chamber view. For orientation, see the small image (above). From the maximum velocity of the flow signal (downward; here about 5 m/s with mild mitral insufficiency), the pressure difference between the two heart chambers can be determined. The upward flow signal reflects mitral inflow with an initial E- and a second A-wave

- **Color-coded Doppler sonography**

Color-coded Doppler sonography is a combination of B-mode and Doppler technique, resulting in a sectional image with a flow profile. In colour-coded Doppler sonography, different flow directions and velocities are represented by different colors (◘ Fig. 2.11). Physically, as the name implies, it is based on the Doppler effect, which describes the changes in frequency of an ultrasound wave reflected by a moving object, in this case blood or blood cells (see also physics textbooks).

- **Tissue Doppler Imaging**

Tissue Doppler Imaging (TDI, ◘ Fig. 2.12), also called Tissue Doppler, is an ultrasound technique in which the velocity of the tissue (and not the blood, as in color-coded Doppler sonography), particularly of the myocardium, is measured and displayed. It allows, among other things, the assessment of myocardial contractility and ventricular relaxation (= diastolic function) as well as the synchrony of wall movements (▶ Sect. 13.2).

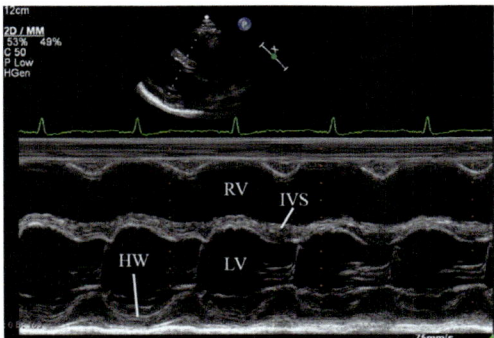

◘ **Fig. 2.9** M-mode through the basal section of the left ventricle in the parasternal long axis view. For orientation, see the small image (above) and ◘ Fig. 2.4. (*IVS*: interventricular septum, *PW*: posterior wall, *LV*: left ventricle, *RV*: right ventricle)

Strain Imaging (Global Longitudinal Strain/GLS)

The GLS describes the shortening or thickening of a myocardial segment as a dimensionless deformation parameter, which is given in percent. This method does more justice to the complex contraction and relaxation movements of the myocardium (◘ Fig. 2.13).

3D Echocardiography

3D echocardiography (◘ Fig. 2.14) is a method of echocardiography that enables a three-dimensional, spatial representation of the organ, but requires significantly higher technical prerequisites.

Stress Echocardiography

A special form of echocardiography is stress echocardiography, which is mainly used when coronary artery disease is suspected and occasionally for the assessment of aortic stenosis or exercise-induced pul-

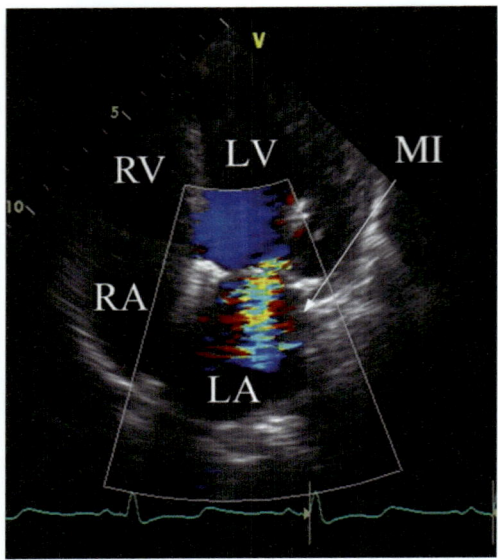

◘ **Fig. 2.11** Color Doppler in the apical 4-chamber view showing mild to moderate mitral regurgitation (MR). *LA*: left atrium, *LV*: left ventricle, *RA*: right atrium, *RV*: right ventricle)

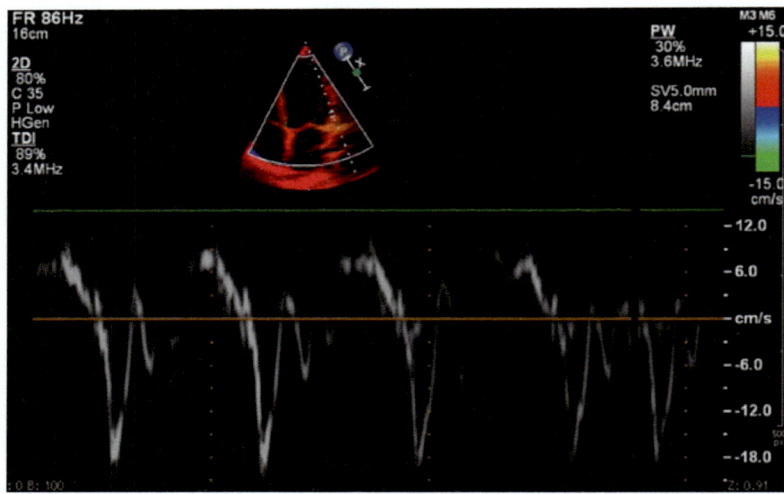

◘ **Fig. 2.12 Tissue Doppler in the basal left ventricle (lateral wall).** For orientation, see small image (above). From the maximum velocity of the Doppler profile (here approx. 18 cm/s), the velocity of the left ventricular longitudinal movement can be determined

Cardiological Diagnostics

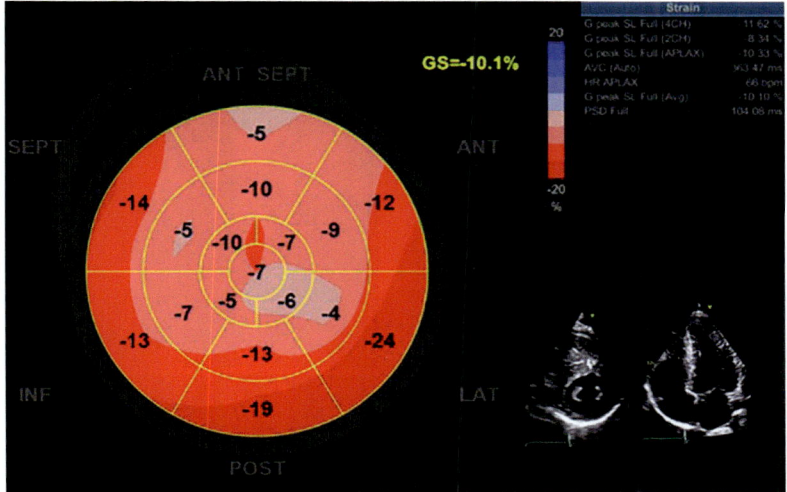

Fig. 2.13 **Strain Imaging** in hypertrophic cardiomyopathy (right window) with reduced GLS

monary hypertension. Stress echocardiography is technically demanding and only makes sense for patients who have good acoustic quality, as the diagnostic yield is otherwise significantly reduced.

In stress echocardiography, the patient performs a bicycle or treadmill ergometry, or a pharmacological stress (e.g., i.v. dobutamine, adenosine, or dipyridamole infusion) is induced, during which ultrasound images are recorded in various standard projections and compared with the images at rest. Stress echocardiography allows the assessment of ventricular function, newly appearing regional wall motion abnormalities, and valve function under stress.

In the case of an underestimated severity of aortic stenosis (e.g., with severely im-

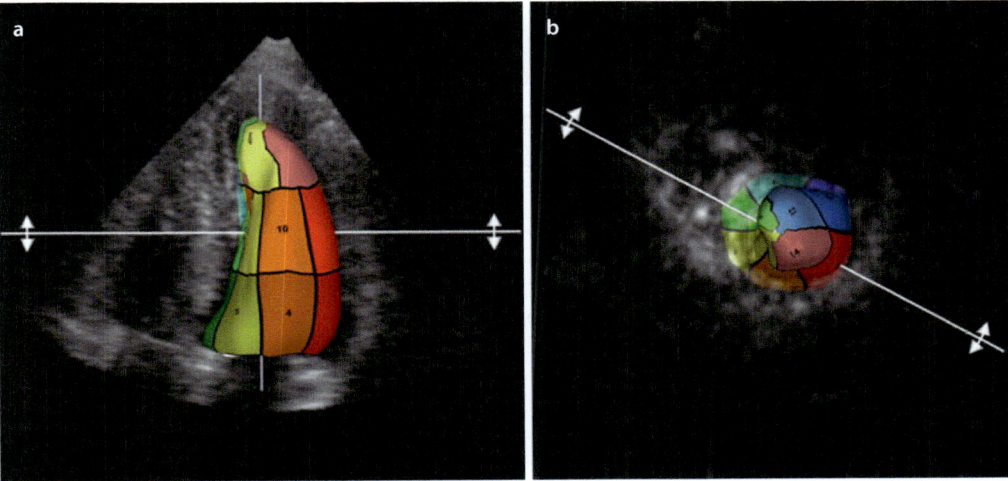

Fig. 2.14 a, b **3D echocardiography of the left ventricle. a** In the apical 4-chamber view (Fig. 2.6), **b** in the parasternal short axis (Fig. 2.4)

paired left ventricular function, so-called *low flow—low gradient* aortic stenosis; ▶ Sect. 9.1), the gradient across the valve increases significantly under stress. In exercise-induced myocardial ischemia, systolic and diastolic wall motion abnormalities occur under stress, which can be displayed.

2.4 Laboratory

The laboratory tests are primarily used in cardiology for
- diagnosis of myocardial infarction (CK, myoglobin, but primarily troponin, ▶ Sect. 7.5),
- diagnosis of cardiovascular risk factors (serum lipids, glucose, HbA1c, hsCRP, etc., ▶ Sect. 3.3, ▶ Chap. 6, ▶ Sect. 7.1),
- assessment of the progression of heart failure (natriuretic peptides; ▶ Sect. 13.3),
- assessment of secondarily involved organs (creatinine and eGFR for kidney function, INR, AST, ALT and bilirubin for liver function),
- assessment of the extent of oral anticoagulation with vitamin K antagonists (INR/Quick measurement; e.g., in atrial fibrillation ▶ Sect. 12.5).

2.5 Non-invasive Imaging Techniques

For the radiological examination of the heart, conventional X-ray, computed tomography (CT), magnetic resonance imaging (MRI), and nuclear medicine techniques are used.

2.5.1 Conventional Radiology

Despite the widespread use of echocardiography and the increasing availability of CT and MRI, conventional X-ray remains a standard diagnostic procedure when

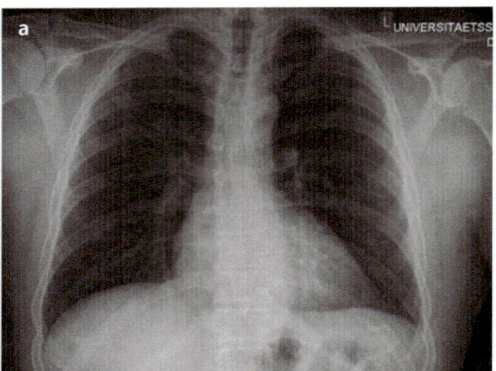
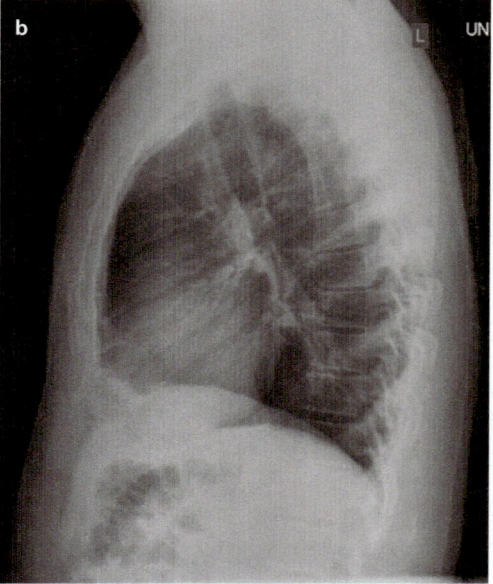

◘ Fig. 2.15 a, b Conventional chest X-ray. a In the pa, b in the lateral projection. Compensated heart-lung findings

heart disease is suspected in many institutions as it is inexpensive, quickly available, and highly reproducible. Nevertheless, the conventional chest X-ray has significantly lost importance. The standing X-ray is performed in 2 standard projections: the chest overview image (◘ Fig. 2.15) in the dorsoventral (= posteroanterior, pa) projection, which, depending on the question, is supplemented by a lateral projection, provides information about the dimensions of the heart (heart-lung ratio) and adjacent struc-

Cardiological Diagnostics

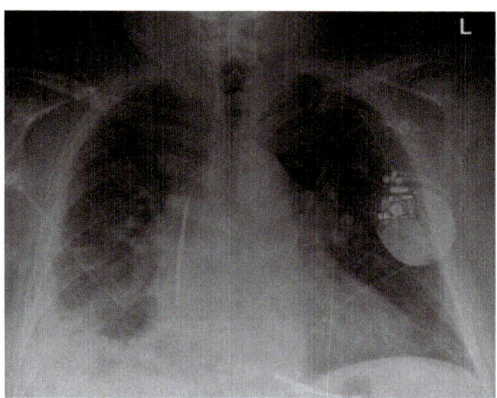

Fig. 2.16 Conventional X-ray (ap, supine position) with typical signs of decompensated heart failure such as dominant pulmonary vessels and a right-sided pleural effusion. Incidentally, an ICD is implanted in the left pectoral region with the correct position of the electrode tip at the base of the right ventricle

tures, such as the large vessels, lungs, diaphragm, and mediastinum.

From a cardiological perspective, chest X-rays are primarily useds to detect cardiopulmonary congestion (usually visible in the form of basoapical redistribution of blood flow in left heart decompensation, possibly with pleural effusion, ◘ Fig. 2.16).

In addition, indirect statements regarding any potential cardiac issues can be made based on the cardiac and mediastinal contours.

Overview
- A **cardiomegaly** can be identified by an increased transverse diameter. This should not exceed half of the thoracic diameter in standing position during inspiration in the pa projection (heart-lung ratio >0.5).
- A displacement of the heart apex to the left caudal in the pa projection or a displacement of the heart contour against the spine (>2 cm extending over the inferior vena cava) in the lateral projection indicates an **enlargement of the left ventricle**.
- An **enlargement of the left atrium** can be present if there is a so-called core shadow, spreading of the carina of the major bronchi (X-ray pa), or dorsal esophagus displacement (X-ray lateral).
- The **right ventricle** appears stressed in the presence of a cardiact enlargement to the left with elevation of the cardiac apex or an enlargement of the cardiact silhouette to the right (pa projection). This suspicion is supported by a reduction of the retrosternal space (contact of the heart over more than 1/3–1/2 of the sternum length) and a displacement of the left ventricle dorsally (distance to the inferior vena cava maintained) in the lateral X-ray.
- A **dilation of the right atrium** is likely if the right heart contour exceeds more than 1/3 of the hemithorax diameter (pa) or by a reduction of the retrosternal space, similar to the right ventricle (lateral).

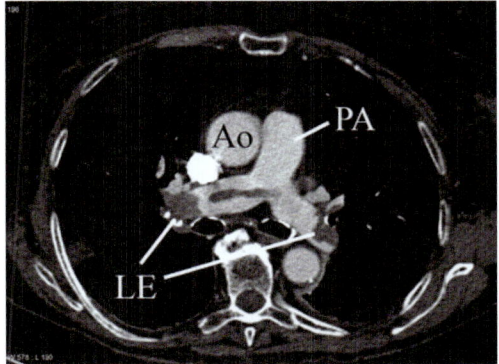

Fig. 2.17 Computed tomography of the thorax with contrast medium. Large bilateral paracentral pulmonary embolisms (*PE*) are visible in the right and left pulmonary artery. *Ao*: Aorta, *PA*: Main pulmonary trunk. (Courtesy of Thomas Frauenfelder, University Hospital Zurich)

2.5.2 Computed Tomography (CT)

In cardiology, CT is primarily used to clarify aneurysms/dissections of the aorta or large arteries, cardiac and vascular tumors, pulmonary embolisms (◘ Fig. 2.17), as well as other structural changes in the vessels, myocardium, and heart valves (CT prior to a TAVI procedure; ▶ Sect. 9.1). Newer devices also allow visualization of the coronary arteries, the so-called **CT coronary angiography**. The most recent phono counting CT provides the best spatial resolution (150um). By intravenous (i.v.) administration of radiopaque contrast medium, soft tissue structures (mostly vessels such as pulmonary arteries, aorta, large arteries, or coronary arteries) are better delineated from the surrounding tissues.

Advantages of CT coronary angiography (◘ Fig. 2.18) over other imaging techniques include good availability, simple and rapid execution, and (with good image quality) high diagnostic value. Prerequisites for good image quality in CT coronary angiography are a low and regular heart rate (<70/min, ideally <65/min). If necessary, this is achieved by i.v. administration of beta-blockers. Pronounced calcifications in the coronary arteries and intracoronary stents can cause artifacts that complicate interpretation, but is much less an issue with photon counting CT. Radiation exposure has been significantly reduced and, in experienced centers with modern equipment, is in the same range as diagnostic invasive coronary angiography (2–3 mSv). Novel photon counting CT (pcCT) provides much better resolution of the coronary arteries.

> ❗ The use of contrast medium for a CT can worsen pre-existing renal failure. In cases of impaired—and especially severely impaired—renal function, the benefits and risks of administering contrast medium must be weighed against each other.

2.5.3 Magnetic Resonance Imaging (MRI)

The Magnetic Resonance Imaging is characterized compared to other modalities by a high resolution of anatomical details and—due to the different magnetic properties of various tissues—by a high soft tissue contrast. It is therefore particularly suitable for examining the morphology of the heart and the large arteries and pathological changes of the myocardium. MRI is mostly used to clarify pericardial diseases, cardiomyopathies, inflammatory or infiltrative myocardial diseases, congenital heart ddisease, and tumors of the heart as well as in aortic diseases (e.g. aortic dissection and aneurysms). MRI (◘ Fig. 2.19) has the advantage over CT and nuclear scans that it does not involve radiation exposure. The main disadvantages are the limited availability and the higher costs of an examination.

The **Perfusion MRI** with contrast agent (Gadolinium) allows for the diagnosis of ischemia or viabilitys in suspected coronary

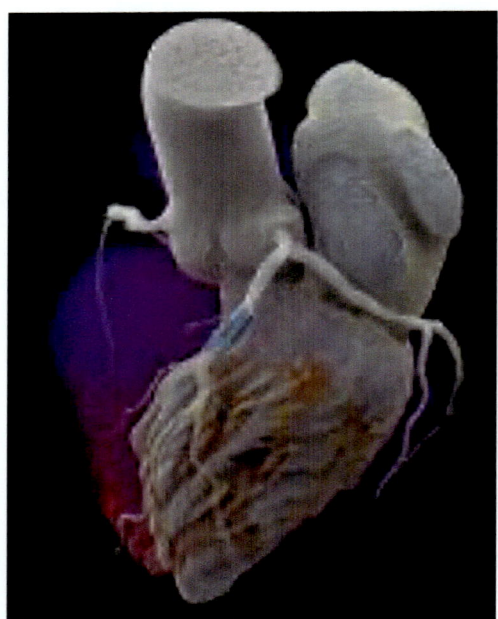

◘ Fig. 2.18 **PCCT coronary angiography** of a healthy individual with patent coronary arteries without significant stenoses

Cardiological Diagnostics

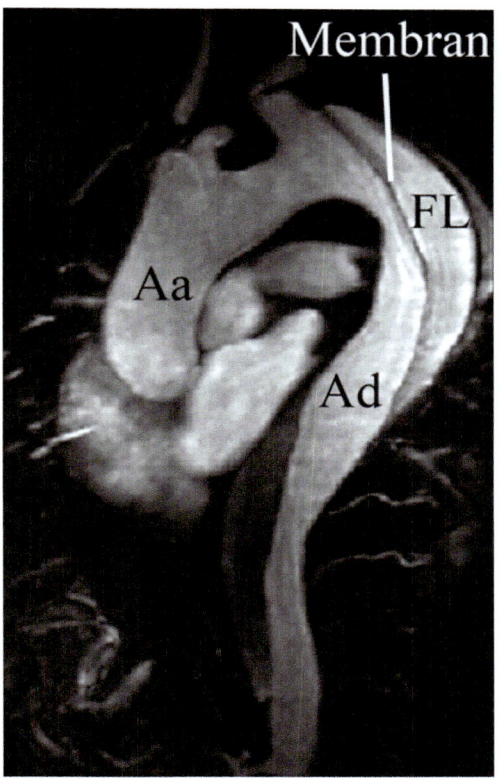

Fig. 2.19 MRI showing an aortic dissection. (*Aa* = ascending aorta, *Ad* = descending aorta, *FL* = false lumen)

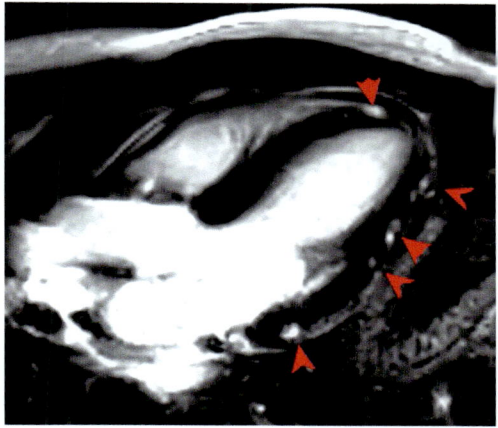

Fig. 2.20 Late Gadolinium Enhancement in myocarditis with different white spots in affected myocardial segments. (Red arrows at the lateral wall and apex of the left ventricle)

artery disease (CAD). After the initial "first pass" of the contrast agent through the coronary arteries, gadolinium preferentially distributes in the interstitium of the heart muscle. In the case of an enlargement of the interstitial space, such as in the context of an myocardial scar after myocardial infarction or due to edema in inflammatory myocardial disease, there is increased uptake in the affacted myocardial segment, which can be visualized by delayed uptake ("Late Enhancement"; Fig. 2.20). Caution is also advised with gadolinium-containing contrast agents in cases of impaired renal function.

❗ For implanted intracardiac defibrillators (ICD) or pacemakers, it must be ensured that they are approved for MRI and that the patient is not pacemaker dependent. Otherwise, MRI should only be performed on these patients with vital indication and with professional medical and technical support. Heart valve prostheses and newly placed vascular clips are relative contraindications.

2.5.4 Nuclear Medicine Procedures

For nuclear scans, radioactively labeled molecules are introduced into the metabolism of the myocardium. The myocardial uptake of radioactivityn can be visualised, and the distribution space as well as the distribution density of the radionuclides can be quantified. The visual representation of the distribution of the radionuclides is called **scintigraphy**.

The scintigram is not primarily used not to depict exact anatomical structures, but rather for functional diagnostics. Scintigraphy is associated with a slightly higher radiation exposure than CT coronary angiography.

In cardiology, two procedures are mainly used, SPECT (i.e. *single photon emission computed tomography*) and PET (i.e. positron emission tomography).

- **Single-Photon Emission Computed Tomography (SPECT)**

In **myocardial perfusion SPECT**, a small dose of a radioactively labeled perfusion tracer is administered. Nowadays, a ^{99m}technetium-labeled substance (^{99m}Tc-MIBI or ^{99m}Tc-tetrofosmin) is mostly used, which is taken up by the mitochondria of myocardial cells. Occasionally, the older ^{201}thallium chloride is used, which, similar to the potassium ion, is taken up into the cell via the energy-dependent sodium-potassium ATPase. ^{201}thallium, in contrast to the ^{99m}Tc nuclide, has a longer half-life (72 h vs. 6 h) and is therefore associated with higher radiation exposure. The advantage of ^{201}thallium, however, lies in the redistribution of the tracer from healthy to underperfused but viable myocardium, which allows its use in viability diagnostics.

The radionuclides accumulate in the myocardium depending on the blood flow of the different myocardial segments. Their distribution pattern allows the relative assessment of myocardial perfusion at rest as well as under physical (e.g., bicycle ergometer) or pharmacological stress (e.g. i.v. infusion of adenosine, dipyridamole or dobutamine). The regional distribution of the radionuclide is recorded by gamma-ray detectors. For SPECT scans, the gamma detectors (usually at a 90° angle) are positioned close to the heart and describe a semicircle movement around the heart during an acquisition, so that image information is captured from different projections and processed three-dimensionally, allowing an accurate assessment of the relative perfusion of all wall segments of the left ventricle.

SPECT scans (◘ Fig. 2.21) are used to examine myocardial perfusion. It is therefore indicated in suspected CAD, but also in proven CAD to detect the presence or extent of myocardial ischemia or infarction. It is performed at rest and under stress. The latter can be done either pharmacologically (usually i.v. injection of adenosine) or by ergometry. In myocardial areas supplied by a stenotic coronary artery, perfusion increases slightly less or may even decrease under pharmacological stress compared to normally perfused myocardial areas. This creates a discrepancy between normal and ischemic areas. Medium to large ischemias (>10% of the left ventricular myocardium) pose a particularly high risk for myocardial infarction or death and should promptly lead to cardiac catheterization. Unlike other procedures, myocardial perfusion SPECT scans are safe in renal failure or irregular rhythm (e.g. atrial fibrillation; ▶ Sect. 12.5). However, the increased radiation exposure (approx. 9–10 mSv with ^{99m}technetium-labeled substances) must be considered, especially in younger patients.

In **radionuclide ventriculography**, ^{99m}technetium-labeled erythrocytes are administered i.v. as a bolus to visualize the heart chambers and cardiac pump function. Due to the more readily available other imaging methods today, radionuclide ventriculography is hardly used.

- **Positron Emission Tomography (PET)**

PET is based on the emission of 2 photons (which move away from each other at an angle of 180°) that are produced during the collision of a positron with an electron (annihilation reaction). By the simultaneous impact of two photons on opposite points of the PET detector ring (coincidence circuit), the exact position of the radionuclide can be determined. PET thus has a higher spatial resolution than SPECT and is primarily used in cardiac diagnostics (similar to SPECT) to assess myocardial ischemia and viability used. Myocardial perfusion

Cardiological Diagnostics

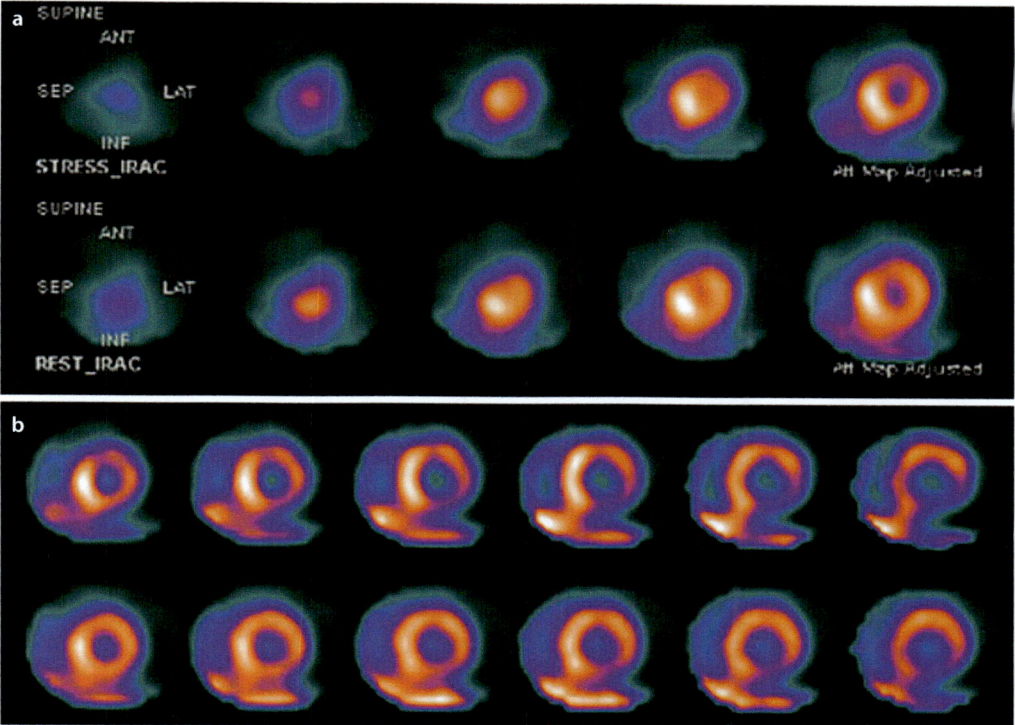

Fig. 2.21 **a**, **b** ^{99m}technetium-tetrofosmin SPECT of the left ventricle from apical (left) to basal (right). **a** Images at rest and **b** under stress. Under stress, a clearly inferolateral reduced uptake is seen from midventricular to basal. (Courtesy of Philipp A. Kaufmann, University Hospital Zurich)

is determined by the injection of radioactive ammonia ($^{13}NH_3$), water ($H_2^{15}O$), or radioactive rubidium (^{82}Rb). To determine viability, ^{18}Fluorodeoxyglucose (^{18}FDG) is injected as a bolus intravenously (after dietary preparation of the patient). The scintigraphic assessment of myocardial viability via glucose metabolism is considered the gold standard for diagnosing myocardial viability.

> PET provides absolute values of myocardial perfusion (while SPECT only measures relative values), so that even in balanced coronary artery disease, i.e., affecting all 3 coronary vessels equally, perfusion deficits can be diagnosed.

Disadvantages of PET include high acquisition costs and high examination costs. Additionally, most perfusion tracers ($^{13}NH_3$, water ($H_2^{15}O$)) contain very short-lived nuclides, so only centers with direct access to a cyclotron can produce and use these substances.

▪ Hybrid Imaging

In cases of intermediate stenosis grade of several coronary arteries or complex coronary anatomy, e.g., after bypass surgery, the combination of anatomical and functional information, i.e., CT coronary angiography and perfusion studies (SPECT, PET, or MRI), can occasionally be helpful. This is referred to as hybrid imaging (Fig. 2.22). This allows for a better assignment of

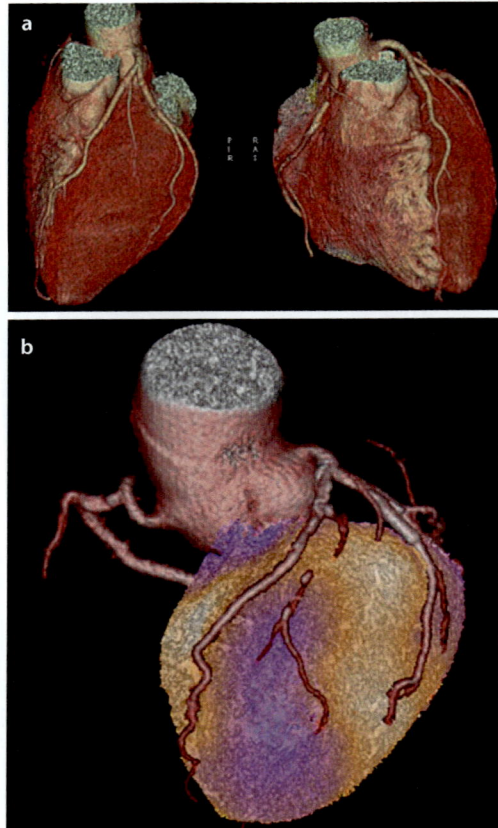

Fig. 2.22 a, b Modern Cardiac Hybrid Imaging. a 3D reconstruction of the left ventricle, **b** hybrid imaging. By fusing SPECT and CT data, functional and anatomical relationships can be superimposed. *Violet:* ischemic area, under-supplied due to the high-grade stenosis in the diagonal branch of the LAD. (Courtesy of Phillip A. Kaufmann, University Hospital Zurich)

which lesion is functionally relevant, i.e., causing ischemia and should be revascularized.

2.6 Coronary Angiography and Left Heart Catheterovation

With **coronary angiography** (Fig. 2.23), a direct visualization of the lumen of coronary arteries is achieved. Under local anesthesia, a catheter is usually advanced radially (via puncture of the the radial artery at the wrist of the right arm) or alternatively via the femoral artery retrogradely through the aorta to the right and left coronary ostium. After selective injection of contrast medium, the coronary arteries can be visualized in various planes using X-ray fluoroscopy.

The coronary angiography can be combined with a complete **left heart catheter examination**. For this purpose, a catheter, usually a so-called pigtail catheter (which is coiled at the end like a pig's tail), is placed retrogradely through the aortic valve into the left ventricle. With a specially connected pressure sensor, complete invasive hemo-

Cardiological Diagnostics

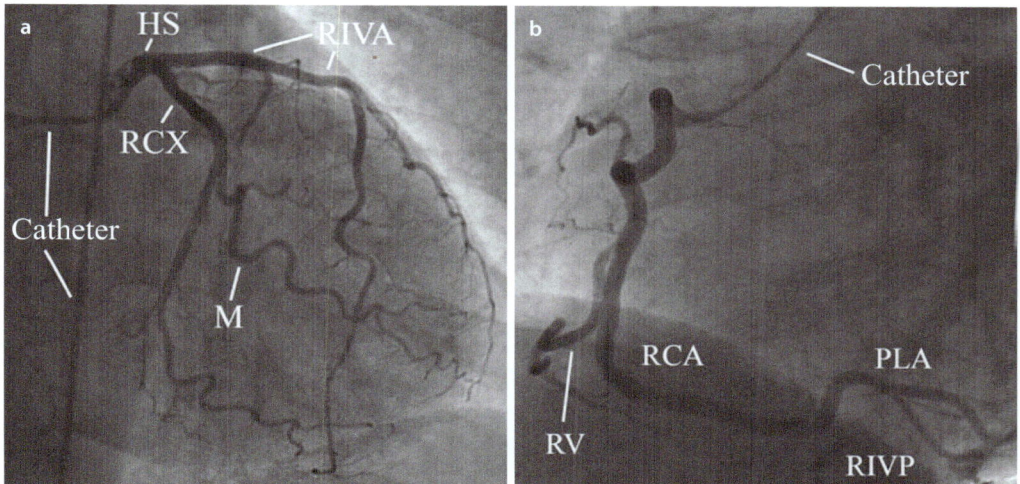

Fig. 2.23 a, b **Coronary Angiography.** a Left and b right coronary artery without significant stenoses. (*LM*: left main, *M*: marginal branch (or posterolateral branch), *RCA*: right coronary artery, *PLA*: posterolateral branch, *LAD*: left anterior descending artery, *PDA*: posterior descending artery, *RV*: right ventricular branch, *LCX*: Left circumflex coronary artery)

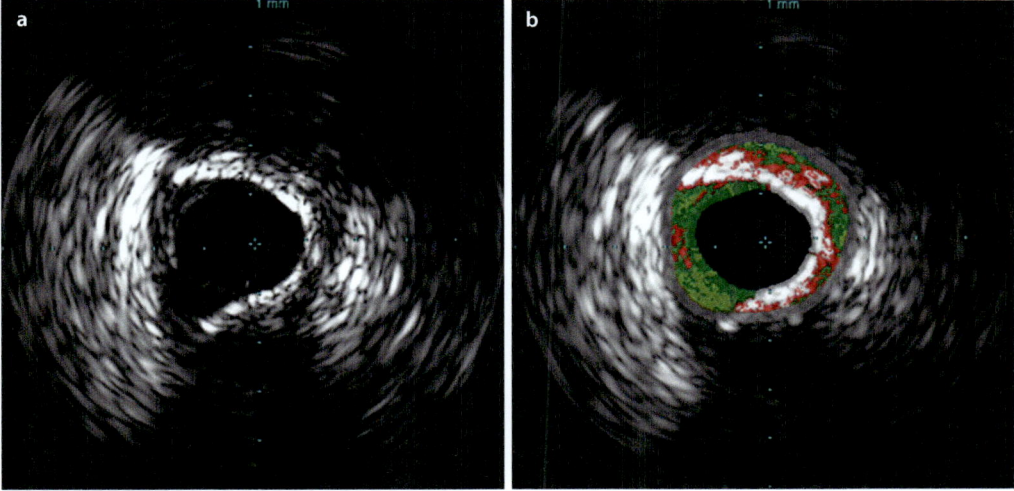

Fig. 2.24 a, b Long 50% main stem lesion. a Ostial part of the LAD with heavily calcified plaque, b Diagnosis of plaque components using *Virtual Histology IVUS*

dynamics can be performed (▶ Chap. 1, ◘ Fig. 1.4). By rapid injection of contrast medium into the left ventricle (**ventriculography**), the heart size as well as valve and ventricular function can be assessed.

During coronary angiography, primarily coronary stenoses and plaques, vascular occlusions (chronic or acute, as in acute myocardial infarction, ▶ Sect. 7.5), coronary dissections, or vascular spasms can be

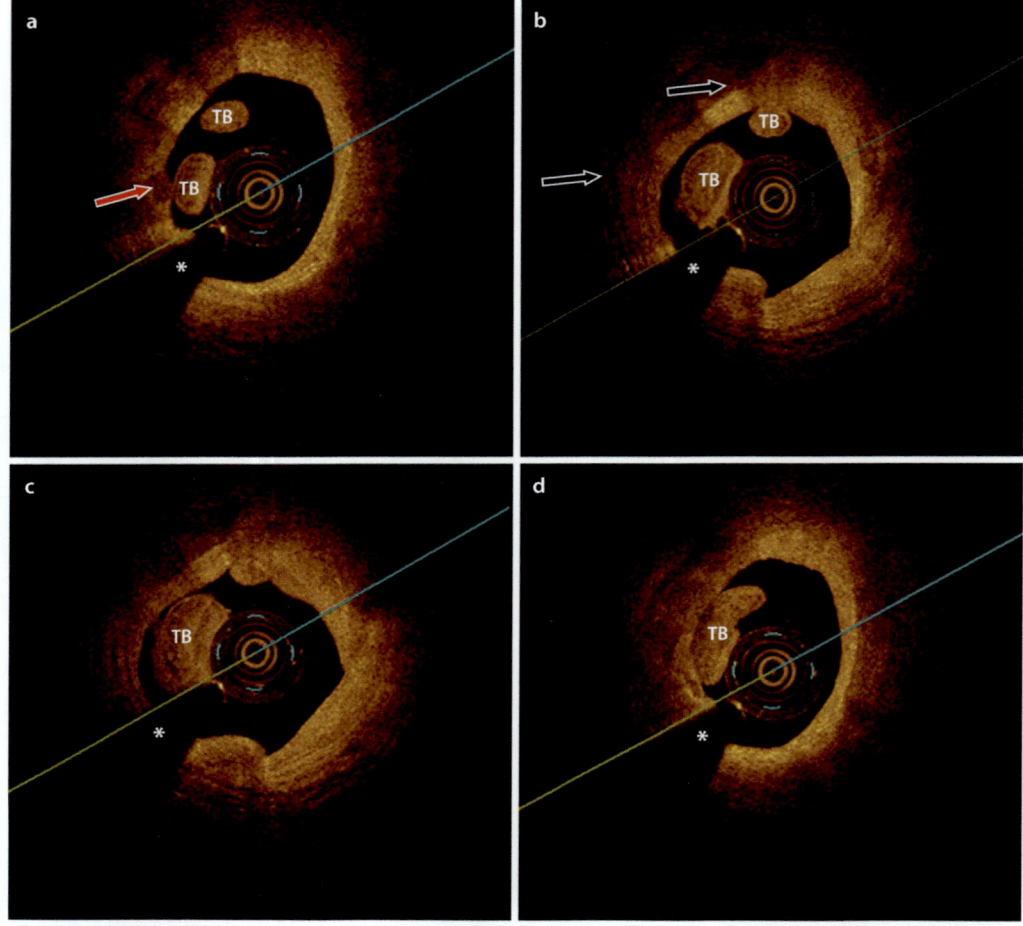

Fig. 2.25 a–d OCT: Red thrombus in a patient with non-STEMI (proximal LCX). Red arrows—plaque rupture; black arrows—shadow of the red thrombus; *TB* = thrombus; * = optical shadow caused by the guidewire

visualised. Anatomical variants (e.g., coronary origin anomalies, coronary fistulas, and myocardial bridges) are also visible, if present.

Types of supply
- If a strong posterolateral branch of the right coronary artery arises supplying the diaphragmatic branches of the left ventricle is present, it is referred to as a righty dominant type (70–75%).
- If it arises from the LCX, is iconsidered a balanced dominance type (15%).
- In the left dominant type (approx. 10%), the RCA is small and supplies only the right atrium and ventricle, while the myocardium of the left ventricle is completely supplied by the LAD and LCX.

Cardiological Diagnostics

- **Supplementary Intravascular Procedures during Coronary Angiography**

Fractional Flow Reserve (FFR)

FFR (fractional flow reserve) is used to evaluate the hemodynamic relevance of a coronary stenosis, i.e., whether it leads to a restriction of blood flow during stress. For this purpose, a coronary wire, which is equipped with a miniaturized pressure sensor at its tip, is placed distal to a stenosis. By comparing the pressure values distal and proximal to the stenosis after i.v. or i.c. administration of adenosine it can be determined whether a coronary stenosis leads to a relevant reduction in blood flow and should be revascularized or not.

Intravascular Ultrasound (IVUS)

IVUS is a high-resolution ultrasound procedure that provides a cross-sectional view of a coronary artery. The high resolution allows visualization of the different layers of the arterial wall (intima, media, adventitia) and is helpful if coronary angiography does not provide sufficient information (e.g., in plaque ruptures, coronary dissections, heavily calcified vessels, after stenting or complex interventions). The *Virtual Histology IVUS* enables differentiation of lipid-rich, fibrotic, and calcified components of a coronary plaque (◘ Fig. 2.24).

Optical Coherence Tomography (OCT)

OCT, like IVUS, provides cross-sectional images of a coronary artery. Unlike IVUS, OCT uses electromagnetic waves in the infrared range, achieving a higher resolution than IVUS (approx. 10–20 µm). However, for an OCT, the blood must be displaced by an optically less dense medium (usually contrast medium or saline solution). The applications for OCT are largely similar to those for IVUS (◘ Fig. 2.25).

2.7 Right Heart Catheterization and Cardiac Output Determination

By means of a **right heart catheterization**, the pressure values in the various compartments of the right heart as well as the pulmonary circulation (◘ Fig. 1.4 ► Chap. 1) can be determined. For this purpose, a catheter is advanced through a large vein (V. brachialis, femoralis, subclavia, or jugularis), then through the V. cava into the right atrium and ventricle up to the pulmonary artery. This is facilitated by an inflatable balloon at the end of the catheter (i.e. Swan-Ganz catheter), which allows "floating" into the pulmonary artery (◘ Fig. 2.26). If the balloon remains wedged in a lower branch of the pulmonary

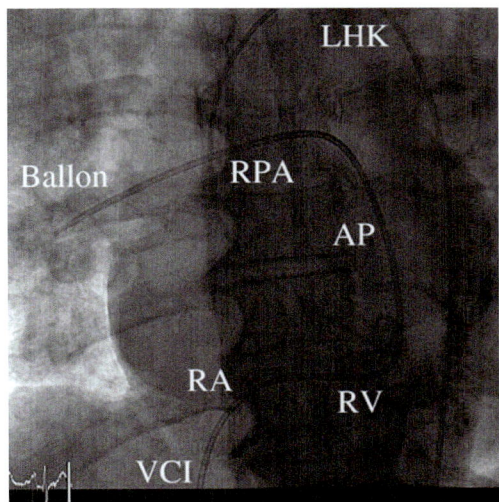

◘ **Fig. 2.26 Right heart catheter in wedge position with inflated balloon.** The right heart catheter is advanced through the V. cava inferior (*IVC*) through the right atrium (*RA*) and the right ventricle (*RV*) into the pulmonary artery (*PA*). *RPA*: right pulmonary artery, *LHC*: left heart catheter. (Pigtail, in the left ventricle for simultaneous left ventricular pressure measurement)

artery, the pulmonary capillary wedge pressure (Wedge-Pressure) can be determined, which approximately corresponds to the pressure in the left atrium.

The **cardiac output** can be determined in two different ways: In the thermodilution method, cold saline solution is rapidly injected through the proximal lumen of a special right heart catheter (modified Swan-Ganz catheter) located in the right atrium or V. cava. A thermosensor at the distal end of the catheter records the temperature change as a function of time, and the cardiac output is extrapolated. Although more or less prone to error depending on the situation, this method has proven particularly useful in intensive care for hemodynamic monitoring. In the cardiac catheterization lab, cardiac output can be calculated using the Fick equation with simultaneous pulse oximetry or with a simultaneously placed central arterial catheter. With known cardiac output, systemic blood pressure, pulmonary arterial pressure values, wedge pressure, and central venous pressure, systemic and pulmonary arterial resistances can be calculated (see also physiology textbooks).

Epidemiology and Prevention

Martin Halle and Thomas Münzel

Contents

3.1 Incidence and Prevalence of Non-Communicable Diseases – 34
3.1.1 Incidence – 35
3.1.2 Prevalence – 35
3.1.3 Mortality – 35

3.2 Cardiovascular Prevention – 35

3.3 Cardiovascular Risk Factors (CVRF) – 37
3.3.1 Arterial Hypertension – 37
3.3.2 Hypercholesterolemia – 37
3.3.3 Overweight – 41
3.3.4 Diabetes – 42
3.3.5 Smoking – 42

3.4 Environmental Factors – 43
3.4.1 Air Pollution – 43
3.4.2 Transport Noise – 44
3.4.3 The Exposome Concept – 44

3.5 Exercise and Sport – 45

References – 47

© The Author(s), under exclusive license to Springer-Verlag GmbH, DE, part of Springer Nature 2025
T. F. Lüscher and U. Landmesser (eds.), *Cardiovascular System*,
https://doi.org/10.1007/978-3-662-70152-2_3

Prevention is of extraordinary importance, because it is said that *"prevention is better than cure"*—and this is especially true for cardiovascular diseases, which are not only common but can also be largely prevented through appropriate lifestyle and therapeutic measures.

3.1 Incidence and Prevalence of Non-Communicable Diseases

Non-Communicable Diseases (NCDs) cause more than 38 million deaths each year, accounting for almost 70% of the total mortality worldwide. Among these deaths, over 14 million adults, who according to the World Health Organization (WHO) *"die too young,"* i.e., between the ages of 30 and 70 years. The vast majority of deaths among NCDs are due to cardiovascular diseases. This trend is increasing. In the *Global Burden of Disease* (GBD) data collection (2020), the number of cardiovascular deaths steadily increased from 12.1 million in 1990 to 18.6 million in 2019 (Fig. 3.1).

› Cardiovascular diseases therefore continue to dominate the death statistics in Western countries.

In just 3 decades of global mortality accounting, there has been a significant shift from communicable diseases (e.g., infectious diseases) to NCDs, with cardiovascular diseases, diabetes (▶ Chap. 6) and arterial hypertension (▶ Chap. 4) predominating (Fig. 3.1).

It should be noted that the forecast for 2030 does not take into account the impact of the COVID-19 pandemic (during which CVD patients had the highest mortality). Despite the pronounced awareness of the growing health and economic consequences of NCDs, the significant contribution of the environment as a cause of NCDs is not sufficiently recognized. This is surprising, as ambient air pollution consistently ranks among the top 5 causes of global mortality (*Global Burden of Disease* Lancet 2017).

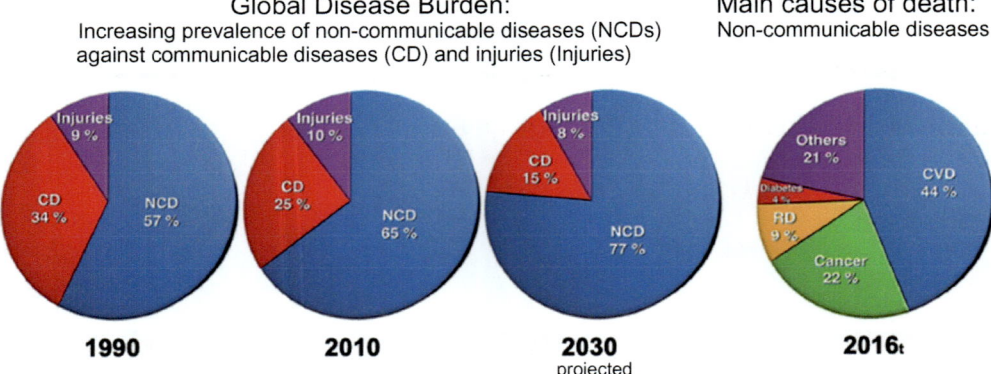

Fig. 3.1 Global Burden of Disease (GBD) and Non-Communicable Diseases (*NCD*). The proportional distribution of global deaths attributable to *communicable diseases* (*CD*) and *NCD* and *injuries* for the years 1990, 2010, and projected for 2030 (left half of the image). Estimation of the most common causes of death by various NCDs (WHO 2024). The category "Others" includes neurological and musculoskeletal diseases, congenital anomalies, digestive disorders, endocrine/blood/immune and urogenital diseases, and rare conditions. *CVD:* Cardiovascular Diseases, *RD:* (Respiratory Diseases). (Modified from *Cardiovasc. Res.* 2022)

3.1.1 Incidence

The age-standardized incidence (i.e., the number of new cases during a specific period) of cardiovascular diseases per 100,000 inhabitants in Europe showed a slight decline from 898 (IQR 766–1033) in 1990 to 748 (IQR 558–972) in 2019. The decline was generally small, and slight increases were recorded in middle-income countries. In 2019, women were more affected than men in European countries (6.5 million vs. 6.1 million), whereas the age-standardized rates were lower for women than for men (*European Society of Cardiology: Cardiovascular Disease Statistics* 2021).

3.1.2 Prevalence

Between 1990 and 2019, the mean age-standardized **prevalence estimates** (i.e., total number of disease cases at a given time) for cardiovascular diseases per 100,000 inhabitants remained stable. In 2019, more women than men lived with cardiovascular diseases in European countries (60 vs. 53 million). However, the mean age-standardized prevalence estimates per 100,000 people were lower for women than for men.

The frequency of cardiovascular diseases varies greatly in **different countries**, likely due to different lifestyles, eating and smoking habits, physical activities, air and noise pollution, genetic predisposition, and more (◌ Fig. 3.2).

In the last 30 years, the decline in age-standardized incidence of cardiovascular diseases in countries on the European continent has been slight and dependent on the average income of the countries. The age-standardized incidences for the main components ischemic (or coronary) heart disease (CHD) and stroke are twice as high in middle-income countries as in high-income countries. Thus, both diseases have also declined by over 25% in high-income countries in the last 30 years. Nevertheless, the ongoing impact of CHD and stroke on population health remains dramatic for both women and men. Indeed, these diseases are estimated to cost 70 million disability-adjusted life years (DALYs) (*European Society of Cardiology: Cardiovascular Disease Statistics* 2021).

3.1.3 Mortality

Cardiovascular diseases are the leading cause of death in European countries, with coronary heart disease (CHD ▶ Sect. 7.2) accounting for 45% of these deaths in women and 39% in men. The age-standardized mortality rates for cardiovascular diseases have decreased by 47% in men and 42% in women since 1990. However, this is quite heterogeneous, with a significantly higher decline in high-income countries (50% compared to low-income countries: <15%). The total number of deaths far exceeds the number of cancer deaths in both genders. In high-income countries, however, cancer diseases also predominate, with a gender distribution unfavorable to men, who have higher cancer mortality. Income is also significant regarding premature deaths (<70 years) from cardiovascular diseases. Here, gender also plays a role. In middle-income countries, women die twice as often from cardiovascular diseases as in high-income countries (36% versus 16%). For men, the corresponding figures are 36% and 24% in middle-income and high-income countries, respectively.

3.2 Cardiovascular Prevention

Prevention is the prevention of cardiovascular diseases ("*Prevention is better than cure*"). Three strategies can be distinguished (although the transition is fluid):

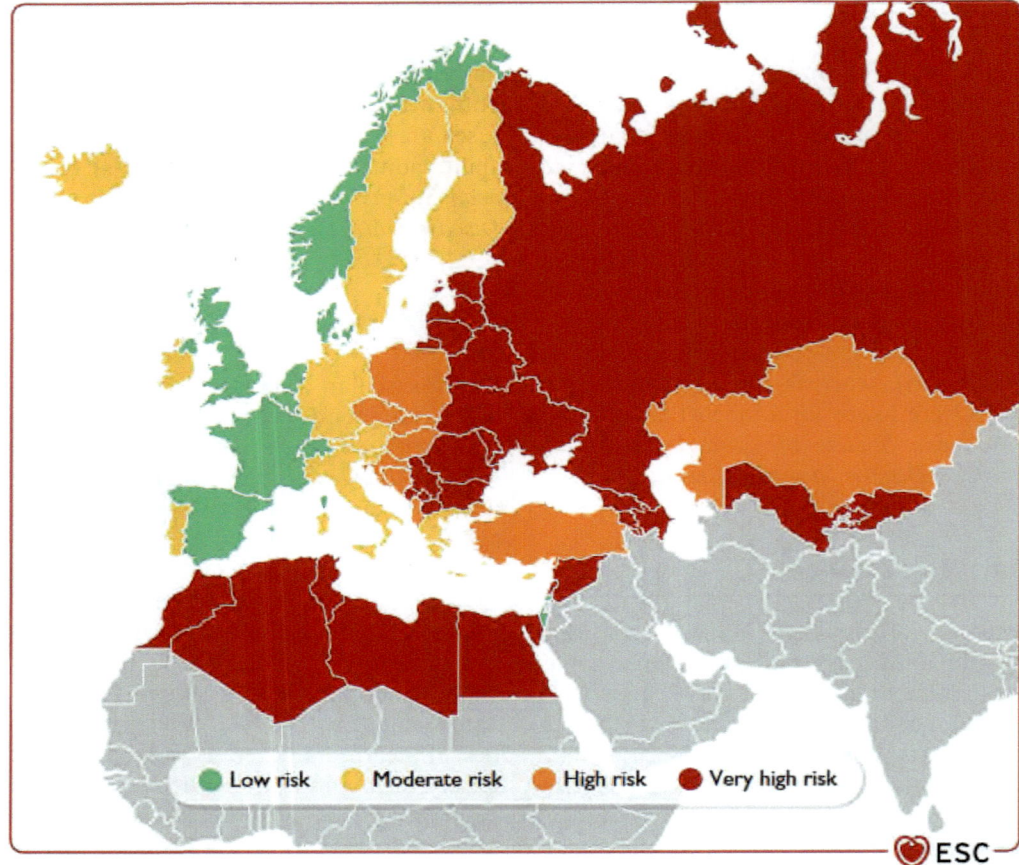

Fig. 3.2 Risk regions, based on data on 10-year morbidity and mortality from cardiovascular diseases. (From Visseren et al. 2021)

- primordial prevention,
- primary prevention, and
- secondary prevention.

Primordial Prevention aims at the prevention of cardiovascular risk factors (e.g., overweight, hypertension, diabetes, lipid metabolism disorders, etc.). This prevention begins with conception and extends into old adulthood—the concept of *"life-long prevention."*

The measures primarily include improvements in lifestyle (i.e., nutrition, exercise, smoking cessation, etc.). In addition to weight normalization through calorie reduction (quantitative dietary recommendations), the main dietary goal, positive cardiovascular effects can also be achieved through qualitative dietary changes. A so-called Mediterranean diet (lots of vegetables and fruits, olive oil, and fish or white meat) with a high proportion of unsaturated fatty acids and low salt consumption is crucial.

Risk factors can be physical, psychological, or environmental factors that increase the risk of the occurrence of a disease, the incidence. A distinction is made between modifiable (e.g., smoking, physical activity) and non-modifiable risk factors (e.g., age, gender, or genetic predisposition).

Primary Prevention of cardiovascular diseases consists of targeted measures for the detection of cardiovascular risk factors as well as their prevention, manifestation, and influence through lifestyle or medication in still healthy individuals without heart diseases such as CAD (▶ Sect. 7.2), heart failure (▶ Chap. 13), arrhythmias such as atrial fibrillation (▶ Chap. 12), peripheral arterial occlusive disease (▶ Sect. 7.6) or stroke (▶ Sect. 7.7).

Whether and to what extent a risk exists in patients and the urgency and type of a preventive intervention can be calculated, among other things, using risk scores, e.g., with the SCORE2 (**S**ystematic **Co**ronary **R**isk **E**stimation) or SCORE2-OP (OP for "**O**lder **P**ersons") (◘ Fig. 3.3)—a risk assessment model of the ESC (*European Society of Cardiology*) for estimating the 10-year risk of morbidity and mortality from cardiovascular diseases in different regions in Europe.

Secondary Prevention includes preventive measures for those already affected, e.g., in patients with CAD or after a myocardial infarction (Sects. 7.2 or 7.5), heart failure (▶ Chap. 13), arrhythmias, (▶ Chap. 12) with peripheral arterial occlusive disease (▶ Sect. 7.6) or after a stroke (▶ Sect. 7.7).

3.3 Cardiovascular Risk Factors (CVRF)

Cardiovascular risk factor (KVRF), are not only associated with an increased risk for cardiovascular events (i.e., myocardial infarction, stroke, premature death etc.), but whose modification leads to a reduction in cardiovascular risk. In addition, there are so-called *innocent bystanders* such as homocysteine, which predicts cardiovascular risk, but whose reduction does not lead to a decrease in cardiovascular risk. Psychological stress or environmental factors are risk modifiers that also increase cardiovascular risk. CVRFs interact with each other and potentiate the risk (◘ Fig. 3.4).

3.3.1 Arterial Hypertension

The rates for **high blood pressure** ($\geq 140/90$ mmHg; ▶ Chap. 4) have decreased by 35% in European countries over the past 35 years, but almost 1 in 4 individuals are still affected. Systolic blood pressure is higher in men than in women. Income also has an influence here. In middle-income countries, the incidence is higher than in high-income countries. Observational studies over the past 40 years show that the incidence of arterial hypertension has increased very significantly in low-income countries. High blood pressure is the leading risk factor for cardiovascular diseases worldwide. There is a continuous linear relationship between blood pressure values and the risk of stroke, myocardial infarction, and premature death. Treatment to lower blood pressure offers significant protection against cardiovascular events, with increasing benefit from intensive treatment in patients with higher overall risk (accompanying vascular disease ▶ Sect. 4.6) such as patients with kidney disease or diabetes (▶ Chap. 6).

As a result, there are increases in disability-adjusted life years (DALYs) and deaths. Population-based interventions are as necessary as additional pharmacological treatment for patients with high blood pressure to address the global burden of hypertension and particularly to reduce clinical events in poorer countries.

3.3.2 Hypercholesterolemia

Cholesterol, especially the fraction of Non-HDL (*non high density lipoprotein*) cholesterol (nonHDL-C), LDL (*low-density lipoprotein*) and VLDL cholesterol with very low density (*very low density lipoprotein*) are

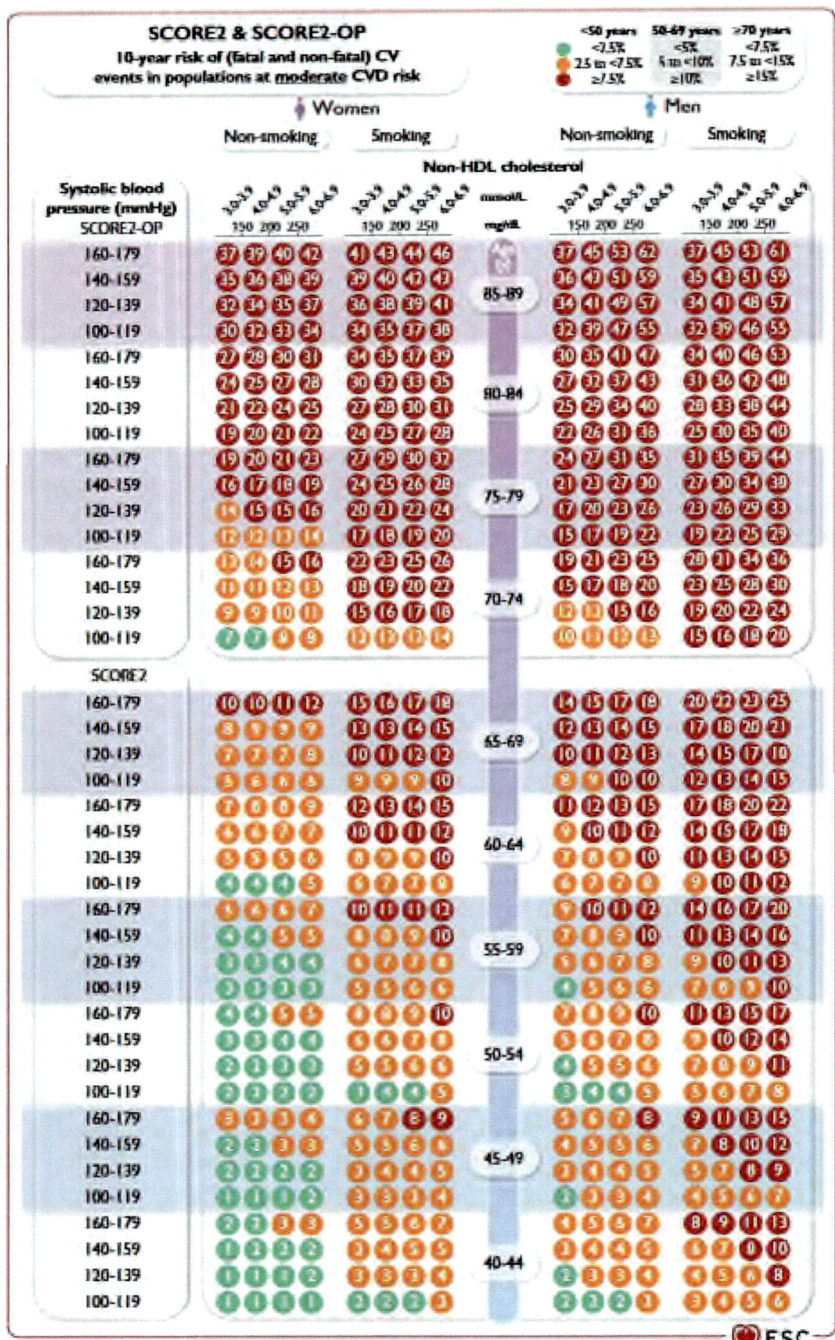

Fig. 3.3 SCORE2 and SCORE2-OP. Risk table for cardiovascular diseases in countries with moderate risk (Austria, Cyprus, Finland, Germany, Greece, Iceland, Ireland, Italy, Malta, Portugal, San Marino, Slovenia, and Sweden). The numbers indicate the 10-year morbidity and mortality of cardiovascular diseases. (From Visseren et al. 2021)

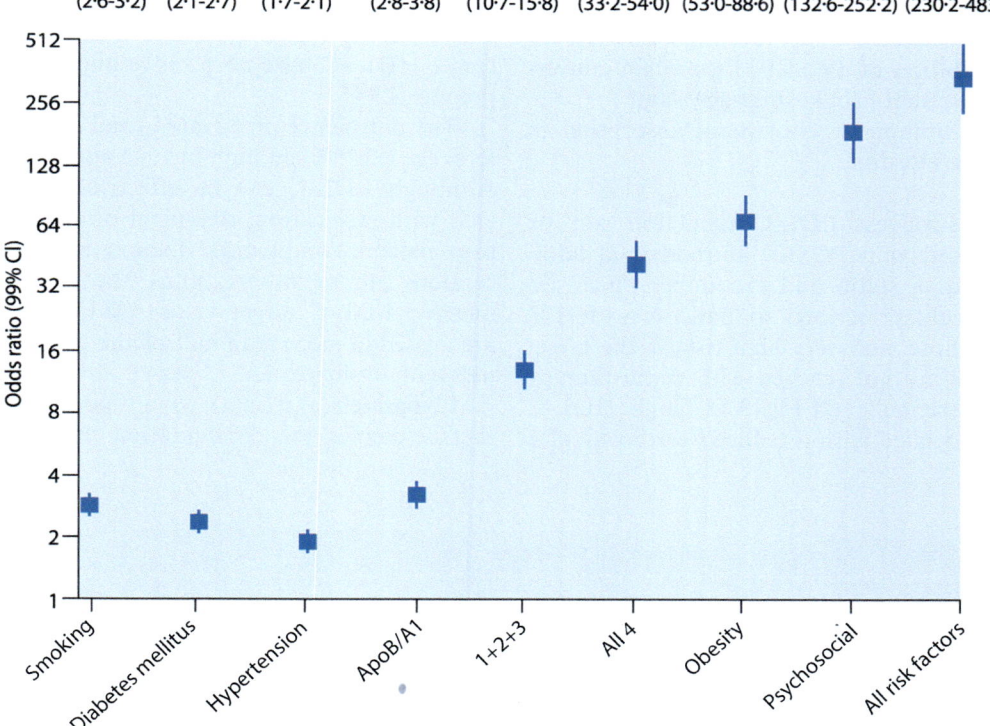

Fig. 3.4 Risk in heart attack when multiple risk factors and modifiers coincide. (Modified according to data from Yusuf et al. 2024)

major determinants of cardiovascular risk. The "vascular load" is an expression of the temporal exposure of LDL-C to the vascular walls with cumulative exposure from childhood to young and older adulthood. Lowering LDL-C or nonHDL-C reduces the vascular load and demonstrably lowers death, heart attack, and stroke.

Hypercholesterolemia is often familial with heterozygous disposition in about 1:500 in the general population. This mutation is associated with a significant increase in serum cholesterol concentrations (often >8.0 mmol/L) with a considerable risk for premature myocardial infarction, occasionally already in young adulthood. **Familial hypercholesterolemia** (FH) remains a clinical diagnosis but can be confirmed by genetic tests (e.g. mutations on the LDL-C receptor, PCSK9 among others). After the diagnosis of an index case is made, cascade screening (lipids or gene analysis) of all first-degree relatives is mandatory. Hypercholesterolemia is also a major target in primary prevention programs for risk reduction, as statin therapy in individuals without cardiovascular disease can reduce the risk of vascular death by 15% if LDL-C can be lowered by 1 mmol/L.

- **Cholesterol-lowering agents and target values**

Cholesterol levels, particularly LDL-C and nonHDL-C, can be lowered in 3 ways (◘ Table 3.1):

- Inhibition of cholesterol synthesis,
- Increase of LDL receptors through inhibition of PCSK9 (Proprotein convertase subtilisin/kexin type 9) and
- Inhibition of cholesterol absorption in the intestine.

The strongest LDL-C reduction can be achieved with PCSK9 antibodies in addition to a statin and ezetimibe, which are routinely prescribed to patients with FH and those with very high risk, if the target values are not reached with statin therapy and ezetimibe (◘ Fig. 3.1). High HDL-C is associated with a reduced cardiovascular risk, but does not have a causally protective effect. Accordingly, medications that increase HDL-C have no positive impact on prognosis.

The prevalence of elevated total cholesterol exceeds 50% in high-income countries. Although LDL-C can be effectively lowered with medication, treatment often fails (e.g. patient compliance, doctors misconceptions among others); thus, the recommended LDL-C target values (◘ Fig. 3.5) are missed in more than half of the individuals with dyslipidemia.

Lipoprotein(a) (Lp(a)) is a lipoprotein that resembles the configuration of plas-

◘ Table 3.1 Most important cholesterol-lowering medications

Medication	Metabolic pathway	Mechanism	Comment
Statins – Atorvastatin – Rosuvastatin – Simvastatin	Reduction of cholesterol synthesis	Inhibition of HMG-Coenzyme A reductase	LDL-C reduction up to 50% Reduction of death and infarction (+ + +)
Bempedoic acid	Reduction of cholesterol synthesis	Inhibition of ATP-citrate lyase	LDL-C reduction around 25% Reduction of death and infarction (+)
PCSK9 inhibitors (antibodies) – Alirocumab – Evolocumab	Increase of LDL cholesterol uptake from the blood	Antibodies against PCSK9 prevent the degradation of LDL receptors and thereby increase the clearance of LDL-C	LDL-C reduction by 60% in addition to statin Reduction of infarction and partly death (+ +)
PCSK9 inhibitors (RNA interference) – Inclisiran	Increase of LDL cholesterol uptake from the blood	Direct inhibition of PCSK9 protein synthesis through RNA interference in the RISC, which reduces the translation of mRNA for PCSK9 into a protein.	LDL-C reduction by 50% in addition to statin Prognostic effect is being investigated
Ezetimibe	Inhibition of cholesterol absorption in the intestine	Inhibition of Niemann-Pick-C1 transporter (NPC1L1)	LDL-C reduction 18% in addition to statin Prognosis (+)

LDL-R = LDL receptor on hepatocytes; + − + + + = extent of evidence for prognostic effect; 1 = one randomized study; + + = 2 randomized studies; + + + = multiple studies. RISC = RNA-induced silencing complex.

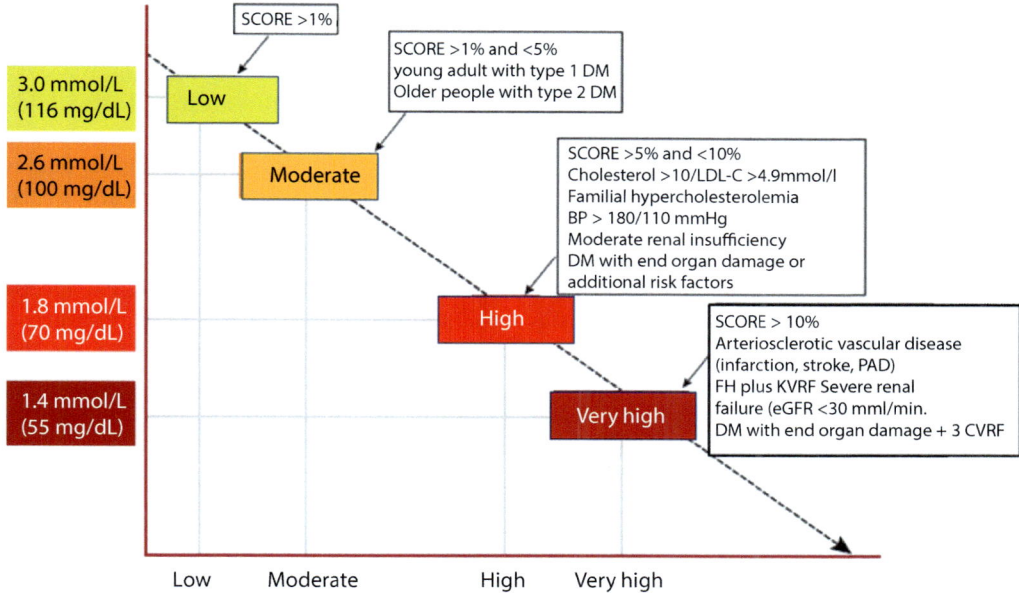

Fig. 3.5 Recommended LDL-C target values according to different risk categories. (Modified after Mach et al. 2020)

minogen and thus blocks fibrinolysis. An elevated Lp(a) level is strongly genetically determined and increases the risk of coronary heart disease, especially with simultaneously elevated LDL-C, although its role as a risk factor has not yet been definitively clarified, as effective medications to lower it are currently lacking or still pending approval. However, Mendelian randomization studies suggest a causality.

Elevated **triglycerides** are frequently observed in diabetes mellitus and obesity, but fundamentally have a lesser pathological role and are dealt with there (▶ Chap. 6).

a further decline in cardiovascular mortality. The prevalence of obesity is now more significant worldwide and in most regions of the world than malnutrition and underweight. The obesity epidemic has been largely caused by global trade liberalization, economic growth, and rapid urbanization, which have impacted lifestyle and food intake, with a trend towards more consumption of animal fat and added sugars in foods. In 2016, the meta-analysis of the *Global BMI Mortality Collaboration* reported that in overweight and obese people living in the European region, mortality increases by 39% for every 5 kg/m² increase in BMI.

3.3.3 Overweight

The prevalence of overweight and obesity, defined by a body mass index (BMI) of ≥ 25 kg/m² and ≥ 30 kg/m² respectively, is increasing in both industrialized and developing countries and threatens to become one of the major factors preventing

Body weight categories
- Underweight < 20 kg/m²
- Normal weight 20–25 kg/m²
- Overweight > 25–< 30 kg/m²
- Obesity > 30 kg/m²

Pharmacological treatment options have recently been developed and allow for sustained weight reduction with glucagon-like peptide-1 (GLP-1) receptor agonists (e.g., liraglutide, semaglutide) or combined GLP-1/GIP (Glucose-dependent insulinotropic polypeptide). GLP-1 Agonism reduces not only weight, but also the the severity or risk for type 2 diabetes, the risk of heart and renal failure and other cardiovascular diseases. Bariatric surgery is significantly more effective in weight reduction, leading also to a reduction in diabetes and mortality. However, the focus of efforts to address the obesity epidemic in the population should be on lifestyle changes and political initiatives to promote exercise and healthy diet and living starting from childhood.

3.3.4 Diabetes

Obesity is an independent modifier of cardiovascular risk, but its main impact lies in its contribution to the epidemic of type 2 diabetes (▶ Chap. 6), which today is estimated to affect 422 million people worldwide, over 60 million of whom live in European countries. The prevalence of diabetes is also increasing in European countries across all age groups, mainly due to high-calorie diets and lack of physical activity, and the successive increase in overweight and obesity. Having diabetes doubles the risk of death compared to people without diabetes. At least half of these deaths are caused by cardiovascular diseases, usually due to a heart attack or stroke. For this reason, the WHO Director-General referred to obesity and diabetes as two of the greatest global health crises of the twenty-first century, from the WHO's perspective, the result of a world where food is abundant and exercise is optional. This development is not only driven by the consumption of high-calorie foods but rather a failure of governments to regulate food and promote recreational physical activity and a healthy lifestyle from childhood.

Regulating blood sugar levels in diabetes is one of the central therapeutic goals, but so far this has only led to a slight reduction in cardiovascular risk. The new blood sugar-lowering drugs such as GLP-1 receptor agonists and SGLT-2 (sodium-glucose transporter type 2) inhibitors have for the first time been able to demonstrate a significant reduction in mortality and the occurrence of heart failure (▶ Chap. 6 and ▶ Sect. 13.4). Obesity surgery is also effective in achieving significant weight loss and controlling metabolic risk factors or even cure type 2 diabetes. Nevertheless, it must be questioned whether these novel pharmacological and surgical interventions can serve as strategies to reduce cardiovascular risk at the population level (e.g. costs, unknown longterm effects). Much more crucial is prevention at the population level through political initiatives that create an environment in which people are empowered to choose a cardio-metabolically healthy lifestyle to protect themselves from obesity and its harmful effects on glucose metabolism, blood pressure, and blood lipids. Political initiatives with proven benefits in this direction include sugar taxes and traffic light labeling of foods and beverages and healthy cities (e.g. pedestrian zones, bicycle lanes among others).

3.3.5 Smoking

It is important to note: There is no smoking without increased cardiovascular risk. Light smokers who consume only one cigarette per day still have almost half the risk of developing cardiovascular diseases compared to heavy smokers (20 cigarettes/day).

Passive smokers are also at risk, and if passive exposure is significant, it is associated with a similar relative risk for cardiovascular diseases as light active smoking exposure. Smokers who quit smoking can reduce their risk of cardiovascular diseases by 39% within 5 years, but it takes at least 15 years for the cardiovascular risk to reach the level of a person who has never smoked in their life.

Smoking cessation after a myocardial infarction (secondary prevention) is particularly important, as this can halve subsequent mortality. E-cigarettes have been proposed as a safer alternative or as a temporary measure for smoking cessation, but the data is not clear. Due to the lack of robust longitudinal data, the evidence is considered insufficient by guideline groups to recommend the use of e-cigarettes to reduce tobacco consumption. Additionally, the use of e-cigarettes among adolescents and young adults is associated with an increased risk of later cigarette smoking. Overall, survey data show that after a temporary decline, smoking rates are currently rising again. This, combined with the increased use of e-cigarettes, will increase cardiovascular risk again in the future.

> Tobacco consumption has been described by the Directorate-General for Health and Food Safety of the European Commission as "the greatest avoidable health risk in the EU." For nicotine cessation, various medications have been developed in addition to behavioral therapy measures, which have a moderate success rate. Both measures should be used in combination.

Medications for Nicotine cessation
- Varenicline (partial nicotine receptor agonist)
- Transdermal nicotine patches

3.4 Environmental Factors

Air pollution and noise are responsible for over 75% of the disease burden attributable to environmental factors. Each year, an estimated 48,000 new cases of CHD due to environmental noise exposure occur across Europe. According to WHO, about 58% of air pollution-related mortality is caused by CHD and stroke. Migrant studies further support the role of the environment as a risk factor by showing that South Asians living in the United Kingdom have a higher cardiovascular risk than those living in South Asia. Furthermore, Finnish twins living in Sweden have lower cardiovascular event rates than their co-twins living in Finland, which again confirms that environmental changes influence risk independently of genetic factors.

3.4.1 Air Pollution

Pollution from particulate matter and gases has various causes, including private and commercial energy use, agriculture, land transport, and power generation. Over 90% of the pollutant mass in the air mixture of urban environments comes from gases or compounds in the vapor phase and secondary pollutants, including ozone (O_3), nitrogen dioxide (NO_2), volatile organic compounds (including benzene), carbon monoxide (CO_2), and sulfur dioxide (SO_2). Combustion residues containing fine particles or PM 0.1 (PM = particulate matter <0.1 μm in diameter) show increased cardiovascular toxicity due to characteristics such as high particle number, large surface-to-mass ratio, oxidative stress potential, high solubility, and charge, leading to effective penetration in the airways and likely systemic penetration.

Air pollution poses a major health risk, responsible for 7.6% of global DALYs and associated with approximately 6.5–8.8

million premature deaths per year, which rivals the health impacts of smoking, high blood pressure, and physical inactivity.

Premature deaths related to exposure to fine particulate matter (PM 2.5) are attributed to cardiovascular diseases. Accordingly, the European Union has set an air quality standard for PM 2.5 of <25 μg/m^3, while the World Health Organisation (WHO) has lowered the new guidelines to 5 μg/m^3 or less. This means that well over 95% of the world's population lives above the limit set by the WHO, and the European guidelines are not accepted worldwide. The adverse effects of air pollution on public health are undisputed, with cardiovascular diseases primarily dominating. Recent figures estimate a total of 780,000 additional deaths per year due to PM 2.5, with 40% attributed to CHD, 8% to strokes, and 32% to other NCDs including diabetes and arterial hypertension. It is estimated that air pollution reduces the average life expectancy in Europe by about 2.9 years, with an annual attributable per capita mortality rate in Europe of 133/100,000 people per year.

The United Nations' sustainable development goals developed in 2016 include air pollution as an urgent issue, and the WHO monitors pollution indicators, including air pollution-related mortality, access to clean energy in households, and air quality in cities. Meanwhile, European environmental policy, based on the principles of precaution, prevention, and pollution elimination, gives cause for optimism that the challenges posed by pollution are high on the political agenda.

3.4.2 Transport Noise

Transport noise refers to noise generated by cars, airplanes, and rail vehicles. Noise can increase cardiovascular risk, especially for people living in densely populated urban areas near busy roads or train stations. It is estimated that noise pollution is responsible for 48,000 new cases of coronary heart disease (CHD) per year and 12,000 premature deaths in Europe. In Western Europe alone, 1.6 million healthy life years are lost annually, mostly due to sleep disturbances and annoyance reactions.

The EU has set permissible noise levels in residential areas at 55 and 50 dB during the day and night, respectively. These limits are often exceeded, and noise levels above 55 dB affect up to 40% of the EU population. Noise causes stress and disrupts sleep, predisposing individuals to CHD, with the risk increasing by 6% for every 10 dB increase in day-night noise. These adverse cardiovascular effects of noise are caused by slight increases in blood pressure, triglycerides, and glycosylated hemoglobin, which occur at exposures >65 dB. It is estimated that a reduction in ambient noise by 5 dB in the USA would reduce the number of cases of hypertension and cardiovascular diseases by 1.2 million and 279,000 cases per year, respectively. New observations are interesting, indicating that transport noise activates the limbic system, specifically the amygdala nuclei in the brain. The activity of the amygdala, determined using ^{18}Fluorodeoxyglucose in PET/CT, correlated within 5 years with the extent of aortic inflammation and cardiovascular complications such as death from heart attack, non-fatal heart attacks, coronary and peripheral revascularizations. Thus, "annoyance" over noise is an important stress factor that significantly increases the incidence of cardiovascular diseases. Conversely, pronounced resilience has a positive effect on the development of cardiovascular diseases.

3.4.3 The Exposome Concept

Unfortunately, environmental risk factors and their disease burden in the population are not mentioned in the WHO's 2013

Epidemiology and Prevention

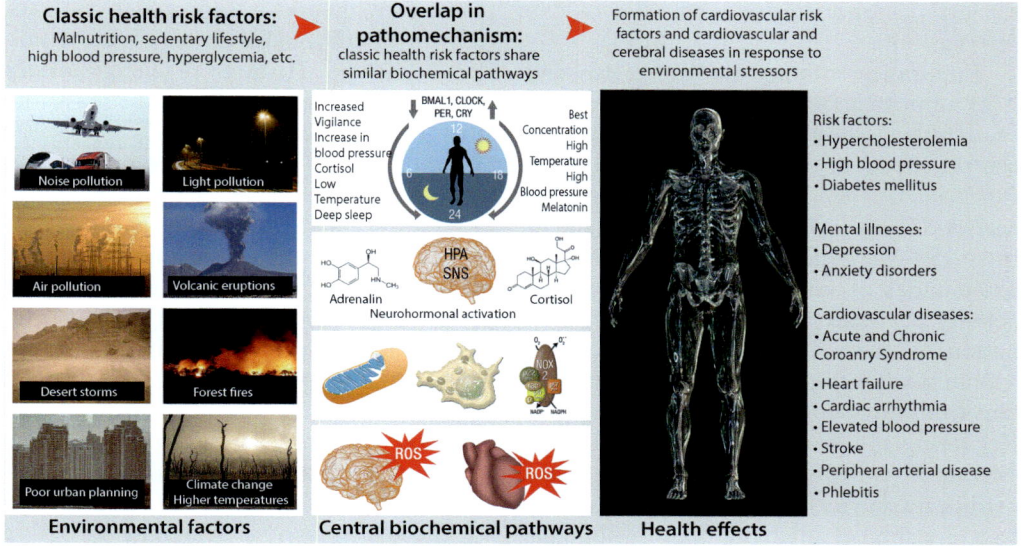

Fig. 3.6 The Exposome Concept. Exposure to environmental risk factors (= external exposome) leads to changes in key biochemical metabolic pathways with health impacts. These include 1. changes to circadian clock genes, leading to impaired rhythmicity and phase shifts, 2. increased release of stress hormones (cortisol and catecholamines, etc.), 3. increased formation of reactive oxygen species by mitochondria and NADPH oxidase, and 4. the release of activated immune cells. This leads to inflammation with tissue infiltration by immune system cells and oxidative damage in various organs. Since classical health risk factors activate similar mechanisms, people with diabetes, hyperlipidemia, or hypertension may suffer additional negative health effects when exposed to environmental risk factors. *HPA:* Hypothalamic-pituitary-adrenal axis, *NOX-2:* phagocytic NADPH oxidase (isoform 2), *ROS:* reactive oxygen species, *SNS:* sympathetic nervous system. (Modified after Münzel et al. CVR 2022; ▶ https://doi.org/10.1093/cvr/cvab316 with permission)

global action plan for NCDs. This dramatic gap is now receiving more attention through the emerging research field of "exposome," which examines the lifelong integral impacts of all environmental exposures on biochemical metabolic pathways and health outcomes (◘ Fig. 3.6) as well as campaigns for "healthy cities".

3.5 Exercise and Sport

Physical inactivity is one of the most important modifiable risk factors for global mortality, especially from cardiovascular diseases. Inactive people have a 20–30% higher risk of dying prematurely compared to physically active people. Regular physical activity can reduce the incidence of CHD (▶ Sect. 7.2), heart failure (▶ Chap. 13), and atrial fibrillation (▶ Sect. 12.5).

Regular exercise units lead to an increase in cardiopulmonary performance, a central indicator of a good prognosis. Accordingly, numerous positive effects on the cardiovascular system are induced, such as an improvement in cardiovascular risk factors (▶ Sect. 3.3), noticeable by a reduction in systolic and diastolic blood pressure, an optimization of glucose and lipid metabolism, and a reduction in chronic inflammation. The latter is particularly supported by additional weight loss in obese individuals. Physical training also induces structural changes in the cardiovascular system, improving endothelial function of the arteries and diastolic function of the myocardium.

Endurance training **Endurance training** is of utmost importance in the prevention of cardiovascular diseases, as it improves central effects on metabolism and vascular function. Current guidelines from the *European Society of Cardiology* recommend at least 150–300 minutes of moderate or 75–150 minutes of intense physical endurance activity per week, or an equivalent combination of these. This illustrates a dose-response relationship, meaning that higher intensities and volumes have greater effects. Regarding the duration of a training session, even short units of 10–15 minutes are cardioprotective. These are particularly effective at higher intensity because they induce a stronger cardiopulmonary and peripheral muscular stimulus.

Even a reduction in daily **sitting** time has preventive effects. This also implies the importance of everyday-based interventions at or to the workplace or educational institution. Although 10,000 steps per day, equivalent to about 8 km of walking, are generally recommended, epidemiological data show maximum effects already at 4500 steps per day, equivalent to about 3 km, which corresponds to 30 minutes of walking per day. Volumes of physical activity beyond this have only marginally higher effects.

Strength training **Strength training** has comparable effects to endurance training when performed as strength-endurance training, i.e., many repetitions with low weights. However, the overall effect size is smaller. Strength training is recommended at least twice a week in addition to endurance training (Visseren et al. 2021) and is particularly important for older patients, e.g., with additional diabetes or heart failure, due to the activation of energy metabolism and the increase in muscle mass and strength for fall prevention.

Training stimuli to **improve glucose metabolisms** are optimal, if applied every 2–3 days because one of the pathophysiological mechanisms of insulin resistance, the impaired activity of the glucose-4 transporter regulating insulin-dependent glucose uptake in the muscle membrane, is enhanced, and this effect lasts about 2–3 days. Vascular effects, which also positively affect blood pressure, are best observed when the training stimulus is applied every day or every other day.

The **activation of skeletal muscles** during physical exertion seems to play a key role. It functions like an "endocrine organ," from which bioactive substances (the so-called myokines) are secreted, especially during muscle contraction, which are responsible for metabolic and functional adaptations (see ◘ Fig. 3.7). Thus, the regular activation of this system through combined endurance and strength training is crucial in cardiovascular prevention.

Due to the **concept of "vascular load"** of risk factors, i.e., the height and duration of interaction time between risk factors and the vascular system and myocardium, early prevention starting in childhood and adolescence is of central importance. Especially obese and physically inactive children and adolescents already show pathophysiological changes in the vascular system, such as impaired endothelial function early on, which, however, are completely reversible through appropriate lifestyle interventions (◘ Fig. 3.7).

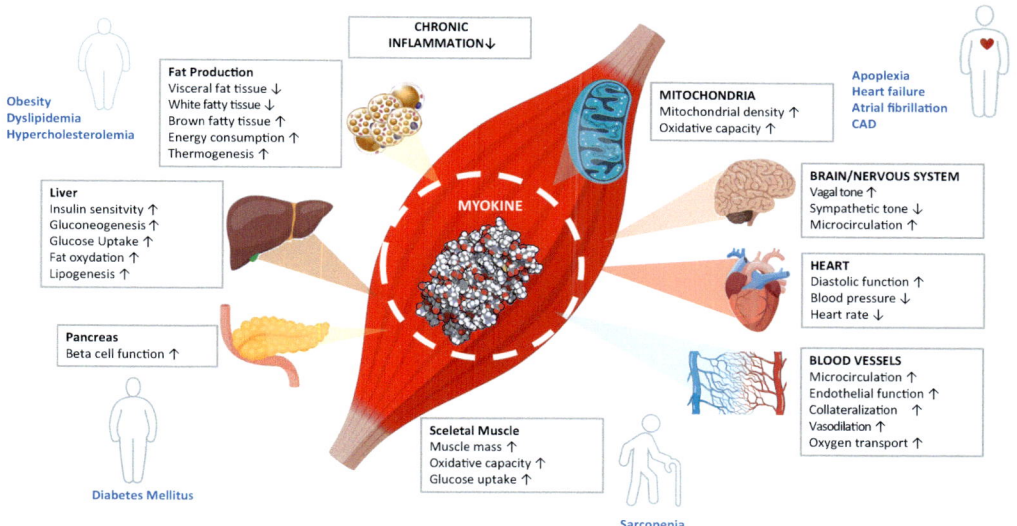

 Fig. 3.7 Effects of physical activity on the cardiovascular system—central role of myokines for regulation and adaptation of metabolic, vascular, and myocardial function

References

Global Burden of Disease (2020) Global burden of 369 diseases and injuries in 204 countries and territories, 1990–2019: a systematic analysis for the Global Burden of Disease Study 2019. Lancet 396(10258):1204–1222. ► https://doi.org/10.1016/s0140-6736(20)30925-9

Mach F, Baigent C, Catapano AL, Koskinas KC, Casula M, Badimon L, Chapman MJ, De Backer GG, Delgado V, Ference BA, Graham IM, Halliday A, Landmesser U, Mihaylova B, Pedersen TR, Riccardi G, Richter DJ, Sabatine MS, Taskinen M-R, Tokgozoglu L, Wiklund O (2020) 2019 ESC/EAS Guidelines for the management of dyslipidaemias: lipid modification to reduce cardiovascular risk. Eur Heart J 41:11–188

Münzel T, Hahad O, Sørensen M, Lelieveld J, Duerr GD, Nieuwenhuijsen M, et al (2022) Environmental risk factors and cardiovascular diseases: a comprehensive expert review. Cardiovasc Res 118(14):2880–2902. ► https://doi.org/10.1093/cvr/cvab316

Visseren FLJ, Mach F, Smulders YM, et al (2021) ESC Guidelines on cardiovascular disease prevention in clinical practice. Eur J Prev Cardiol. ► https://doi.org/10.1093/eurjpc/zwab154

Yusuf S, Hawken S, O'unpuu S, Dans T, Avezum A, Lanas F, McQueen M, Budaj A, Pais P, Varigos J, Lisheng L (2024) on behalf of the INTERHEART Study Investigators. Effect of potentially modifiable risk factors associated with myocardial infarction in 52 countries (the INTERHEART study): case-control study. Lancet. ► http://image.thelancet.com/extras/04art8001web.pdf

World Health Organization (2024) Global Health Estimates: Life expectancy and leading causes of death and disability. ► https://www.who.int/data/gho/data/themes/mortality-and-globalhealth-estimates

Arterial Hypertension

Felix Mahfoud, Roland Schmieder and Thomas F. Lüscher

Contents

4.1 Definition and Epidemiology – 50

4.2 Primary Hypertension – 50

4.3 Secondary Hypertension – 51

4.4 Pathogenesis – 52

4.5 Diagnostics – 53

4.6 Therapy – 55

Earlier versions of this chapter also involved Isabella Sudano, Jan Steffel, and Georg Noll.

© The Author(s), under exclusive license to Springer-Verlag GmbH, DE, part of Springer Nature 2025
T. F. Lüscher and U. Landmesser (eds.), *Cardiovascular System*,
https://doi.org/10.1007/978-3-662-70152-2_4

Arterial hypertension is one of the most common, modifiable cardiovascular risk factors. At the initial diagnosis, especially in younger patients, a secondary cause should be considered before diagnosing primary arterial hypertension. In addition to lifestyle modification, treatment usually involves combination therapy with ACE inhibitors or angiotensin receptor blockers, calcium channel blockers or diuretics, and possibly beta-blockers.

risk factor. The average prevalence in adults in Europe is about 25%, over 50% in those over 50 years old, and up to 75% in obesity. Approximately 1.3 billion people between the ages of 30 and 79 worldwide have hypertension, and only 1 in 5 achieve the recommended target values.

Etiology Arterial hypertension is divided into two groups based on etiology: primary (formerly: essential) and secondary hypertension. This classification is crucial for diagnosis and subsequent therapy.

4.1 Definition and Epidemiology

Definition Arterial hypertension refers to an elevated blood pressure in the systemic circulation. A blood pressure of 140/90 mmHg in clinical or practice measurements and 135/85 mmHg in ambulatory self-measurement is considered the threshold. Hypertension is classified into different grades depending on the extent (◘ Table 4.1).

Epidemiology Arterial hypertension is the most common cardio- and cerebrovascular

4.2 Primary Hypertension

Primary hypertension, also known as primary hypertension, refers to arterial hypertension without an underlying primary disease. Primary hypertension accounts for over 90% of all hypertension cases. Several factors are etiologically possible, and the cause is usually multifactorial:
- **Genetic factors**: In about 60% of cases, primary hypertension is inherited. Various gene mutations can trigger this, e.g., the GNB3–825T mutation.

  > In general, the more relatives have hypertension, the greater the individual risk of developing the condition.

- **Salt sensitivity**: Some hypertensive patients exhibit increased salt sensitivity and develop hypertension even with so-called "normal" salt consumption.
- **Diet**: Hypertension is strongly associated with metabolic syndrome. In Central Europe, obesity, alongside genetic factors, is the main trigger for hypertension. Excessive consumption of alcohol, licorice, or sodium salt, as well as a lack of potassium-rich foods like vegetables and fruits, and a high intake of saturated fatty acids, also promote elevated blood pressure levels.
- **Lifestyle**: An unhealthy lifestyle with physical inactivity and smoking can

◘ **Table 4.1** Definitions and classification of blood pressure values (mmHg)

Category	Systolic	Diastolic
Ideal	<120	<80
Normal	120–129	80–84
High normal	130–139	85–89
Grade 1 hypertension (mild)	140–159	90–99
Grade 2 hypertension (moderate)	160–179	100–109
Grade 3 hypertension (severe)	≥180	≥110
Isolated systolic hypertension	≥140	<90
Isolated diastolic hypertension	<140	≥90

contribute to the development of hypertension.
- Stress-induced **sympathetic hyperactivity** can also play a pathophysiological role.

4.3 Secondary Hypertension

Secondary hypertension, also known as secondary hypertension, refers to hypertension caused by an underlying primary disease. Less than 10% of hypertension cases fall into this category. The most common primary diseases are:

> **Secondary Hypertension: Primary Diseases**
> **Kidney diseases**
> - **Renal insufficiency**: A decrease in kidney function increases the activity of the sympathetic nervous system and the renin-angiotensin-aldosterone system.
> - **Renal artery stenosis**: Prevalence increases with age, caused by atherosclerotic changes (mainly in older patients) or fibromuscular dysplasia (mainly in younger patients)
> - **Renal parenchymal diseases:** e.g., polycystic kidney disease, glomerulonephritis, chronic pyelonephritis
> - Kidney tumors (hypernephroma, etc.)
>
> **Endocrine diseases**
> - Primary hyperaldosteronism (Conn's syndrome, bilateral adrenal hyperplasia)
> - Pheochromocytoma
> - Cushing's syndrome (central pituitary or adrenal disease)
> - Acromegaly
> - Adrenogenital syndrome
> - Hyperthyroidism
>
> **Others**
> - Obstructive sleep apnea syndrome
> - Pregnancy-induced hypertension
> - Aortic coarctation
> - Medications (oral contraceptives, anabolic steroids, steroids, NSAIDs, cyclosporine, etc.)
> - Foods (licorice, alcohol)

In the **kidney**, hypoperfusion leads to increased renin secretion, which in turn increases the production of angiotensin and aldosterone (activation of the renin-angiotensin-aldosterone system, RAAS, ◘ Fig. 4.1) and thus leads to hypertension (◘ Fig. 4.2). All renal parenchymal diseases can, especially due to vascular loss, trigger hypertension. An increase in organ mass (in polycystic kidney disease or malignancies) also leads to an increase in renin production or activation of the sympathetic nervous system.

A pheochromocytoma is a benign catecholamine-producing neoplasm of the chromaffin cells of the adrenal medulla or the paraganglia (Zuckerkandl's organ) in ~90% of cases. It typically results in pulsatile adrenaline secretion, leading to episodes of headaches (hypertension), tachycardia, cold sweats, and feelings of anxiety. Diagnostic determination involves measuring normetanephrines in plasma and/or urine.

Approximately 10% of pregnant women develop **hypertension** during the course of pregnancy. It usually manifests in the 2nd trimester and resolves after childbirth. Young first-time mothers are more frequently affected.

> **Phenotyp of Patients with secondary hypertension**
> - Young patients
> - Very high blood pressure values, sudden onset
> - Lack of nocturnal blood pressure drop

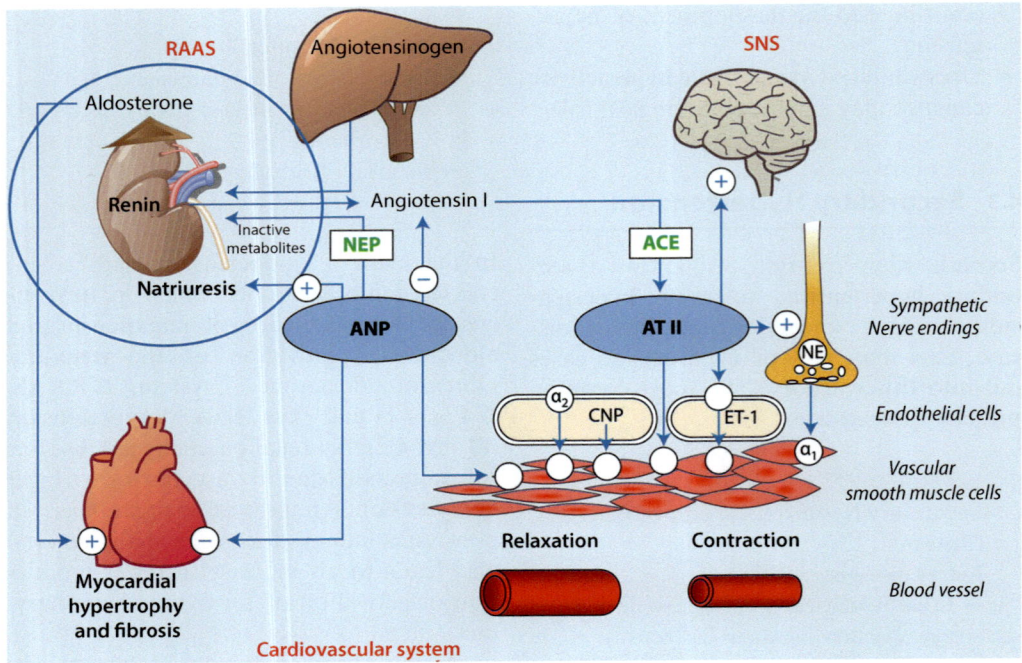

Fig. 4.1 Interaction of the renin-angiotensin-aldosterone system (RAAS) and the sympathetic nervous system (SNS) with the cardiovascular system in blood pressure regulation. (*ACE:* angiotensin-converting enzyme, *ANP:* atrial natriuretic peptide, *AT II:* angiotensin II, *NE:* norepinephrine, *NEP:* neural endopeptidase)

- Poor response to antihypertensive therapy
- Deterioration of previously well-controlled hypertension
- Hypokalemic hypertension
- In the presence of suggestive accompanying symptoms, e.g., moon face in Cushing's syndrome, paroxysmal hypertensive crises in pheochromocytoma

4.4 Pathogenesis

The physiological cause of any hypertension is either an increase in cardiac output, a rise in total vascular resistance, or a combination of both factors:

› Blood pressure = cardiac output × peripheral resistance

The regulation of blood pressure is a complex process, which is primarily determined by the interaction of the autonomic nervous system, the renin-angiotensin-aldosterone system, and the vascular musculature itself (Figs. 4.1, 4.2). Numerous mediators are responsible for the regulation of vascular resistance. An increase (and thus a rising blood pressure) occurs on the basis of an imbalance between vasoconstrictive (angiotensin II, endothelin, thromboxane, etc.) and vasodilatory substances (nitric oxide, NO; prostacyclin, natriuretic peptides, etc.).

Clinical Findings In most cases, arterial hypertension does not cause clinical symptoms. This is treacherous both in the context of diagnosis (often missing the diagnosis for many years) and in terms of therapy, as the lack of symptoms means there is no suffering pressure, and thus medication adherence is problematic for many patients.

> About a quarter of hypertensive patients do not know that they have high blood pressure. Of the known hypertensive patients, a quarter are not treated at all, and another quarter are inadequately treated.

Typical signs that may occasionally occur are headaches, dizziness, dyspnea, decreased exercise tolerance, tinnitus, nervousness, sleep disturbances in nocturnal hypertension, and nosebleeds.

All clinical manifestations of arteriosclerosis occur more frequently and earlier in hypertensive patients than in normotensive patients. An increase in diastolic blood pressure by 5 mmHg results in an increase in the likelihood of a cerebrovascular insult (CVI) by about 33% or a myocardial infarction by 20–25%. Additionally, the risk of cerebral hemorrhages is significantly increased (Fig. 4.3). Although hypertension represents a significant cardiovascular risk factor (Fig. 4.4) and antihypertensive therapy has been proven to reduce cardiovascular risk, this risk factor is often neglected: Hypertension is frequently not recognized, and when it is diagnosed, it is often not adequately treated.

4.5 Diagnostics

An important goal of diagnostics is to identify potentially treatable secondary forms. Therefore, both the clinical and subsequent instrumental diagnostics are oriented towards the findings characteristically expected in the aforementioned secondary forms of hypertension.

Clinical History

The first step of any hypertension diagnostics is a comprehensive anamnesis.
- Family history:

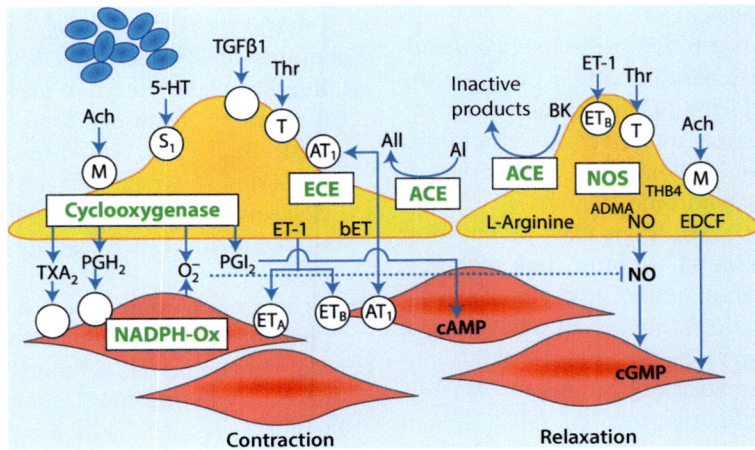

Fig. 4.2 **Vascular regulation.** (*5HT:* serotonin, *ACE:* angiotensin-converting enzyme, *Ach:* acetylcholine, *ADMA:* asymmetric dimethylarginine, *AI:* angiotensin I, *AII:* angiotensin II, *AT1:* angiotensin receptor 1, *bET:* big endothelin, *BK:* bradykinin, *cAMP:* cyclic adenosine monophosphate, *cGMP:* cyclic guanosine monophosphate, *ECE:* endothelin-converting enzyme, *EDCF:* endothelium-derived contracting factor, *ET-1:* endothelin-1, *ETA:* endothelin-A receptor, *ETB:* endothelin-B receptor, *NADPH-Ox:* NADPH oxidase, *NO:* nitric oxide, *NOS:* nitric oxide synthase, *PGH2:* prostaglandin H2, *PGI2:* prostacyclin, *TGF-β1:* transforming growth factor β1, *THB4:* tetrahydrobiopterin, *Thr:* thrombin, *TXA:* thromboxane)

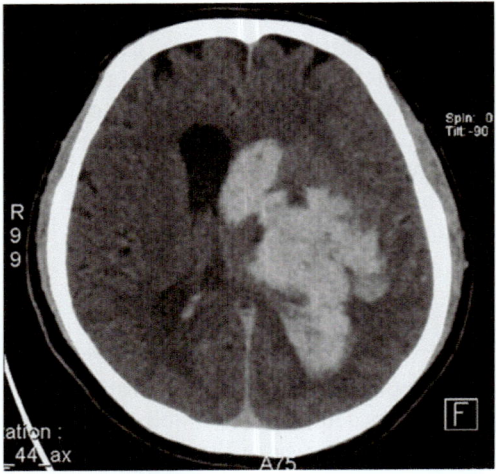

Fig. 4.3 MRI of an intracerebral mass hemorrhage with ventricular breakthrough

- Kidney diseases, diabetes mellitus, cardiovascular diseases, dyslipidemia, stroke, Recklinghausen's disease, multiple endocrine adenomatosis
- **Patient history:**
  - Abdominal trauma, kidney diseases, edema, flank pain → suspicion of renal hypertension
  - Crisis-like blood pressure spikes, sudden paleness, sweating, tachycardia → suspicion of pheochromocytoma
  - Noticeable weakness in extremities, cramps, polyuria → suspicion of Conn's syndrome
  - Weight loss, diarrhea, nervousness (restlessness), tremor, and tachycardia → suspicion of hyperthyroidism
  - Medications: contraceptives, steroids, cyclosporine A, nonsteroidal anti-rheumatics, erythropoietin, etc.
  - Foods: licorice, alcohol, salt
  - Other cardiovascular risk factors

Clinical Examination

A thorough clinical examination follows:
- **Aspect**: Moon face, striae, and buffalo hump in central obesity → suspicion of Cushing's syndrome, also iatrogenic (steroids)
- **Weight, height, BMI** (= body weight in kg/body height in m²)
- **Blood pressure measurement**: 3 times sitting, 1 time lying, 1 time standing, right and left
- **Heart**: Pulse differences upper/lower extremities → suspicion of aortic coarctation; pulse rhythm, heart enlargement, heart murmurs
- **Lungs**: Congestion sounds, bronchospasm
- **Abdomen**: Abnormal aortic pulsation, auscultation (flow sounds), palpation
- **Extremities**: Peripheral pulses (ABI), flow sounds, edema, temperature, skin trophic
- **Thyroid**: Palpation (enlargement, nodules?)
- **Fundus of the eye**: only from stage II
- Caliber fluctuations of the arteries
- Changes in the retina and/or papilla (edema, exudates, hemorrhages) → emergency and end-organ damage (specialist ophthalmological assessment)

Laboratory Examinations

Laboratory examinations include:
- **Routine laboratory:** Plasma glucose (preferably fasting), total cholesterol, LDL and HDL cholesterol, triglyceride serum (fasting), uric acid, creatinine, electrolytes (especially sodium, potassium, calcium), hemoglobin, and hematocrit
- **Urine examination:** Urine dipstick (supplemented with examination of urine sediment), microalbuminuria (absolutely necessary in diabetics), quantitative proteinuria (if urine dipstick is positive)
- **Special examinations** depending on the clinical situation, including aldosterone-renin ratio (in case of suspicion of Conn's syndrome; caution: influenced by antihypertensive medication), HbA1c, TSH, measurement of plasma

metanephrines (in case of suspicion of pheochromocytoma).

Further imaging and special diagnostics follow depending on the clinical suspicion (e.g., duplex of the renal arteries in case of suspicion of renal artery stenosis, CT or MRI in case of suspicion of aortic coarctation, etc.).

4.6 Therapy

The basic therapy for any hypertension consists of measures to modify lifestyle.

> A consistent implementation of lifestyle changes can lead to a reduction in blood pressure and, in individual cases, make drug therapy unnecessary for mild forms of hypertension.

Basic Therapy

The most important measure is the normalization of body weight, which can lead to an average reduction in blood pressure of up to 15 mmHg systolic and 10 mmHg diastolic per 10 kg of weight loss in obese patients. A reduced intake of salt (<6 g/day) and alcohol also lowers blood pressure. Endurance sports (jogging, swimming, walking, cycling, etc.) can also lower blood pressure. In cases of secondary hypertension, the underlying disease is treated whenever possible (e.g., stenting of a renal artery stenosis, surgery for an adrenal or pituitary adenoma, etc.).

Drug Therapy

In cases of severe hypertension or when target values are not achieved with the aforementioned measures, drug therapy represents the second cornerstone of treatment. The choice of a particular substance group is significantly influenced by any existing comorbidities or the patient's risk profile. In most cases, an initial fixed combination therapy, i.e., two substance classes in one tablet, is administered. If blood pressure control is not achieved under this therapy, it is escalated to a triple fixed combination. Exceptions to this are patients with grade 1 hypertension (especially with systolic blood pressure <150 mmHg), low cardiovascular

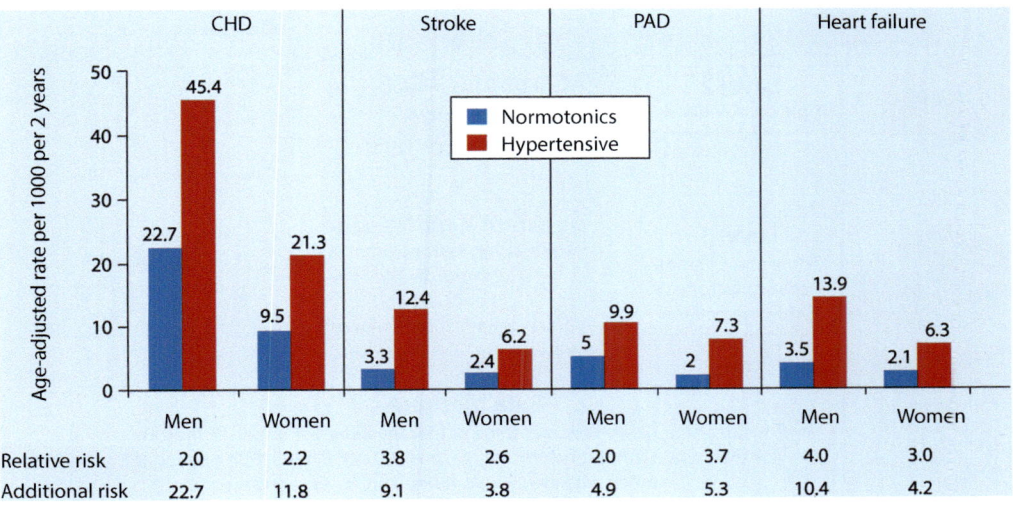

Fig. 4.4 Increase in the risk of CHD, stroke, PAD, and heart failure in normotensive (blue) and hypertensive (red) individuals. (Mod. after data from Kannel WB 1996)

risk, as well as very old (≥80 years) or frail patients, for whom monotherapy is initiated.

The most commonly used classes of medications (◘ Fig. 4.5) are:

■ ACE Inhibitors

ACE inhibitors are currently the most frequently prescribed substances in hypertension therapy. They are characterized by good blood pressure reduction and a low rate of side effects. Their mechanism of action is based on the inhibition of the angiotensin-converting enzyme (ACE), which converts angiotensin I into the vasopressor angiotensin II (◘ Fig. 4.6). Additionally, the production of aldosterone is inhibited. About 10% of patients experience a dry cough after taking ACE inhibitors, which is mediated by bradykinin (whose breakdown is also inhibited by the blocking of ACE). Very rarely, the use of ACE inhibitors can lead to the development of potentially life-threatening angioneurotic edema.

Typical representatives of ACE inhibitors are lisinopril (e.g., Zestril®), enalapril (Reniten®), ramipril (Delix®), or captopril (Lopirin®). A calcium antagonist or a thiazide/thiazide-like diuretic are ideal combination therapies for this class of substances.

> ACE inhibitors reduce cardiovascular risk and significantly extend life expectancy in hypertensive patients (and diabetics).

■■ Angiotensin II Receptor Blockers (ARB)

ARBs (◘ Fig. 4.6) act similarly to ACE inhibitors and are usually better tolerated. Their target, the angiotensin II receptor, is competitively blocked. Unlike ACE inhibitors, no dry cough occurs as a side effect due to the mechanism of action (lack of ACE inhibition). Typical representatives are losartan (Cozaar®), valsartan (Diovan®), irbesartan (Aprovel®), candesartan (Blopress®), or telmisartan (Kinzal®, Micardis®).

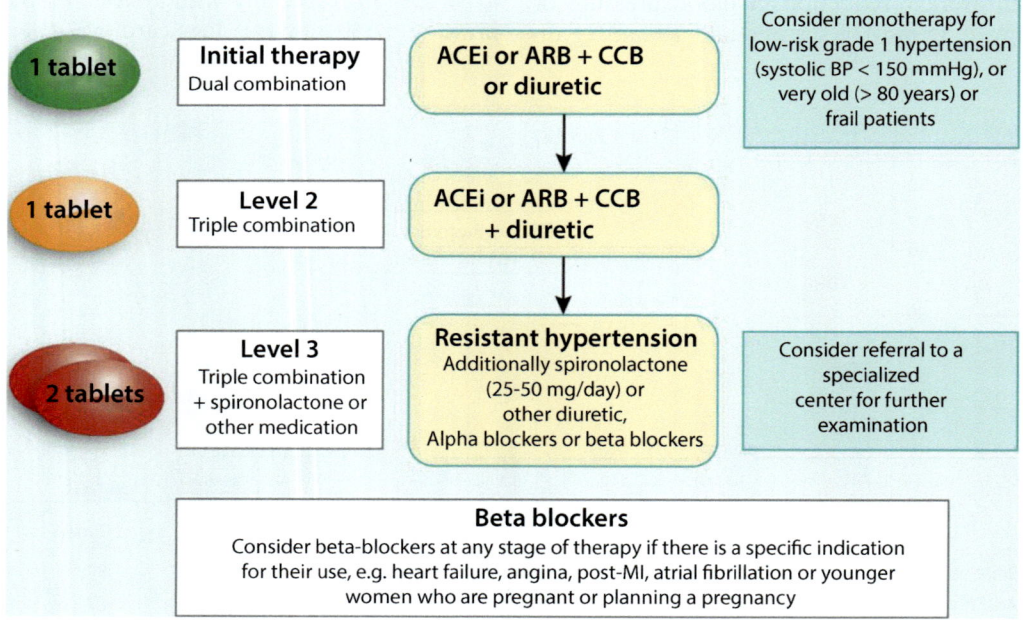

◘ Fig. 4.5 Basic drug strategy for uncomplicated hypertension. (Pocket guideline of the German Society of Cardiology)

> ARBs represent excellent first-line medications that positively influence patient adherence to therapy due to their good tolerability.

■ Thiazides and thiazide-like diuretics

Thiazide diuretics are the oldest antihypertensives currently in use (hydrochlorothiazide). They represent a good first-line medication and an ideal combination therapy drug, whose benefits are especially documented in a large long-term study. Typical representatives of thiazide-like diuretics are chlorthalidone (Hygroton®), indapamide (Fludex SR and in fixed combination preparations), hydrochlorothiazide (Esidrex), and xipamide (Aquaphor). Due to their longer half-life and the proven reduction of hypertensive end-organ damage, thiazide-like diuretics should be preferred. The mechanism of action of diuretics is not entirely clear: their intake leads to a decrease in peripheral vascular resistance, which could be responsible for the blood pressure reduction. However, increased excretion of sodium and water with a decrease in circulating blood volume does not fully explain the blood pressure reduction. In cases of significantly impaired renal function, loop diuretics should be used (torasemide, Torem®).

■■ Beta-blockers

Beta-blockers are no longer recommended by the current European guidelines for the initial primary therapy of hypertension. They are antihypertensives that are primarily indicated for coronary heart disease, atrial fibrillation, and/or heart failure. Their mechanism of action is based on inhibiting the effects of the sympathetic nervous system (direct negative inotropic effect and inhibition of β-receptor-mediated renin release in the kidney). Typical representatives are metoprolol (Beloc®), bisoprolol (Concor®), or nebivolol (Nebilet®).

■■ Calcium antagonists

The antihypertensive efficacy of calcium antagonists is excellent and documented in numerous studies. Disadvantages include the tendency to peripheral edema, the worsening of existing heart failure (especially with negatively inotropic diltiazem, Dilzem®, verapamil, Isoptin®), and reflex sympathetic activation with a tendency to reflex tachycardia, especially with short-acting dihydropyridines. Typical representatives of long-acting dihydropyridines are amlodipine (Norvasc®) or lercanidipine (Carmen®).

■■ Aldosterone antagonists

If ACE inhibitors/ARBs with or without diuretics and calcium channel blockers have not led to sufficient blood pressure reduction, aldosterone antagonists are preferably used. Renal function (eGFR $\geq$ 45 ml/min) and serum electrolytes (potassium $\leq$ 4.5 mmol/l) must be considered. They block the binding of aldosterone to its cytoplasmic receptor in the tubule and collecting duct. The result is reduced sodium and water retention in the kidney. Typical representatives are spironolactone (Aldactone®) and eplerenone (Inspra®).

! Aldosterone antagonists can lead to deterioration of renal function and hyperkalemia (particularly in patients with renal disease and with high dosages).

■■ Vasodilators

This group includes nitrates, dihydralazine, and minoxidil, whose use is reserved for specific indications and after careful consideration in therapy-resistant patients.

■■ Central sympatholytics

Central sympatholytics are second-line medications that are only used in combination therapy for refractory hypertension. However, additional blood pressure reduction is often accompanied by pronounced central side effects such as fatigue or dry

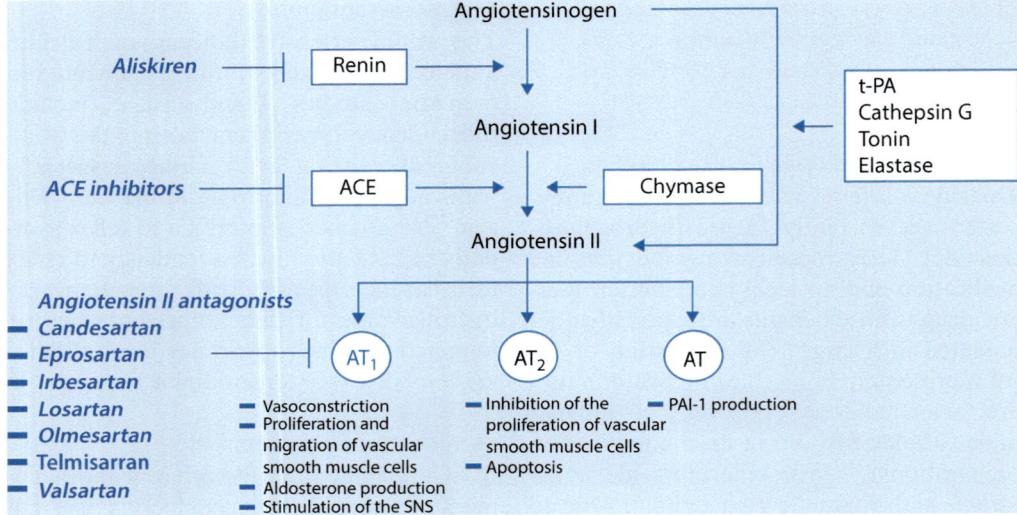

Fig. 4.6 Targets of ACE inhibitors and angiotensin II receptor blockers in the RAAS. (*t-PA:* Tissue Plasminogen Activator, *ACE:* Angiotensin-converting Enzyme, *AT1:* Angiotensin Receptor 1, *AT2:* Angiotensin Receptor 2, *PAI-1:* Plasminogen Activator Inhibitor 1)

mouth. Typical representatives are clonidine (Catapresan®) and moxonidine (Physiotens®). Alpha-methyldopa is the first-line medication for treating hypertension during pregnancy, not least because there is extensive experience with this preparation regarding effectiveness and safety for both mother and child (alternatives in this situation are nifedipine and beta-blockers).

❗ ACE inhibitors and ARBs, on the other hand, are contraindicated during pregnancy; alpha-methyldopa is the most suitable option.

Consequences for Practical Application
Which antihypertensive should be preferred for which comorbidity?
- Hypertension without comorbidity: ACE inhibitors, angiotensin II receptor blockers, diuretics, or calcium antagonists
- Isolated systolic hypertension: diuretics, calcium antagonists
- Hypertension and angina pectoris: beta-blockers, calcium antagonists (verapamil, diltiazem)
- Hypertension and atherosclerosis: ACE inhibitors, ARB
- Hypertension and nephropathy: ACE inhibitors, ARB
- Hypertension and heart failure: diuretics, ACE inhibitors; beta-blockers; spironolactone/eplerenone
- Diabetics: ACE inhibitors, ARB, beta-blockers
- Secondary prevention of cerebrovascular infarction (CVI): ARB, ACE inhibitors, diuretics, calcium antagonists

Combination Therapy
Most patients will require combination therapy to achieve target values. Since sensible combinations not only have an additive but also a partially potentiating effect on blood pressure (e.g., ACE inhibi-

tors block the RAAS activated by thiazide diuretics), monotherapy should not be exhausted to the maximum, but rather a combination with initially low dosage should be used. Common 2- and 3-drug combination therapies are ACE inhibitors/ARB, calcium antagonists, and thiazide diuretics.

> ❗ Due to the poor adherence of many patients with arterial hypertension, the therapy regimen should be as simple and effective as possible!

- **Renal Denervation for Difficult-to-Control Hypertension**

The overactivity of the sympathetic nervous system contributes to the development and progression of arterial hypertension and is associated with an increased cardiovascular risk. In cases of difficult-to-control hypertension, there is the option to perform a percutaneous renal nerve ablation. Hypertension is classified as difficult-to-control if blood pressure is ≥140/90 mmHg despite 3 antihypertensives in adequate dosage including a diuretic. Excluding secondary hypertension before renal nerve ablation is advisable.

In renal denervation, a special catheter (radiofrequency or ultrasound catheter) is placed via the femoral artery into the renal artery, with which the afferent and efferent sympathetic nerves are modulated (◘ Fig. 4.7). The blood pressure reduction after the procedure mainly depends on the initial blood pressure level and averages about 10–15 mmHg systolic and 8–10 mmHg diastolic after 6 months. In the long term, the blood pressure-lowering effect can further increase. Unlike the effect of antihypertensive medications, the effect of renal denervation is independent of adherence, medication timing, and pharmacokinetics. The complication rate of the procedure, especially injuries to the renal vessels, is very low. Minor local hematoma formation at the puncture site is possible. Renal denervation should only be performed in experienced centers.

Indications for Renal Denervation
— Therapy-resistant hypertension
— Intolerance to antihypertensive medication
— Proven non-adherence to medication therapy

- **Target blood pressure values**

A therapy indication exists for blood pressure values above 140 mmHg systolic or 90 mmHg diastolic (for those under 60 years, 130/80 mmHg). For nearly all patients, a target range of 120–129 mmHg systolic blood pressure applies. Excluded from this are patients over 65 years, for whom, if tolerable, a systolic target blood pressure between 130 and 140 mmHg should be aimed for. The diastolic blood pressure should be lowered to <80 mmHg for all patients, regardless of age and comorbidities. This recommendation is based on evidence that the risk for cardiovascular endpoints, particularly cardiovascular death and heart failure, is lowest at a blood pressure range of 120–129 mmHg systolic and 70–79 mmHg diastolic.

Prognosis The prognosis of hypertension significantly depends on the severity and any accompanying comorbidities. Especially in high-risk cases, good management is of crucial importance. However, even

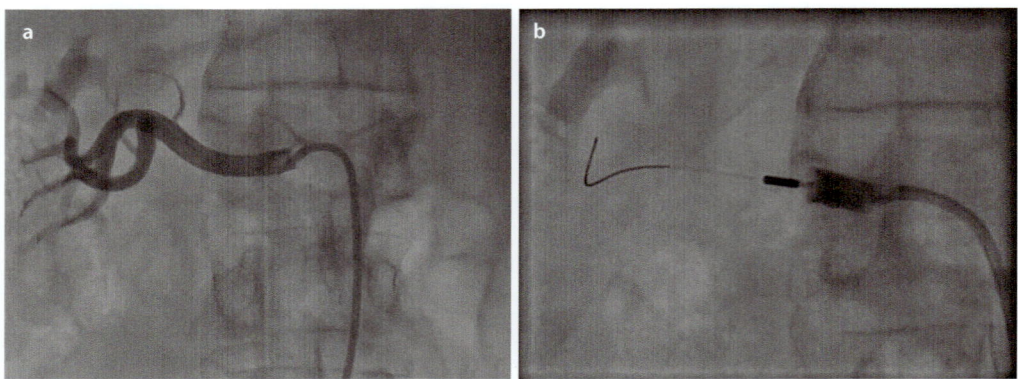

Fig. 4.7 a, b After creating an angiogram a, a special ultrasound balloon is placed and inflated b (in the system used here). Subsequently, ultrasound energy is delivered, thus modulating the afferent and efferent sympathetic nerve fibers

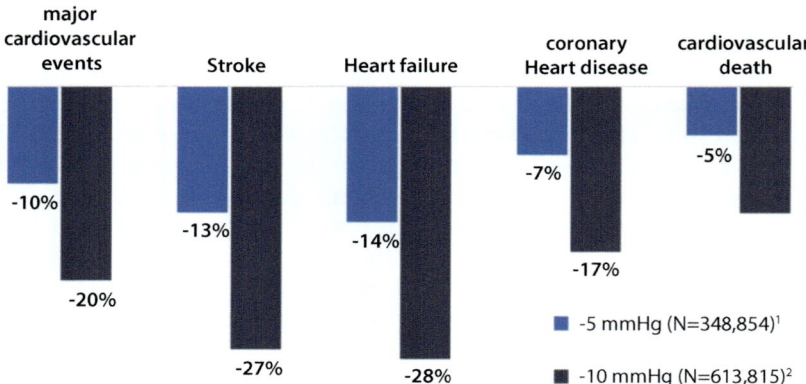

Fig. 4.8 Relative risk reduction by lowering office blood pressure by 5 or 10 mmHg. (Ettehad and Lancet. 2016)

with only a low risk, controlling high blood pressure is worthwhile, as cardiovascular sequelae can be largely avoided in these cases. Even moderate blood pressure reductions can lead to a drastic reduction in complications (Fig. 4.8).

Pulmonary Hypertension

Irene M. Lang and Stephan Rosenkranz

Contents

5.1 Definition and Classification – 62

5.2 Epidemiology and Pathogenesis – 66

5.3 Diagnostics – 67

5.4 Management – 69

Pulmonary hypertension is defined as an increase in the mean blood pressure >20mmHg and/or peripheral resistance >2 Wood Units in the pulmonary circulation due to various causes such as left heart failure, lung or systemic diseases, which eventually lead to an overload of the right heart with subsequent shortness of breath, tricuspid regurgitation, ascites, and peripheral edema, and if undetected and untreated, is often associated with a poor prognosis and premature death.

> **Facts**
> - Pulmonary hypertension (PH) is a complex disease. PH is defined by an increase in the mean pressure in the pulmonary circulation >20 mmHg during invasive measurement.
> - Echocardiographically, the threshold has been defined as a tricuspid regurgitation velocity of >2.8 m/s (corresponding to a pulmonary systolic pressure of 35mmHg assuming an right atrial pressure of 4mmHg)for the likelihood of pulmonary hypertension .
> - Therapies for PH are based on vasodilating substances, which are mostly used in combination.
> - Risk scores determine the choice of initial therapy. Chronic thromboembolic pulmonary hypertension (CTEPH) is primarily treated with mechanical therapies (surgical pulmonary endarterectomy, PEA, or balloon pulmonary angioplasty BPA) and often supported by pharmacological therapies.

5.1 Definition and Classification

Pulmonary hypertension (pulmonary hypertension, PH) describes an increase in pressure and/or resistance in the pulmonary circulation (◘ Fig. 5.1), which can occur as a primary pulmonary vascular disease (◘ Fig. 5.1a, b and d, e) or in the context of various heart (◘ Fig. 5.1c), lung (◘ Fig. 5.1d), or systemic diseases (◘ Fig. 5.1f).

Hemodynamic phenotypes of pulmonary hypertension and the typical clinical diagnostic groups are schematically represented in ◘ Fig. 5.1a–f. The confirmation of the PH diagnosis is achieved through invasive hemodynamic measurement. PH is defined by a mean pulmonary arterial pressure (mPAP) >20 mmHg in a resting supine position. This new definition, which lowered the threshold from 25 mmHg to 20 mmHg, is based on the observation from large hemodynamic databases that in an unselected population, an mPAP starting from a threshold of 20 mmHg was abruptly associated with poorer survival time. A pulmonary arterial wedge pressure (PAWP) ≤15 mmHg and a pulmonary vascular resistance (PVR) >2 Wood units define a precapillary PH, as seen, for example, in pulmonary arterial hypertension (PAH) (◘ Fig. 5.1b). In contrast, postcapillary PH is defined by an mPAP >20 mmHg and a PAWP >15 mmHg. In the *2022 ESC (European Society of Cardiology) Guidelines* for the diagnosis and treatment of PH, pulmonary hypertension under exercise was also newly defined by an increase in the mPAP/CO slope >3 mmHg/L/min.

The clinical classification of PH is presented in the following overview: Group 1 corresponds to pulmonary arterial hypertension (PAH, ◘ Fig. 5.1b), Group 2 to PH associated with left heart disease (◘ Fig. 5.1c), Group 3 to PH associated with lung diseases with/without hypoxia (◘ Fig. 5.1d), and Group 4 to chronic thromboembolic PH (CTEPH, ◘ Fig. 5.1e). Group 5 encompasses other pathologies and is often a combination of pre- and postcapillary changes (◘ Fig. 5.1f).

Pulmonary Hypertension

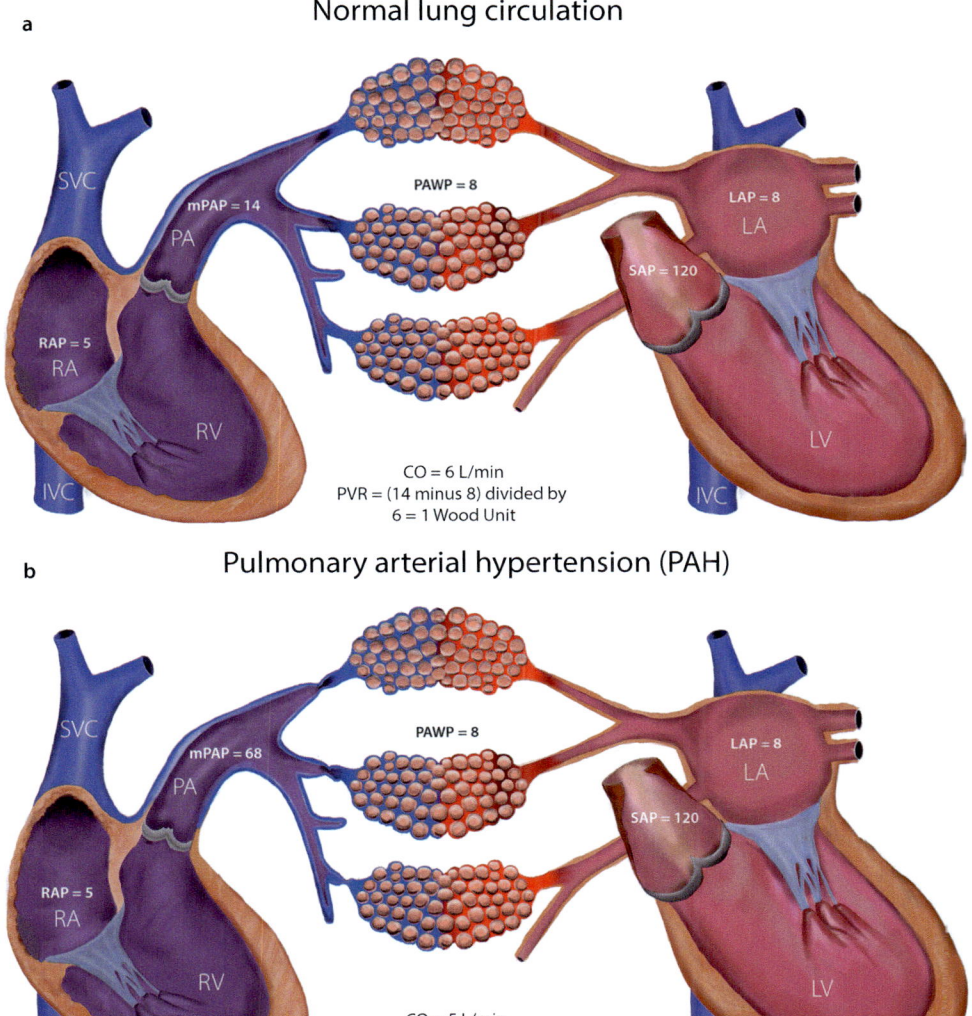

Fig. 5.1 a–f Classification of pulmonary hypertension (PH). Hemodynamic phenotypes of pulmonary hypertension and the clinical diagnostic groups. The color shades indicate the degree of oxygen saturation. The calculation of pulmonary vascular resistance for each representative example is given for each hemodynamic PH type. **a** Normal pulmonary circulation, **b** Pulmonary circulation in pulmonary arterial hypertension (PAH), **c** Pulmonary circulation in pulmonary hypertension associated with left ventricular failure, **d** Pulmonary circulation in pulmonary hypertension associated with lung diseases with/without hypoxemia, **e** Pulmonary circulation in chronic thromboembolic pulmonary hypertension, **f** Pulmonary circulation in combined post- and precapillary pulmonary hypertension as an example of diagnostic group 5. Pulmonary hypertension with unclear and/or multifactorial mechanisms, where different hemodynamic phenotypes of pulmonary hypertension can occur. SVC: superior vena cava, IVC: inferior vena cava, RA: right atrium, RAP: right atrial pressure, RV: right ventricle, PA: pulmonary artery, mPAP: mean pulmonary arterial pressure, PAWP: pulmonary arterial wedge pressure, CO: cardiac output, PVR: pulmonary vascular resistance, SAP: systemic arterial pressure, LV: left ventricle, LA: left atrium, LAP: left atrial pressure, all pressure values are given in mmHg

c Pulmonary hypertension associated with left ventricular heart disease

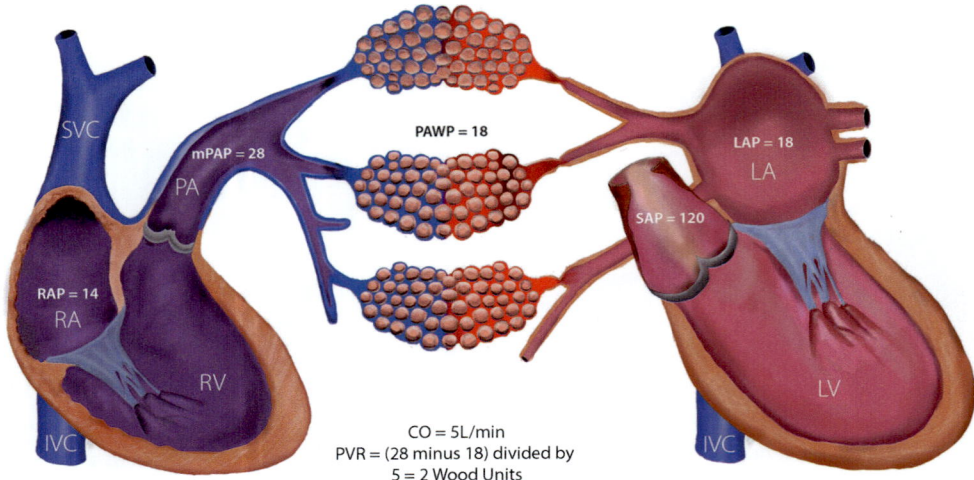

d Pulmonary hypertension in lung diseases with/without hypoxemia

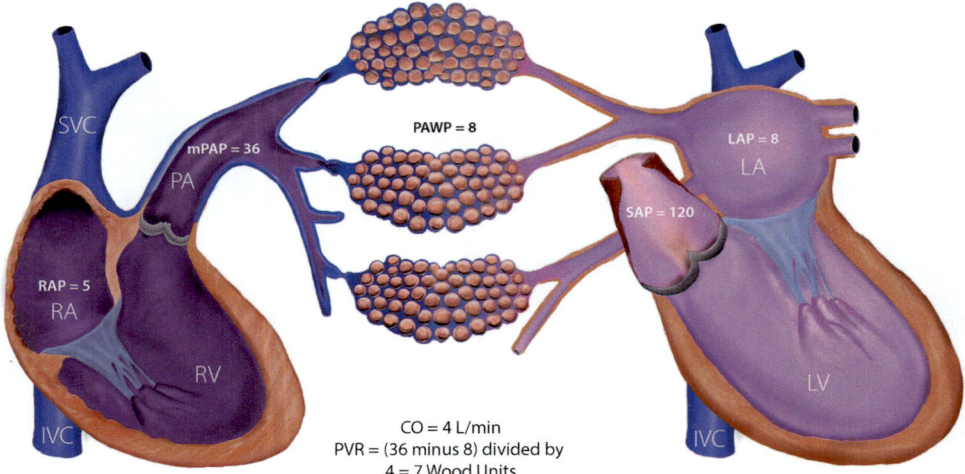

Fig. 5.1 (continued)

e
Pulmonary hypertension associated with pulmonary vascular obstruction

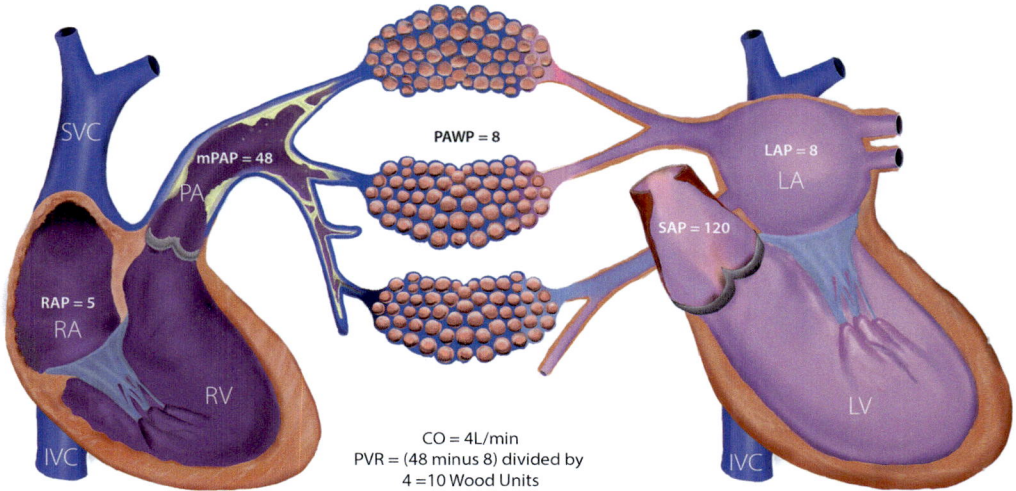

f
Pulmonary hypertension with unclear and/or multifactorial mechanisms

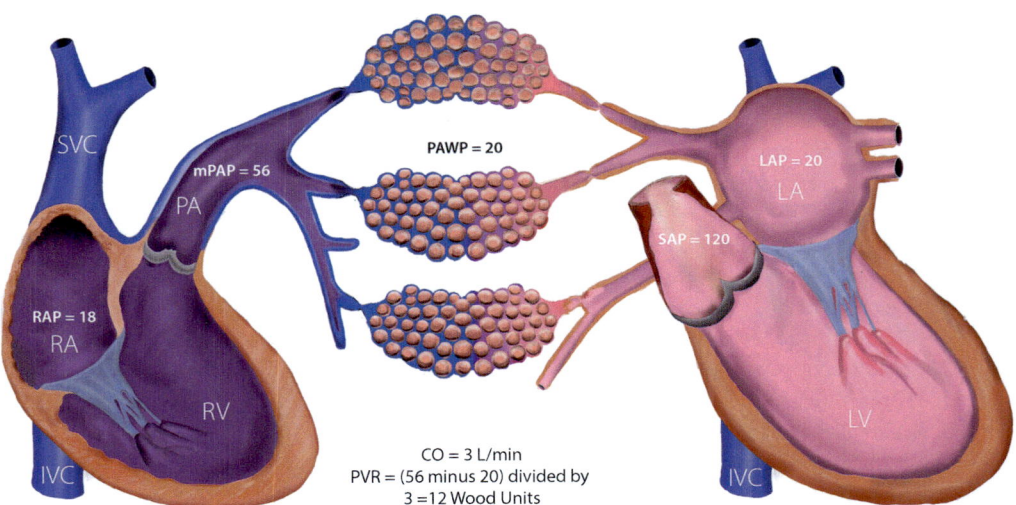

Fig. 5.1 (continued)

Clinical Classification of Pulmonary Hypertension
1. **Pulmonary Arterial Hypertension (PAH)**
   - 1.1. Idiopathic PAH (IPAH)
     - 1.1.1. Non-responder in the vasoreactivity test
     - 1.1.2. Responder in the vasoreactivity test
     - 1.1.3 Drug/Toxin induced PAH (*move below 1.2*)
   - 1.2. Heritable PAH
     - 1.2.1. BMPR2 mutation
     - 1.2.2. ALK-1, ENG, SMAD9, CAV1, KCNK3
     - 1.2.3. Other mutations
   - 1.4. PAH associated with
     - 1.4.1. Collagenoses
     - 1.4.2. HIV infection
     - 1.4.3. Portal hypertension
     - 1.4.4. Congenital heart disease
     - 1.4.5. Schistosomiasis
   - 1.5. PAH with characteristics of pulmonary veno-occlusive disease (PVOD) and/or pulmonary capillary hemangiomatosis (PCH)
   - 1.6. Persistent pulmonary hypertension of the newborn
2. **Pulmonary Hypertension associated with left heart disease**
   - 2.1. Heart failure
     - 2.1.1. with preserved ejection fraction (HFpEF)
     - 2.1.2. with reduced or mildly reduced ejection fraction (HFmEF or HFrEF)
   - 2.3. Valvular heart disease
   - 2.4. Congenital/acquired heart diseases associated with postcapillary pulmonary hypertension
3. **Pulmonary Hypertension associated with lung diseases with/without hypoxemia**
   - 3.1. Obstructive lung diseases or emphysema
   - 3.2. Restrictive lung diseases
   - 3.3. Other lung diseases with mixed restrictive and obstructive patterns
   - 3.4. Hypoventilation syndromes
   - 3.5. Hypoxia without lung disease (e.g., chronic high-altitude exposure)
   - 3.7. Developmental abnormalities
4. **Pulmonary Hypertension associated with pulmonary vascular obstruction**
   - 4.1 Chronic thromboembolic pulmonary hypertension (CTEPH)
   - 4.2. Other obstructions of the pulmonary arteries
5. **Pulmonary Hypertension with unclear and/or multifactorial mechanisms**
   - 5.1. Hematologic diseases: chronic hemolytic anemia, myeloproliferative disorders, splenectomy
   - 5.2. Systemic diseases: sarcoidosis, pulmonary Langerhans cell histiocytosis, lymphangioleiomyomatosis, neurofibromatosis, vasculitis
   - 5.3. Metabolic diseases: glycogen storage disease, Gaucher, thyroid diseases
   - 5.4. Chronic kidney disease with or without dialysis
   - 5.5. Thrombotic tumor microangiopathy of the pulmonary vessels
   - 5.5. Fibrosing mediastinitis

5.2 Epidemiology and Pathogenesis

The **incidence** of idiopathic PAH (iPAH) is estimated in the population at 1–2 cases per million. The highest prevalence is between the ages of 20 and 40 years. While both genders are equally affected in childhood, this ratio shifts towards the female gender in adulthood, with women being twice as likely to develop the condition. For the associated forms of PH, the prevalence is 10–20% for patients with systemic sclerosis, 10–20% for patients with congenital heart disease, 2–4% for patients with portal hypertension, and 0.5% for HIV patients.

The consequences of increased pulmonary arterial pressure and PVR are right heart hypertrophy and eventually dilation due to right heart strain, ultimately leading to right heart failure.

The **pathogenesis** of PH is complex and multifactorial. Gene mutations of the *bone morphogenetic protein receptor 2* (BMPR2) gene from the *transforming growth factor beta* (TGFb) family have been identified in 70% of patients with hereditary PAH and in 11–40% of patients with idiopathic PAH. Additionally, there are "modifier genes" (e.g., the serotonin transporter, the endothelin receptor, or caveolin), and exogenous disease triggers such as herpes viruses, appetite suppressants, and amphetamines or circulating autoantibodies are also suspected.

The histopathological picture is very similar in all forms of PH and consists of intimal hyperplasia, smooth muscle cell hypertrophy, and adventitial fibrosis of the precapillary pulmonary vessels (◘ Fig. 5.1b, d and f). The current disease concept is that, in addition to vasoconstriction, remodeling of the pulmonary vessel wall occurs with histological changes in all layers of the vessel wall, in-situ thromboses, and the formation of so-called plexiform lesions as collaterals of vascular occlusions.

The hemodynamic changes of precapillary PH (◘ Fig. 5.1b, d, f) are fundamentally different from those of postcapillary PH (◘ Fig. 5.1c, f). CTEPH usually presents as precapillary PH (◘ Fig. 5.1e), but it can also occur in combination with postcapillary PH.

5.3 Diagnostics

Due to the scant clinical symptoms in the early stages of the disease, PH is still often only recognized at an advanced stage. The use of screening programs for the early detection of PH (screening of scleroderma patients or family members and gene carriers of patients with hereditary PAH, pulmonary embolism screening, splenectomy screening, etc.) is limited to targeted patient groups and specialized PH centers. Referral to expert centers is important and a justified demand of international guidelines.

▪ Clinical Findings

The clinical symptoms are nonspecific. The early stage is characterized by heavy legs and fatigue, while in the advanced stage, dizziness, chest pain, palpitations, hemoptysis, or syncope on exertion occur. The limitation of exercise capacity is classified according to the WHO/NYHA functional stages (I–IV). Leg edema and hemoptysis are typical for CTEPH, while syncope is more common in PAH. The severity of PAH in stable patients should be reevaluated every 3–6 months using clinical examination, exercise testing, biomarkers, echocardiography (▶ Sect. 2.5) and hemodynamic measurement (▶ Sect. 2.7).

▪ Physical Examination

The clinical-physical signs of the disease are only recognizable in the advanced stage. On auscultation of the heart, tachycardia, a loud split second heart sound, and/or a systolic murmur as an indication of tricuspid insufficiency and occasionally a diastolic murmur as an expression of pulmonary insufficiency can be detected. Other findings include lip cyanosis, distended jugular veins, hepatomegaly, ascites, and peripheral edema.

▪ Electrocardiogram (ECG)

Due to an increase in pressure in the pulmonary arteries and enlargement of the right ventricle, ECG signs of PH can include a right axis deviation, an incomplete or complete right bundle branch block, and T-wave inversions in the precordial leads V1–V4 (*"right ventricular strain pattern"*).

Chest X-ray

An unremarkable chest X-ray does not rule out PH. A chest X-ray can show dilated central pulmonary arteries ("prominent pulmonary segment") with loss of vascular markings in the lung periphery as well as enlargement of the right atrium and ventricle.

Transthoracic Echocardiography (TTE)

Transthoracic echocardiography (▶ Sect. 2.5) is the most suitable method for the non-invasive evaluation of patients suspected of having PH. The parameters that serve to substantiate a suspicion of PH are the systolic pulmonary arterial pressure (PASP), estimated from the peak tricuspid regurgitant velocity jet (TRVJ) calculated as $4 \times TRVJ^2$ plus the estimated right atrial pressure, the right ventricular size and function, the movement of the tricuspid annular plane (*tricuspid annular plane systolic excursion*; TAPSE) as a parameter of right heart function, right ventricular ejection fraction (RVEF), and the eccentric flattening of the interventricular septum (so-called *D-Sign*), which moves "paradoxically" from right to left during systole. The TTE also allows the detection of shunt defects (▶ Sect. 14.2) or the exclusion of other causes of PH or right heart enlargement such as valvular defects (▶ Chap. 8), diastolic ventricular dysfunction (▶ Sect. 13.3) and left ventricular hypertrophy (▶ Chap. 4).

Right Heart Catheterization

To confirm the diagnosis of PH, right heart catheterization is necessary (▶ Sect. 2.7). The invasive hemodynamic measurement serves, on the one hand, to measure the systolic, diastolic, and mean pulmonary arterial pressure (mPAP). On the other hand, it distinguishes whether the pressure increase is due to an increase in filling pressure in the left ventricle (postcapillary PH; ◘ Fig. 5.1c) or as a result of pathological vascular changes in the pulmonary circulation (precapillary PH, PAH; ◘ Fig. 5.1b). To differentiate, the pulmonary arterial wedge pressure (PAWP) or the left ventricular end-diastolic pressure (LVEDP) is measured. Up to a PAWP value of ≤ 15 mmHg, it is referred to as precapillary PH (e.g., PAH; ◘ Fig. 5.1b). A PAWP value >15 mmHg, on the other hand, defines postcapillary PH (◘ Fig. 5.1c), usually as a result of left heart disease. The difference between mPAP and PAWP is referred to as the transpulmonary gradient (TPG). In addition to pressure recording, cardiac output (CO) or cardiac index (CI) is routinely measured. From the TPG and cardiac output, the pulmonary vascular resistance (PVR) is calculated (◘ Fig. 5.1). A PVR > 2 Wood units (WU) defines precapillary PH or precapillary disease in postcapillary PH (◘ Fig. 5.1f). Other parameters such as stroke volume index (SVI) and right atrial pressure indicate the functional status of the right ventricle. Finally, the measurement of mixed venous O_2 saturation serves, on the one hand, to determine the severity of PH, and on the other hand, to detect or exclude a shunt defect (if necessary, step oximetry is performed, i.e., repeated measurement of O_2 saturations at defined points in the right heart and pulmonary circulation, e.g., in the right atrium, left atrium, superior and inferior vena cava).

Vasoreactivity Testing

In patients with suspected idiopathic (iPAH), hereditary (hPAH), or drug-induced PAH, an acute test with a rapidly acting pulmonary vasodilator, such as inhaled nitric oxide (NO) or iloprost, is recommended as part of the diagnostic right heart catheterization. Alternatively, intravenous epoprostenol (both prostaglandin analogs) can also be used. The test is considered positive if the mPAP – with constant cardiac output – falls by at least 10 mmHg and to below 40 mmHg. Such patients are called vasoresponders, and they are treated with high-dose Ca^{2+} antagonists, with an excellent long-term prognosis predictable under this therapy.

Pulmonary Hypertension

- **Ventilation-/Perfusion Scintigraphy of the Lungs**

This examination is used to distinguish between non-thromboembolic forms of PH and CTEPH. The sensitivity of this examination is 96–97%, and the specificity is 90–95%. It should be consistently used in the context of PH clarification, also to reliably exclude CTEPH.

- **Computed Tomography (CT)**

CT is helpful for assessing the lung parenchyma and adjacent anatomical structures to detect possible causes of pulmonary hypertension. Although modern dual-source devices can detect pulmonary embolism with high sensitivity and specificity, they do not allow for a reliable exclusion of CTEPH. A C-arm CT allows for detailed resolution of structures in the vessel wall with a resolution of 2 mm or less.

- **Pulmonary Angiography**

Pulmonary angiography is the method of choice for therapy decisions in CTEPH in terms of surgical (i.e., surgical pulmonary endarterectomy) or interventional therapy (i.e., balloon angioplasty of the pulmonary arteries). Modern injection techniques and digital subtraction make pulmonary angiography a safe, low-contrast examination method even for very sick patients.

- **Biomarkers**

The Brain Natriuretic Peptide (BNP) and the N-terminal pro-brain natriuretic peptide (NT-proBNP) are laboratory parameters used routinely in PH, have prognostic significance, and are part of risk stratification in PAH. However, they are nonspecific in that they can also be elevated in kidney disease or left heart disease. Hyponatremia, which is already established as a marker for poor prognosis in left heart failure, is also associated with PH with right heart failure and consequently poor outcome. A promising biomarker is the endogenous nitric oxide synthase inhibitor ADMA *(Asymmetrical Dimethylarginine)*, which is elevated in patients with idiopathic PAH and CTEPH and represents a prognostic parameter. However, the application of ADMA determination in clinical routine still needs to be established.

Management of Pulmonary Arterial Hypertension The approvals of all currently used substances for PAH (◘ Fig. 5.1b) are based on randomized, double-blind, and placebo-controlled studies that have shown an improvement in exercise tolerance and/or a reduction in morbidity and mortality. Most substances are only approved for pulmonary arterial hypertension (PAH; Group 1 of the classification in the overview in ▶ Sect. 5.1). However, none of the currently available drug treatments can cure PAH. Nevertheless, there are several drug options, from oral to intravenous therapy, which have the following aspects in common: stopping the progression of the disease, stabilizing the patient's health condition, and improving the quality of life, with the target being the reduction of the right ventricular afterload through simple vasodilation.

Pregnancy with PH leads to a mother/child mortality of up to 50% and must be avoided. Risk stratification (◘ Fig. 5.2) is the basis for prescribing the sometimes complex treatments.

5.4 Management

- **Conventional Management**

Oral Anticoagulation

Small thrombotic lesions in the microcirculation of the pulmonary vascular system are frequently observed in patients with PH and constitute the rationale for oral anticoagulation. However, evidence for this therapy could only be obtained in uncontrolled studies, e.g., in a large German

Determinants of the forecast (estimated 1-year mortality)	Low risk (< 5 %)	Intermediary risk (5-20%)	High risk (> 20 %)
Clinical observations and modifiable variable			
Signs of right heart failure	None	None	Available
Progression of symptoms and clinical manifestations	No	Slowly	Fast
Syncope	No	Occasional syncope	Repeated syncope
WHO functional class	I,II	III	IV
6-minute walk test	> 440 m	165–440 m	< 165 m
CPET (cardiopulmonary exercise testing)	Peak VO2 >1 mL/min/kg (>65% pred.) VE/VCO2 Slope < 36	Peak VO_2 11-15 mL/min/kg (35-65% pred.) VE/VCO_2 Slope 36-44	Peak VO_2 < 11 mL/min/kg (<35% pred.) VE/VCO_2 Slope > 44
Biomarker: BNP or NT-proBNP	BNP <50 ng/L NT-proBNP <300 ng/L	BNP 50-800 ng/L NT-proBNP 300-1,100 ng/L	BNP > 800 ng/L NT-proBNP > 1,100 ng/L
Echocardiography	RA area <18cm² TAPSE/sPAP >0.32 mm/mmHg No pericardial effusion	RA area 18-26 cm² TAPSE/sPAP 0.19-0.32 mm/mmHg Minimal pericardial effusion	RA area > 26 cm² TAPSE/sPAP < 0.19 mm/mmHg Moderate or high Pericardial effusion
cardiac MRI	RVEF > 54% SVI > 40 mL/m² RVESVI < 42 mL/m²	RVEF 37-54% SVI 26-40 mL/m² RVESVI 42-54 mL/m²	RVEF < 37% SVI < 26 mL/m² RVESVI > 54 mL/m²
Hemodynamics	RAP < 8 mmHg CI > 2.5 L/min/m² SVI > 38 mL/m² SvO2 > 65%	RAP 8-14 mmHg CI 2.0-2.4 L/min/m² SVI 31-38 mL/m² SvO_2 60-65%	RAP > 14 mmHg CI < 2.0 L/min/m² SVI < 31 mL/m² SvO2 < 60%

Fig. 5.2 Risk stratification of pulmonary arterial hypertension

database, in which anticoagulation was effective only in iPAH and hPAH, but not in systemic sclerosis-associated PAH (SSC-PAH). However, the data on this is overall controversial. According to the *2022 ESC Guidelines*, general anticoagulation in PAH is therefore no longer recommended.

Diuretics

Symptoms such as peripheral edema and ascites occur in advanced stages of the disease and are signs of right heart failure. The use of potassium-sparing diuretics with aldosterone-antagonizing effects (e.g., spironolactone or eplerenone) is preferred. Due to the lack of scientific research results supporting the use of diuretic therapy, the choice of substance class, dosage, and treatment remains at the discretion of the treating physicians.

Oxygen

Currently, there are no study data on the long-term effect of oxygen in patients with PH. However, the general recommendation is to aim for a sustained oxygen saturation above 92%. For symptomatic indication, oxygen is often used in advanced stages.

Positive Inotropic Substances

Positive inotropic substances such as digitalis are given to patients with atrial arrhythmias (Sects 12.3 and 12.5). This is based not on scientific evidence but on clinical experience.

The intravenous administration of dobutamine, milrinone, or levosimendan in advanced stages of decompensated right heart failure is used in many expert centers in intensive care units under full hemodynamic monitoring, albeit based on little controlled data-based evidence.

▪ **Targeted Therapies**

Untreated PAH is characterized by a progressive course with right heart failure. The median survival time without treatment is only 2.8 years. The *2022 ESC/ERS Guidelines* stipulate that therapy decisions should be made based on an individual risk profile (low, intermediate, or high risk) (◘ Fig. 5.2). For patients with low or intermediate risk, a primary oral combination therapy is suggested. The guidelines further recommend a therapy evaluation after 3–6 months, considering a 4-strata risk score that distinguishes low, intermediate-low, intermediate-high, and high risk. If the initial therapy response is inadequate, therapy escalation should occur.

Calcium Channel Blockers

The high-dose use of calcium channel blockers is justified only in hemodynamic responders (see definition above in the section on vasoreactivity testing), who occur in only 1–2% of all patients with PAH. Careful titration of substances such as nifedipine (120–240 mg/day) or diltiazem (240–720 mg/day) is crucial for therapeutic success. Arterial hypotension and peripheral edema are side effects that can complicate therapy. In clinical practice, amlodipine (15–30 mg/day) or felodipine (15–30 mg/day) are also used. The long-term outcome is invasively evaluated after 3–6 months. Patients in NYHA stage I–II with sustained hemodynamic improvement remain on monotherapy.

Synthetic Prostacyclin and Prostacyclin analogs

Prostacyclin is synthesized in endothelial cells and is a potent vasodilator. The reduced expression of prostacyclin synthase in pulmonary arteries of patients with PAH suggests the clinical use of prostacyclin analogs. The side effects of this class of substances, such as blood pressure drop, headaches, flush, diarrhea, jaw pain, joint pain, etc., are occasionally therapy-limiting. An increased dosage requirement over time is considered a characteristic of this class of substances.

- **Epoprostenol**: Epoprostenol is administered intravenously. Its short half-life of 3–5 minutes makes continuous application via infusion pump and permanent central venous catheter (Hickman) indispensable. Placebo-controlled studies have shown that epoprostenol has a favorable effect on performance, hemodynamics, and survival. Mechanical complications with the infusion pump or tubing system can have life-threatening consequences, such as acute right heart failure due to sudden therapy discontinuation, air embolisms, and bleeding. Other feared complications include thrombosis and catheter sepsis.
- **Treprostinil**: Treprostinil is a tricyclic benzidine analog of epoprostenol and can be administered subcutaneously, via inhalation, or intravenously. This substance also led to improved performance and hemodynamics in randomized clinical studies. In addition to the class-typical side effects mentioned above, subcutaneous administration can cause pain at the injection site, which can make continuation of therapy impossible in about 15% of patients.
- **Beraprost**: Beraprost is a chemically stable and orally active prostacyclin analog. Due to its lack of effect on performance beyond the first 3–6 months, the drug is not approved in the USA and Europe, but it is in Japan and South Korea.
- **Selexipag:** The oral prostacyclin receptor agonist Selexipag was investigated in the GRIPHON trial, a Phase III study. A total of 1156 PAH patients were studied over a period of 4.3 years. Selexipag was able to significantly reduce the risk of morbidity and mortality events by 39% compared to placebo, both as monotherapy and in combination with other existing PAH therapies. Selexipag works best in combination and in less severely ill patients.

- **Inhaled Iloprost:** This form of therapy has not established itself as monotherapy in practice but is occasionally used in combination therapies. The disadvantage of this therapy arises from the very short duration of action of only about 45–60 minutes, resulting in 6 to 9 daily inhalations, each lasting 5–10 minutes. As monotherapy, this treatment is primarily used short-term in intensive care units.
- **Inhaled Treprostinil:** The inhalative form of treprostinil therapy is used in combination with endothelin receptor blockers or sildenafil. Administration is 4 times daily at intervals of 4 hours. The inhalative (and also the oral) form of treprostinil is currently only approved in the USA and is still undergoing clinical trials.

■■ **Endothelin Receptor Antagonists (ERAs)**
The effect of endothelin-1 is mediated via the ET receptors ET-A and ET-B, which are expressed on endothelial cells, smooth muscle cells, and also fibroblasts. The binding of ET-1 to ET-A receptors mediates vasoconstriction and proliferation. Activation of the ET-B receptors additionally promotes ET-1 clearance and leads to the release of vasodilative and antiproliferative factors (e.g., NO, prostacyclin). Endothelin receptor antagonists are among the established PAH therapies.
- **Ambrisentan:** This is a highly selective ETA receptor antagonist. Ambrisentan is indicated for the treatment of patients with PAH of WHO functional class II and III and is intended to improve their performance. Ambrisentan has a low hepatotoxic potential. An increase in transaminases was observed in 2.8% of cases.
- **Bosentan:** This is an orally active dual ET-A and ET-B receptor antagonist. It improves performance and hemodynamics. The most important side effect is an increase in transaminases in 7–11% of cases.
- **Macitentan:** This is an orally active dual ET-A and ET-B receptor antagonist. The hepatotoxicity of ERAs is absent in macitentan; additionally, macitentan has a low interaction potential with other substances. An undesirable side effect is a reduction in hemoglobin levels. In a large Phase III study including 742 patients with PAH (SERAPHIN Trial), the risk of a morbidity or mortality event was reduced by 30% and 45% with 3 mg and 10 mg, respectively, compared to placebo over the treatment period (85.3 weeks).

■■ **Phosphodiesterase inhibitors (PDE)**
- **Sildenafil:** This is administered orally and selectively inhibits the enzyme PDE-5, which degrades cyclic guanosine monophosphate (cGMP), thereby increasing the intracellular concentration of cGMP. This leads to relaxation and antiproliferative effects in smooth muscle cells via intracellular calcium. Clinical studies have shown an improvement in performance and hemodynamics.
- **Tadalafil:** This is administered orally and only once a day. It is another selective inhibitor of PDE-5. Clinical studies with patients in WHO functional class II and III have shown an improvement in performance.

■■ **Soluble guanylate cyclase stimulators**
- **Riociguat:** This is an oral stimulator of soluble guanylate cyclase (sGC). When NO binds to the heme domain of sGC or even in the absence of NO, the enzyme catalyzes the synthesis of the signaling molecule *cyclic guanosine monophosphate* (cGMP). cGMP, in turn, plays an important role in regulating cellular Ca^{2+} metabolism and consequently vascular tone, cell proliferation, fibrosis, and inflammation. In two phase III studies in patients with PAH and in patients with inoperable or post-operative persistent CTEPH, a significant and sustained improvement was demon-

strated both in the 6-minute walk test (additional walking distance: 39 m) and in WHO functional classification. Riociguat also showed a good efficacy and safety profile in long-term use.

- **Therapy strategies and combination therapies**

The use of the above-mentioned active substances and therapy strategies is carried out taking into account individual risk stratification. In the AMBITION trial, an initial (*first-line*) combination treatment of PAH with Ambrisentan 10 mg/day and Tadalafil 40 mg/day achieved a significant 50% risk reduction for clinical failure compared to the pooled group of Ambrisentan and Tadalafil monotherapy (hazard ratio = 0.502). The initial combination was also significant for the primary endpoint compared to the individual monotherapy groups. The rate of serious adverse events and adverse events leading to discontinuation of therapy was not different across all treatment arms. A significant hemodynamic reduction of PVR by around 50% and clinical improvement could also be achieved through the initial combination of Macitentan and Tadalafil. Therefore, the initial combination therapy of ERA and PDE5i is recommended in the *2022 ESC/ERS Guidelines* for patients with low and intermediate risk (estimated 1-year mortality 5–20%). High-risk patients (estimated 1-year mortality >20%) should be given combination therapy with parenteral prostanoids.

Following the initiation of initial therapy, PAH patients must be re-evaluated and the medication adjusted every 3 to 6 months.

List of Substances Approved for PAH in Most Western European Countries (Active Substances and Tade Names)
- Epoprostenol (Flolan®)
- Treprostinil sodium (Remodulin®) Trisuva
- Inhaled Iloprost (Ventavis®)
- Parenteral Iloprost (Ilomedin)
- Inhaled Treprostinil Sodium (Tyvaso®)
- Oral Treprostinil (Orenitram®)
- Selexipag (Uptravi®)
- Bosentan (Tracleer®)
- Ambrisentan (Volibris®)
- Macitentan (Opsumit®)
- Sildenafil (Revatio®)
- Tadalafil (Adcirca®)
- Riociguat (Adempas®)

- **Interventional and Surgical Techniques**

Atrial Septostomy
This is a measure to create a right-to-left shunt and is used by some PH centers as palliative bridging to transplantation.

Lung Transplantation
Bilateral lung transplantation or heart-lung transplantation is indicated when medical therapies are exhausted. The 5-year survival rate after lung transplantation in PAH is 45–55%.

Pulmonary Denervation
The interventional denervation of the pulmonary arteries is based on the observation that elevated catecholamine levels are measured in the circulation in pulmonary hypertension. Initial data with an ultrasound-based ablation catheter (Sonivie®) show a decrease in mPAP and PVR after 4 months, which was not sustained.

Management of Pulmonary Hypertension with Left Ventricular Heart Disease Left heart diseases such as heart failure with preserved or reduced LVEF (▶ Sect. 13.2), cardiomyopathies (▶ Chap. 8) or mitral regurgitation (▶ Sect. 9.3, 9.4 and 9.5) are often associated with PH. In fact, group 2 PH is the most common form of PH. Pathophysiologically, there is primarily an increase in left ventricular filling pressures with backflow initially into the left atrium and eventually into the pulmonary circulation (postcapillary PH; ◘ Fig. 5.1c). This is accompanied by pulmonary vasoconstriction, impaired vascular permeability, and pulmonary vascular remodeling. Depending on the extent of these components, different hemodynamic characteristics can result. Therefore, depending on the PVR, isolated postcapillary PH (PVR ≤ 2 WU; ◘ Fig. 5.1c) and combined post- and precapillary PH (PVR > 2 WU; ◘ Fig. 5.1f) are separate entities. This hemodynamic profile impacts on prognosis. A severe precapillary component is defined by a PVR > 5 WU. The focus of PH therapy is on optimized treatment of the left heart disease. In patients with heart failure, the risk of cardiac decompensations and hospitalizations can be substantially reduced by PAP-guided heart failure therapy using implantable pressure sensors (e.g., CARDIOMEMS®) (▶ Chap. 13). PAH medications are not generally indicated for group 2 PH. However, in patients with a PVR > 5 WU, an individualized therapy decision in expert centers is recommended.

Management of Pulmonary Hypertension with Lung Diseases with/without Hypoxemia   Various interstitial or obstructive lung diseases are associated with pulmonary hypertension (◘ Fig. 5.1d). PH in this context is usually only mildly expressed; it is nevertheless prognostically relevant. The etiology involves changes in the airways, lung parenchyma, and pulmonary vessels. Severe PH in lung disease is defined by a PVR > 5 WU and is associated with significantly poorer life expectancy. Such patients should be treated individually in expert centers, taking into account the severity of the lung disease and PH. The INCREASE trial has shown the superiority of inhaled treprostinil compared to placebo in patients with PH and interstitial lung disease (ILD). Additionally, in patients with lung disease and severe PH, therapy with PDE5i can also be considered. The ERA ambrisentan is contraindicated in ILD, and the sGC stimulator riociguat is contraindicated in idiopathic interstitial pneumonia (IIP).

Management of Chronic Thromboembolic Pulmonary Hypertension (CTEPH)   CTEPH (◘ Fig. 5.1e) results from intraluminal obstructions of the pulmonary vessels caused by chronically recurrent thrombi and emboli. Patients with CTEPH must be anticoagulated for life. The therapeutic strategy for CTEPH includes a multimodal approach with medical therapy as well as surgical (pulmonary endarterectomy) and catheter interventional procedures (pulmonary balloon angioplasty; see below). The primary therapy option is surgery.

- **Pharmacological Therapy**

The rationale for pharmacological therapy in CTEPH is vascular dysfunction and remodeling occurring in the peripheral vascular bed. Approved pharmacological therapy options include the sGC stimulator Riociguat as well as subcutaneously or intravenously administered Treprostinil.

- **Surgical and Interventional Techniques**

Pulmonary Endarterectomy (PEA)
In the treatment of CTEPH, the surgical side-selective endarterectomy in deep hypothermia is considered the gold standard of therapy. Pulmonary endarterectomy can cure CTEPH, but it is applicable in only half of all CTEPH cases.

Pulmonary Balloon Angioplasty (BPA)
This interventional method is used to treat inoperable CTEPH or PH after PEA through a balloon angioplasty directed at the pulmonary vessels using the intervention technique established in the coronary arteries (▶ Sect. 7.3).

Japanese groups have established this method since 2001, and BPA is now also available in expert centers in Europe and has substantially changed the treatment algorithm of CTEPH. Thus, an interventional therapy with usually significant clinical improvement can also be offered to patients classified as inoperable. In combination with modern PAH substances, BPA in expert centers is a safe method for patients with distally located pulmonary artery occlusions that are not eligible for surgery or for patients who do not wish surgical treatment or carry an unacceptable surgical risk.

Diabetes Mellitus

Roger Lehmann and Nikolaus Marx

Contents

6.1　Definition and Classification – 78

6.2　Epidemiology – 78

6.3　Diabetic Complications – 79

6.4　Treatment of Type 2 Diabetes – 81

　　　Further Reading – 88

Trailer

The numerous endpoint studies on diabetes mellitus have led to a revolution in therapy recommendations. This chapter explains this simply and step by step.

6.1 Definition and Classification

Definition Diabetes mellitus is present when fasting blood glucose is ≥7.0 mmol/l, the oral glucose tolerance test (OGTT) is ≥11.1 mmol/l, or glycated hemoglobin (HbA1c) is ≥6.5% or ≥48 mmol/mol. The diagnosis of diabetes mellitus can also be made with a random blood glucose ≥11.1 mmol/l and the simultaneous presence of symptoms (weight loss, diuresis, fatigue, excessive hunger, etc.) of diabetes mellitus.

Classification
Initially, 2 types of diabetes are distinguished:
- *Type 1 diabetes*: This is an autoimmune disease in which the β-cells of the pancreas are destroyed by antibodies. This affects about 5% of all diabetics.
- *Type 2 diabetes* is the most common form of diabetes (about 90–95%) and has a complex, multifactorial pathogenesis.

Today, a total of **5 subtypes** of diabetes are distinguished: (1) Type 1 diabetes with antibodies (Anti-GAD, Anti-IA2, or Anti-ZnT8); (2) Insulin deficiency in the absence of typical Type 1 diabetes antibodies; (3) pronounced insulin resistance and high insulin levels, often associated with NAFLD/NASH (see below) and renal complications; (4) obesity-associated diabetes; and (5) diabetes in older patients.

In diabetes with pronounced insulin deficiency, monogenic diabetes, mitochondrial diabetes, or diabetes in chronic pancreatitis may also be present. The proportion of Type 1 diabetes and specific forms of diabetes is 5% each. The pathogenetic mechanism of most specific forms of diabetes (except for the rare MODY 2; *maturity onset diabetes of the young*, which is caused by glucokinase mutations) is insulin deficiency, which is initially treated with insulin in most cases (except MODY 1 and 3 with sulfonylureas) and subsequently with SGLT-2 inhibitors or GLP-1 receptor agonists due to their protective cardiorenal effects (◘ Fig. 6.1).

According to international guidelines, an algorithm for diagnosing the type of diabetes and insulin deficiency has been developed based on age, specific antibodies, family history of diabetes, and C-peptide levels: If the C-peptide is >200 and <600 pmol/l, specific antibodies are negative, and there is no pronounced family history of diabetes, insulin deficiency can be diagnosed. In the early stages, Type 1 diabetes is still possible. In this regard, the determination of C-peptide must be repeated 3 years later. In this situation, treatment with a co-formulated insulin at the main meal or at the two main meals is preferable to monotherapy with an ultra-long-acting insulin because postprandial blood glucose levels are also lowered and the treatment is simpler than a basal-bolus system (same HbA1c levels, but less hypoglycemia).

6.2 Epidemiology

Worldwide, over 370 million people suffer from diabetes mellitus, with an estimated 50% undiagnosed. By 2030, it is predicted that the number could rise to over 550 million. The greatest increase is seen in emerging and developing countries and primarily affects Type 2 diabetes mellitus.

> Furthermore, 80% of diabetes deaths occur in developing countries. Thus, diabetes mellitus accounts for as many victims as HIV and AIDS. Every 10 seconds, a patient with diabetes dies from the

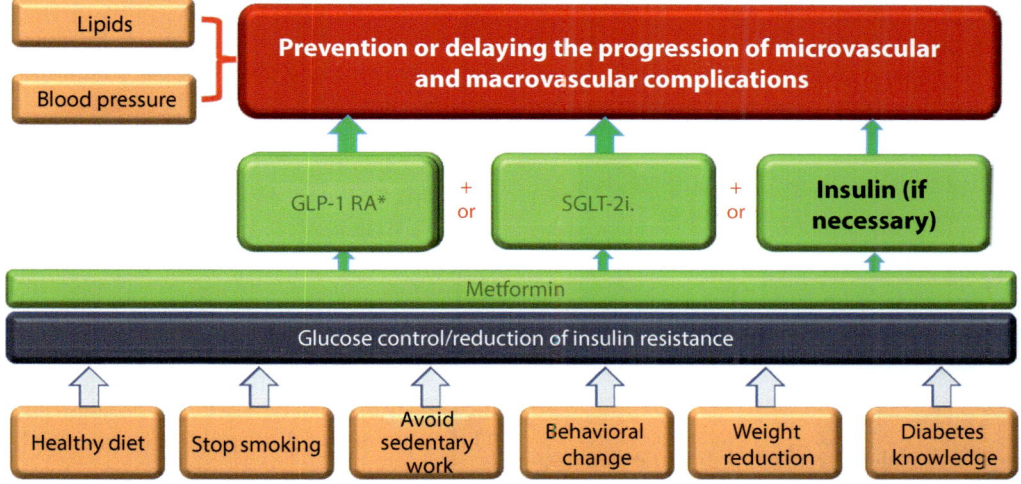

Fig. 6.1 Measures for the prevention of Type 2 diabetes

mainly cardiovascular consequences of the disease.

In industrialized countries of the western world, at least 6–8% of adults suffer from diabetes mellitus, with the number of undiagnosed cases likely to be very high. The prevalence increases sharply with age, already reaching 10% or more among those over 65 years old.

6.3 Diabetic Complications

Causes of Diabetic Complications

Pathophysiologically, in type 2 diabetes, high blood glucose levels lead to changes in endothelial function with increased production of free oxygen radicals, formation of toxic degradation products, and glycosylation of various important proteins in the vascular wall. Furthermore, the permeability of endothelial cells is increased, leading to increased penetration of LDL into the vascular wall and thus to the progression of atherosclerosis and its complications such as heart attack, stroke, and premature death (▶ Sect. 7.2). Chronic hyperglycemia damages tissue through various pathomechanisms, some of which are listed here (◘ Fig. 6.1):

- *Non-enzymatic glycosylation:* Here, glucose binds non-enzymatically to amino groups of proteins (e.g., HbA1c). After the formation of intermediate products, AGEs (*advanced glycosylated end products*) are formed. The altered proteins impair or change tissue function.
- *Disruption of the polyol pathway:* In insulin-independent tissues (nerves, lens, kidney, blood vessels), hyperglycemia leads to an increase in intracellular glucose concentration. Aldose reductase metabolizes excess glucose to sorbitol (and fructose). Due to the accumulation of sorbitol, the cell's osmolarity increases, leading to intracellular edema with cell damage. The intracellular myo-inositol concentration decreases, disrupting the phosphatidyl-inositol metabolism and leading to a decrease in Na^+/K^+-ATPase activity.
- *Formation of hexosamines:* Formation of amino sugars (glucosamine, etc.), which play an important role in the development of insulin resistance.

- Upregulation of signal transduction molecules, especially the *protein kinase C isoforms PKC β and δ*, leading to an enhancement of the pro-inflammatory state at the cellular level.

> The various vascular damaging effects of diabetes mellitus are summarized under the term diabetic angiopathy.

In addition to the cardiovascular system, there are other complications:
- **Retinopathy**: In Europe, about 30% of all cases of blindness are due to diabetes.
- **Glomerulosclerosis and diabetic nephropathy**: About one-third of diabetics are affected. About half of all dialysis patients have diabetes.
- **Neuropathy**: After 10 years of diabetes, about half of diabetics develop mostly sensorimotor polyneuropathy.

Cardiovascular Consequences of Diabetes Diabetes mellitus is the "cancer" of the blood vessels. The impact of diabetes on the cardiovascular system corresponds to premature aging by about 15 years and at the age of 50, a reduction in life expectancy by 6 years.

! The presence of diabetes mellitus doubles the cardiovascular risk in women and doubles to triples it in men. 55% of diabetics die from a heart attack!

In chronic coronary syndromes and acute coronary syndromes (◘ Fig. 6.2), mortality is significantly increased both in the short and long term (Sects. 7.2, 7.3 and 7.5). In addition to myocardial infarction, diabetics also have a significantly increased risk of developing peripheral arterial occlusive disease (PAOD; ▶ Sect. 7.4) or a cerebrovascular insult (CVI; ▶ Sect. 7.5).

Prevention of Type 2 Diabetes
For the treatment of (pre-)diabetes, a change in lifestyle is initially recommended for all age groups. Healthy eating, weight control, and physical activity (▶ Sect. 3.5) play a key role and should ideally be implemented simultaneously (◘ Fig. 6.1):
- Control of **blood sugar**, **blood pressure**, and **LDL-C**
- Achieving and maintaining the desired **body weight**
- Delaying or preventing **diabetic complications** (micro- and macrovascular disease)

With a weight reduction of >15%, a diabetes remission rate of 86% can be achieved. The most important predictor of weight loss is adherence to a specific diet. In individuals with prediabetes and obesity, GLP (glucagon-like Peptide)-1 receptor agonists and recently also GLP-1/GIP (*Glucose-dependent insulinotropic Polypeptide*) receptor agonists have been developed, which in studies achieve significant weight reduction, normalization of blood sugar, and a reduction in cardiovascular events (SELECT Trial). Additionally, in individuals with prediabetes, the onset of type 2 diabetes can be significantly reduced with the help of SGLT-2.

- **Multifactorial Risk Factor Management**

Simultaneous treatment of cardiovascular risk factors such as hyperglycemia, hypertension, LDL cholesterol, and smoking cessation is particularly important in type 2 diabetes. It is crucial to consider the condition and preferences of the patients and to prioritize parameters such as body weight, blood sugar control, and cardiorenal protection based on the individual situation.

- **Lipid and Blood Pressure Management**

To control high LDL-C, a potent statin is the first choice (▶ Sect. 3.2). If the targets are not achieved, ezetimibe is added. If the values are still too high, PCSK-9 inhibitors should be considered.

The target blood pressure should be <130/80 mmHg in younger patients and

Diabetes Mellitus

<140/90 mmHg in those over 65 years (▶ Chap. 4). When choosing medications, a combination of an ACE inhibitor with a calcium channel blocker is recommended for diabetics. If the ACE inhibitor is not tolerated, an angiotensin II receptor blocker can be prescribed. Individuals with diabetes exhibit higher platelet reactivity and turnover, resulting in a prothrombotic status (see ▶ Sect. 7.3). Inhibition of platelet aggregation with aspirin or other medications is generally recommended for patients with established cardiovascular disease, but not in primary prevention.

6.4 Treatment of Type 2 Diabetes

> The treatment of type 2 diabetes aims to lower or normalize blood sugar levels and prevent macro- and microvascular complications (◘ Fig. 6.2).

Not all antidiabetic drugs lower blood sugar equally well, and not all reduce heart attack, stroke, and cardiac death (so-called Major Adverse Cardiovascular Events; MACE) and/or overall mortality. Indeed, some older antidiabetic drugs are associated with an increased risk of mortality. Therefore, it is not only about demonstrating a reduction in blood sugar but also about cardiovascular safety and subsequently a reduction in MACE. Studies with dipeptidyl peptidase-4 (DPP-4) inhibitors demonstrated their cardiovascular safety; however, an additional benefit concerning MACE could not be proven. In contrast, with sodium-glucose co-transporter type 2 (SGLT-2) inhibitors such as empagliflozin, dapagliflozin, and sotagliflozin, MACE, as well as hospitalization due to heart failure, renal endpoints, and overall mortality, could be reduced for the first time. Glucagon-like peptide-1 (GLP-1) receptor agonists such as liraglutide showed a comparable effect concerning MACE as well as combined renal endpoints and overall mortality. Particularly significant is a marked reduction in hospitalizations due to heart failure by SGLT-2 inhibitors, both with reduced and preserved ejection fraction

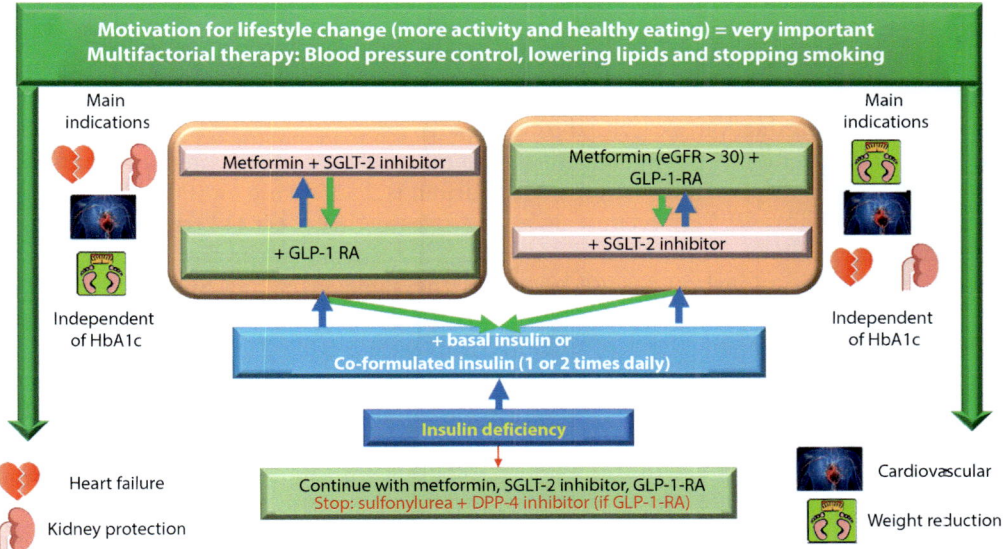

◘ Fig. 6.2 Differential treatment of diabetes

(Sects. 12.2 and 12.4). GLP-1 receptor agonists, on the other hand, showed a reduction in strokes. Against the backdrop of all these studies, new recommendations have emerged (see ◘ Fig. 6.2). ◘ Figure 6.3 providing an overview of the studies and their main results.).

In addition to cardiorenal protection and the prevention or treatment of heart failure by new medications, weight reduction and lowering blood sugar levels remain significant. According to the definition of the *European Society of Cardiology*, all patients with type 2 diabetes inherently have a high or very high cardiovascular risk (▶ Chaps. 3 and 4), the recommendations for cardiorenal protection and the prevention or treatment of heart failure apply equally to all type 2 diabetics (◘ Fig. 6.2).

The first steps in treatment are always lifestyle improvements (◘ Fig. 6.1) and a multifactorial treatment of arterial hypertension (▶ Chap. 4), the reduction of LDL-C (▶ Sect. 3.2), and smoking cessation. The initial pharmacological treatment should always consist of a combination of metformin and an SGLT-2 inhibitor or a GLP-1 receptor agonist (◘ Fig. 6.2). Metformin is maintained as first-line therapy because all cardiovascular endpoint studies were conducted on this basis and because no other antidiabetic drug reduces hepatic glucose production as well. If the initial dual combination is not sufficient for type 2 diabetics, a triple combination with an SGLT-2 inhibitor, GLP-1 receptor agonist, and metformin is recommended. Although this triple combination has not been directly studied, increasing practical experience shows that it represents the best option compared to other combinations to prevent MACE, overall mortality, and heart failure. Compared to the modern triple combination, the combination of metformin and a sulfonylurea (e.g., glibenclamide, tolbutamide, glibornuride, gliclazide, glimepiride) used in the last 60 years has more than 10 times higher mortality and 7 times higher MACE risk and thus should be avoided.

If the triple combination is not sufficient to lower HbA1c to the desired target value, insulin is required, which is necessary in a quarter of all type 2 diabetics. If insulin deficiency is the predominant factor at the onset of type 2 diabetes, the order of medications must be reversed (◘ Fig. 6.2, blue arrows), i.e., insulin first, then medications for cardiorenal protection (SGLT-2 inhibitors, GLP-1 receptor agonists, and metformin).

- **Renal Function and Chronic Kidney Disease**

In patients with chronic kidney disease (*Chronic Kidney Disease*; CKD), i.e., with a reduced glomerular filtration rate (estimated GFR, eGFR) and/or albuminuria, an SGLT-2 inhibitor should be used regardless of blood sugar levels, as these provide cardiorenal protection in type 2 diabetics and even in individuals without diabetes. SGLT-2 inhibitors not only reduce renal and cardiovascular endpoints in patients with CKD but also overall mortality. Although the blood sugar-lowering effect of SGLT-2 inhibitors diminishes or is completely absent with significantly reduced eGFR, the nephroprotective effects remain. Therefore, one should continue with SGLT-2 inhibitors even if the eGFR falls below 30 ml/min. However, metformin must be discontinued due to the risk of lactic acidosis. At an eGFR of 30–45 ml/min, the daily maximum dose of metformin is 2×500 mg or 1000 mg in extended-release form. GLP-1 receptor agonists also have nephroprotective effects, but not to the same extent as SGLT-2 inhibitors. GLP-1 receptor agonists can be used in patients with a BMI > 27 kg/m^2 without dose adjustment, even if their eGFR is significantly reduced or they need dialysis. DPP-4 inhibitors do not have nephroprotective effects but are safe with reduced eGFR and can be given as an alternative to GLP-1 receptor agonists for blood sugar reduction after dose adjustment (except for linagliptin) (e.g., in patients with a BMI < 27 kg/m^2 or who do not tolerate GLP-1 receptor agonists). Sulfonylureas, including gliclazide, should not be used at an eGFR < 30 ml/min due to the increased risk of hypoglycemia. The non-steroidal mineralocorticoid receptor antagonist finerenone reduces the renal endpoint by about a quarter and the combined cardiovascular endpoint by 14% in type 2 diabetics with CKD.

In patients treated with insulin, insulin requirements are reduced and the risk of hypoglycemia is increased as kidney function deteriorates. Therefore, insulin regimens and preparations with the lowest risk of hypoglycemia should be preferred in cases of reduced eGFR.

▪ Heart Failure and Diabetes

Heart failure (▶ Sect. 12.2) is a common complication of diabetes with a prevalence of up to 30% in patients over 65 years old, even in those without cardiovascular risk factors. If there is a clinical suspicion, determination of natriuretic peptides and transthoracic echocardiography (▶ Sect. 2.5) should be performed. However, this is not recommended as routine screening for all patients with diabetes.

SGLT-2 inhibitors are suitable for the prevention or treatment of all forms of heart failure such as HFpEF, HFmrEF, and HFrEF (▶ Sect. 12.2) with and without diabetes.

No randomized studies have been conducted on the risk of heart failure with metformin. However, a meta-analysis of 9 cohort studies with nearly 34,000 subjects suggests that metformin reduces the risk of mortality by about 20% in heart failure compared to the control group and is associated with a lower reduction in hospitalization.

Risk reduction (95% CI) SGLT-2 inhibitors	MACE	CV	Heart Failure	Combined Renal Endpoint	Mortality	Duration of the study (years)
EMPA-REG Empagliflozin	0.86 (0.74, 0.99) NNT 63	0.62 (0.49, 0.77) NNT 45	0.65 (0.50, 0.85) NNT 71	0.54 (0.40, 0.75) NNT 71	0.68 (0.57, 0.82) NNT 38	3.1
CANVAS/R Canagliflozin	0.86 (0.75, 0.97) NNT 94	0.87 (0.72, 1.06)	0.67 (0.52, 0.87) NNT 86	0.60 (0.47, 0.77) NNT 83	0.87 (0.74, 1.01)	3.4
DECLARE-TIMI Dapagliflozin	0.93 (0.84, 1.03)	0.98 (0.82, 1.17)	0.73 (0.61, 0.88) NNT 125	0.53 (0.43, 0.66) NNT 40	0.93 (0.82, 1.04)	4.2
VERTIS CV Ertugliflozin	0.97 (0.85, 1.11)	0.92 (0.77, 1.11)	0.70 (0.54, 0.90) NNT 91	0.81 (0.64, 1.03)	0.93 (0.80, 1.08)	3.5

GLP-1-RA	MACE	CV Death	Stroke	Combined Renal Endpoint	Mortality	Duration of the study (years)
LEADER Liraglutide	0.87 (0.78, 0.99) NNT 53	0.78 (0.66, 0.93) NNT 77	0.86 (0.71, 1.06)	0.54 (0.67, 0.82) NNT 67	0.85 (0.74, 0.97) NNT 71	3.8
SUSTAIN Semaglutide	0.74 (0.58, 0.95) NNT 30	0.98 (0.65, 1.48)	0.61 (0.38, 0.99) NNT 91	0.64 (0.47, 0.77) NNT 43	1.05 (0.74, 1.50)	2.1
REWIND Dulaglutide	0.88 (0.79, 0.99) NNT 71	0.91 (0.78, 1.06)	0.76 (0.62, 0.94) NNT 111	0.85 (0.77, 0.93) NNT 40	0.90 (0.80, 1.01)	5.4
PIONEER Oral semaglutide	0.79 (0.57, 1.11)	0.49 (0.27, 0.92) NNT 100	0.74 (0.35, 1.57)	nk	0.51 (0.31, 0.84) NNT 71	1.3

▫ **Fig. 6.3** Large randomized and controlled studies with SGLT-2 inhibitors and GLP-1 receptor agonists and their results. (*MACE:* Major Adverse Cardiovascular Events (heart attack, stroke, death), *Cv death:* cardiovascular death)

A meta-analysis of GLP-1 receptor agonists suggests that these drugs not only reduce strokes, MACE, and overall mortality but also, although less pronounced than with SGLT-2 inhibitors, the incidence of heart failure.

In contrast, therapy with thiazolidinediones or saxagliptin appears to be associated with an increased risk of heart failure. Thiazolidinediones (glitazones) have definitively shown an increased risk of weight gain and peripheral edema, heart failure, and hospitalization due to heart failure, as well as death in meta-analyses and randomized studies. They also showed a higher cardiovascular risk. Therefore, glitazones, especially pioglitazone, are not recommended for diabetics with heart failure, nor is the DPP-4 inhibitor saxagliptin. However, linagliptin or sitagliptin can be used to lower blood sugar levels if a GLP-1 receptor agonist is not indicated or not tolerated.

- **Regular Examinations during Follow-up**

Adherence to certain regular examinations and laboratory values is of crucial importance for diabetics. Thus, non-compliance with medical standards in long-term care, such as biannual HbA1c determination, ensuring LDL-C is within the target range, annual renal status, and ophthalmological check-ups, are associated with an increased likelihood of future hospitalization.

- **Weight Management in Type 2 Diabetes**

The risk of developing diabetes increases with rising body weight. Almost all patients with type 2 diabetes are obese. In addition to preventing micro- and macrovascular complications, the main goal of diabetes treatment is to reduce body weight. Obesity combined with a sedentary lifestyle is the greatest risk factor associated with increased insulin resistance and type 2 diabetes. Therefore, weight loss and an active lifestyle with physical exercise and strength training are of utmost importance.

> A person's normal weight is defined by a Body Mass Index (BMI) of 18.5–24.9. From 25.0 to 29.9, it is considered overweight. A BMI value over 30 is classified as obesity. The higher the BMI, the greater the risk of diabetes, while weight reduction lowers the risk.

- **Pharmacological Weight Reduction**

Since dietary weight reduction is often unsuccessful, medications have been developed. The weight reduction achievable with GLP-1 and GLP-1/GIP (*Glucose-dependent insulinotropic Polypeptide*) receptor agonists varies between individual molecules and dosages. The GLP-1 receptor agonist with the most pronounced weight reduction is Semaglutide at a dosage of 2.4 mg s.c./week, and the new GLP-1/GIP receptor agonist Tirzepatide (15 mg s.c./week; up to 22% weight reduction) achieves similar results. Since GLP-1 receptor agonists in lower dosages have been shown to reduce cardiovascular endpoints, they are currently preferred. The main limitations in the use of GLP-1 receptor agonists are side effects such as nausea and vomiting. These occur mainly in the first days to weeks and are less pronounced with a slow increase in dose. Sometimes avoiding large portions can reduce nausea symptoms. Although GLP-1 receptor agonists can also be used in severe renal failure (in fact delays the decrease in renal function), but nausea can sometimes be limiting. SGLT-2 inhibitors also have a weight-reducing effect, but to a much lesser extent. Accordingly, GLP-1 receptor agonists should be preferred over SGLT-2 inhibitors. More recent combination drugs mimicking both GLP-1 and Glucose-dependent Insulinotropic Polypeptide (GIP) are even more effective.

- **Weight-Reducing Surgery**

In addition to pharmacological therapy, bariatric surgery should be considered in cases of severe obesity (e.g., Roux-en-Y bypass, sleeve surgery). Such a procedure is considered for poorly controlled type 2 diabetes with HbA1c > 8% and a BMI > 30 kg/m². However, the difference between a bariatric procedure and high-dose Semaglutide or Tirzepatide in terms of weight loss is becoming increasingly smaller.

- **Non-Alcoholic Fatty Liver and Steatohepatitis**

NAFLD (*Non-Alcoholic Fatty Liver Disease*) and especially NASH (*Non-Alcoholic Steatohepatitis*) are associated with an increased risk of liver dysfunction and cardiovascular complications (◘ Fig. 6.4). The management of type 2 diabetics with NAFLD or those with the more advanced NASH should undergo significant weight reduction, which particularly means considering pharmacological and/or surgical approaches for patients with an increased risk of liver fibrosis. GLP-1 receptor agonists appear to be particularly beneficial here. SGLT-2 inhibitors have been shown to reduce elevated liver enzyme levels and liver fat content in NAFLD patients, but they are not currently recommended.

- **Differential therapy of various diabetes subtypes and insulin deficiency**

In certain situations, insulin may be the preferred substance for blood sugar control, especially in cases of severe hyperglycemia (HbA1c > 10%) and particularly when this is associated with normal or underweight individuals with the typical signs of insulin deficiency such as weight loss or ketonuria/ketosis or with acute glycemic dysregulation (e.g., during hospitalization, surgery, or an acute illness; ◘ Fig. 6.4) or when type 1 diabetes is suspected as part of the diagnosis. After the restoration of euglycemia, it is usually possible to discontinue insulin treatment again.

Type 2 diabetes is not a uniform disease. Generally, two pathogenic factors—insulin resistance and relative insulin deficiency—are predominant. Each of these two factors can be dominant and may occur before the other. Insulin resistance is typical in visceral obesity and physical inactivity. In cases of pronounced insulin resistance, the produced insulin is no longer sufficient to ensure glucose homeostasis, even if insulin and C-peptide levels are within the normal range.

- **Target range for blood sugar, HbA1c target, and reduction of hypoglycemia risk**

The main goal of blood sugar control is to keep the HbA1c level as normal as possible while avoiding hypoglycemia, which is associated with an increased risk of arrhythmic death. For most patients, this is an HbA1c level of 7.0%. For younger individuals with a short history of diabetes or patients with microvascular complications, this should be reduced to 6.5% if this can be achieved without repeated hypoglycemia. Regarding hypoglycemia or cardiovascular complications, an HbA1c level <6.5% is not dangerous, provided no insulin or sulfonylurea is used.

For older patients, individuals with severe hypoglycemia, patients with comorbidities (e.g., visual impairments, osteoporosis, autonomic neuropathy), or individuals with a limited life expectancy, a higher HbA1c target of 7–8% is reasonable. In all cases, however, an HbA1c level >8.0% should be avoided because the complications outweigh the potential benefits. Treating physicians should agree on an individual HbA1c target with the patients, which may change over time. To achieve an HbA1c target of 7.0%, most patients need a preprandial blood sugar <7 mmol/l and a postprandial value <10 mmol/l. In most cases, a satisfactory HbA1c level is achieved when patients achieve a value between 3.9 and 10 mmol/l in >70% of the hours in the target range (Time in Range, TIR).

GLP-1 receptor antagonists and SGLT-2 inhibitors do not entail a risk of hypoglycemia and still effectively reduce blood sugar. Among all oral antidiabetics, the highest risk is associated with long-acting sulfonylureas with active metabolites (glibenclamide, glimepiride) and, to a lesser extent, with gliclazide due to its shorter half-life and lack of active metabolites. The highest hypoglycemia rate is seen with intensive insulin therapy (basal-bolus insulin), with or without antidiabetics. When using an ultra-long-acting basal insulin, this rate is significantly lower. The highest hypoglycemia rates occur with insulin in combination with sulfonylurea. Therefore, this should be avoided.

If the HbA1c target is not achieved after administration of a GLP-1 receptor agonist, SGLT-2 inhibitors, or metformin, a basal insulin should be preferred over a sulfonylurea. A basal insulin is easy to use, effectively lowers blood sugar, and is cardiovascularly safe. The higher hypoglycemia risk associated with the newer ultra-long-acting insulins (degludec, glargine 300) is only slightly pronounced when administered as monotherapy. The hypoglycemia risk increases when a basal-bolus regimen is used. In these cases, it is recommended to prescribe a glucagon nasal spray (Baqsimi®), which makes the use of glucagon significantly easier in cases of severe hypoglycemia. It has been shown that with a co-formulated insulin administered twice daily with main meals, the same HbA1c level is achieved as with a basal-bolus regimen, but with significantly lower hypoglycemia rates. When starting insulin, the concomitant administration of SGLT-2 inhibitors, GLP-1 receptor agonists, and metformin should be continued (◘ Fig. 6.1).

Management of Elderly Diabetics Older adults >65 years make up more than half of all diabetics. The prevalence in this group varies between 16 and 30% in Western countries. Longer life expectancy and lifelong exposure to cardiometabolic risk factors are the main reasons for the increase in diabetes prevalence among the elderly. Older diabetics have a higher risk of known geriatric syndromes such as frailty, cognitive impairment and dementia, urinary incontinence, falls and traumatic fractures, disability, and side effects of polypharmacy. All these aspects can have serious impacts on quality of life and impair antidiabetic treatment.

If older people have no appetite, medications with minimal side effects and maximum benefit are to be preferred. SGLT-2 inhibitors are the best choice, also for the

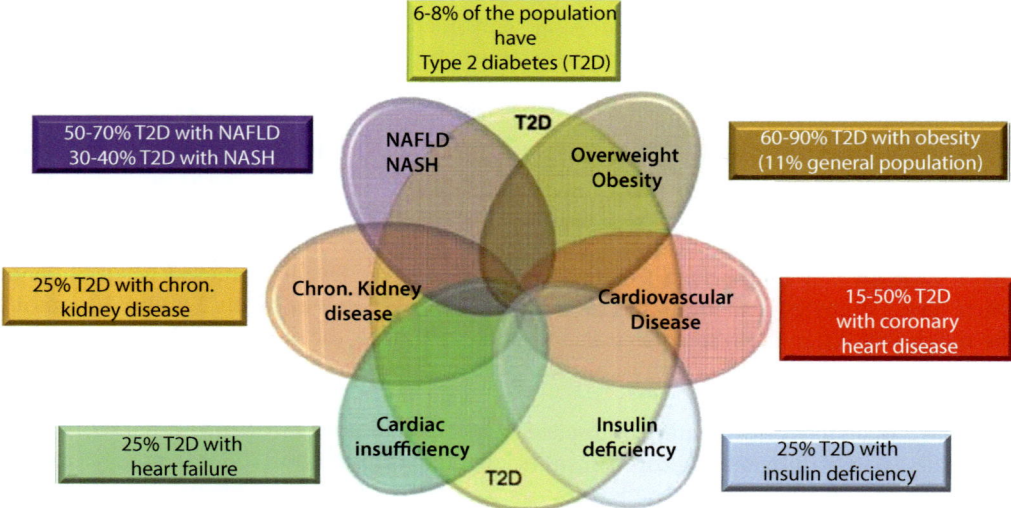

◘ **Fig. 6.4** Spectrum of comorbidities in Type 2 Diabetes

prevention or treatment of heart failure (▶ Sect. 12.2), which affects over a quarter of diabetics over 65 and is characterized by high mortality. In older men with prostate hypertrophy, SGLT-2 inhibitors can cause nocturia. In malnourished patients, GLP-1 receptor agonists should be avoided as they reduce appetite. The alternative would be DPP-4 inhibitors like linagliptin, because they lower HbA1c at any stage of CKD and do not need to be adjusted to eGFR.

Metformin should be used as long as eGFR > 30 ml/min. If nausea occurs, the dose should be reduced to 1000 mg per day, even if eGFR > 45 ml/min. In this case, a sustained-release formulation of metformin (once daily) can be tried.

Caution is advised in older diabetics with impaired eGFR when using insulin secretagogues due to their high risk of hypoglycemia. Short-acting sulfonylureas such as gliclazide or the glinide repaglinide are preferable.

If none of these substances are used, the HbA1c value should be between 6.5–7.0%. For those >80 years old, the HbA1c target value is 7.5–8.0%. However, if insulin or sulfonylurea is used, the HbA1c target should always be <8.0%.

Restrictions in the Use of Antidiabetics The use of different preparations of the same class of medication (e.g., 2 different SGLT-2 inhibitors or 2 DPP-4 inhibitors) is not sensible. Combining a GLP-1 receptor agonist with a DPP-4 inhibitor makes no pharmacological sense. Due to the increased risk of hypoglycemia, insulin and sulfonylureas should never be combined.

In situations where dehydration occurs (diarrhea, fever, vomiting), or food intake is not ensured (nausea, vomiting, perioperative), some antidiabetics must be temporarily discontinued (◘ Fig. 11.4). With metformin, there is a risk of lactic acidosis. An SGLT-2 inhibitor should be discontinued due to the risk of ketoacidosis if carbohydrate intake is not possible (vomiting, prolonged fasting, perioperative, before a stomach or colonoscopy). Insulin and sulfonylureas must be discontinued or their dose adjusted in all situations where carbo-

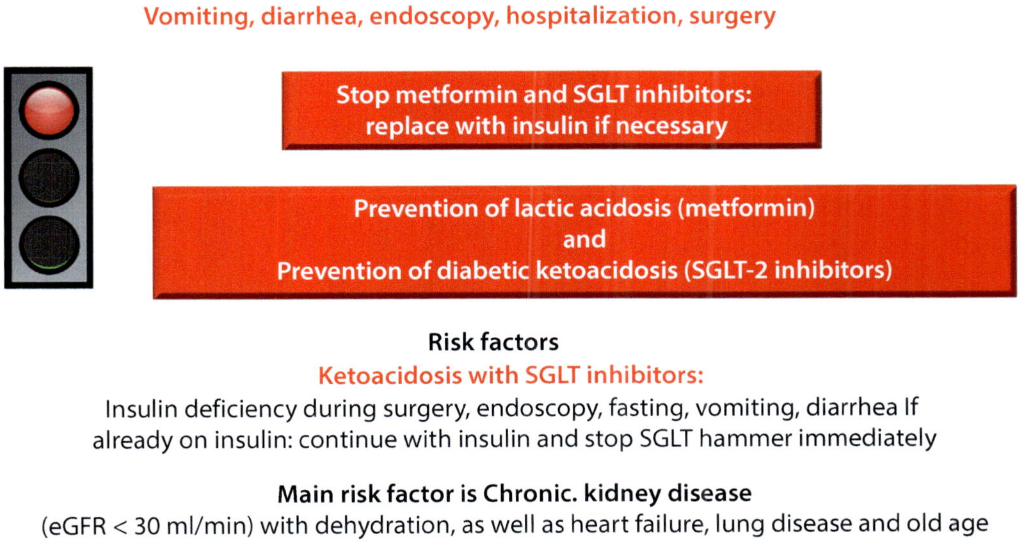

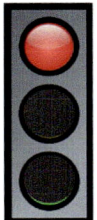

Vomiting, diarrhea, endoscopy, hospitalization, surgery

Stop metformin and SGLT inhibitors: replace with insulin if necessary

Prevention of lactic acidosis (metformin) and Prevention of diabetic ketoacidosis (SGLT-2 inhibitors)

Risk factors
Ketoacidosis with SGLT inhibitors:
Insulin deficiency during surgery, endoscopy, fasting, vomiting, diarrhea If already on insulin: continue with insulin and stop SGLT hammer immediately

Main risk factor is Chronic. kidney disease
(eGFR < 30 ml/min) with dehydration, as well as heart failure, lung disease and old age

◘ **Fig. 6.5** Adjustments of antidiabetic therapy during sick days

hydrate intake is not ensured, especially in insulin therapy (◘ Fig. 6.5).

Costs of Antidiabetics and Cost-Effectiveness Analysis Older antidiabetics like metformin or gliclazide are inexpensive, while DPP-4 and SGLT-2 inhibitors and insulin are more costly. The most expensive antidiabetics are GLP-1 receptor agonists. Several studies indicate that the use of SGLT-2 inhibitors and GLP-1 receptor agonists in addition to metformin therapy may even be cost-saving compared to other antidiabetics.

Further Reading

Davies MJ et al (2022) Management of hyperglycemia in type 2 diabetes, 2022. A consensus report by the american diabetes association (ADA) and the European Association for the Study of Diabetes (EASD). Diabetes Care 45(11):2753–2786

Visseren FLJ et al (2021) 2021 ESC Guidelines on cardiovascular disease prevention in clinical practice. Eur Heart J 42(34):3227–3337

Jensen MH et al (2020) Risk of major adverse cardiovascular events, severe hypoglycemia, and all-cause mortality for widely used antihyperglycemic dual and triple therapies for type 2 diabetes management: a cohort study of all danish users. Diabetes Care 43(6):1209–1218

Dave CV et al (2021) Risk of cardiovascular outcomes in patients with type 2 diabetes after addition of SGLT2 inhibitors versus sulfonylureas to baseline GLP-1RA therapy. Circulation 143(8):770–779

Mori Y et al (2022) Sodium-glucose cotransporter 2 inhibitors and new-onset type 2 diabetes in adults with prediabetes: systematic review and meta-analysis of randomized controlled trials. J Clin Endocrinol Metab 108(1):221–231

Bakris GL et al (2020) Effect of Finerenone on chronic kidney disease outcomes in type 2 diabetes. N Engl J Med 383(23):2219–2229

Atherosclerosis and Sequelae

Andreas Zirlik and Ronald K. Binder

Contents

7.1   Pathogenesis and Risk Factors – 90

7.2   Coronary Heart Disease (CHD) – 92

7.3   Chronic Coronary Syndrome with Stable Angina Pectoris – 93

7.4   Vasospastic Angina Pectoris (Prinzmetal's Angina) – 99

7.5   Acute Coronary Syndrome (ACS) and Myocardial Infarction – 100

7.6   Peripheral Arterial Occlusive Disease (PAOD) – 111

7.7   Cerebrovascular Accident (CVA) – 115

Earlier versions were created with the collaboration of M. Husmann, O. Gämperli, A. Luft, and J. Steffel.

© The Author(s), under exclusive license to Springer-Verlag GmbH, DE, part of Springer Nature 2025
T. F. Lüscher and U. Landmesser (eds.), *Cardiovascular System*,
https://doi.org/10.1007/978-3-662-70152-2_7

Atherosclerotic vascular changes are responsible for a variety of cardiovascular diseases. This includes coronary artery disease (CAD) with its entire clinical spectrum from stable angina pectoris (AP) to acute myocardial infarction, atherosclerotic cerebrovascular insult (CVI), and peripheral arterial occlusive disease (PAOD). Medicinal, invasive, and surgical treatment measures are used for these diseases and have significantly improved their prognosis in recent decades.

Atherosclerosis is a disease of the large arteries characterized by a chronic inflammatory process. Primarily affected are the aorta, the carotids, the coronary arteries, the renal arteries, as well as the pelvic and leg vessels. However, atherosclerosis can affect all arteries of the systemic circulation and must fundamentally be regarded as a generalized disease.

Depending on the **location**, it triggers different disease patterns:
- In the epicardial **coronary arteries**, it leads to coronary heart disease (CHD), which can result in anginal symptoms, heart attack or premture death.
- In the **cerebral arteries**, it results in cerebrovascular occlusive disease with transient ischemic attack (TIA) or cerebrovascular insult (CVI, cerebral infarction or stroke).
- In the **peripheral arteries** of the pelvis and legs, atherosclerosis leads to the development of peripheral arterial occlusive disease (PAOD).

7.1 Pathogenesis and Risk Factors

In atherogenesis, i.e., the development of arteriosclerotic plaques, five phases can be distinguished (◘ Fig. 7.1).

Phase 1 In the first phase, **endothelial dysfunction** is at the forefront. Endothelial cells line the inside of vessels (◘ Fig. 7.2) and regulate both the interaction of the vessel wall with circulating blood cells such as platelets, granulocytes, macrophages, and lymphocytes, as well as the vascular tone and structure by influencing the subendothelial vascular muscle cells. Changes in vascular tone are accompanied by a reduction in endothelial vasodilation due to increased inactivation of nitric oxide (NO) by superoxide anions (O_2^-) and in turn a decreased formation and availability of NO. The predominance of free radicals leads, among other things, to increased oxidation of LDL, which is no longer recognized as such by the LDL receptors of the liver and therefore remains in the plasma and is taken up into the vessel wall via LOX-1

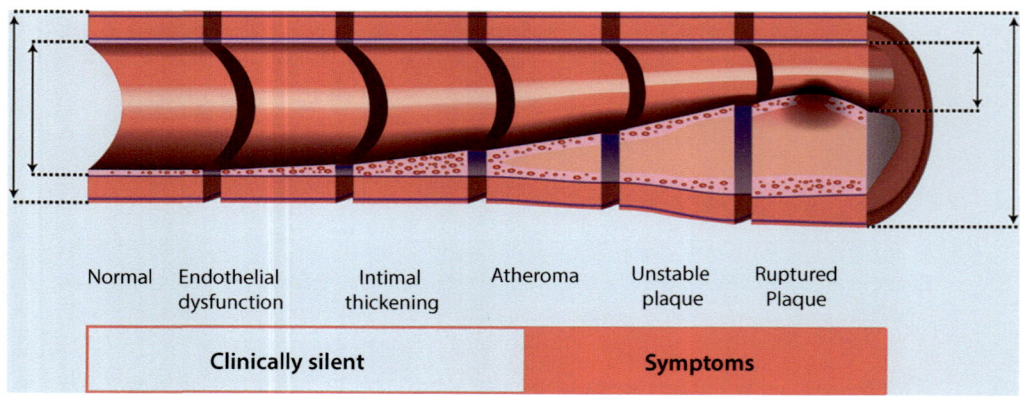

◘ Fig. 7.1 Temporal course of atherogenesis and clinical correlation

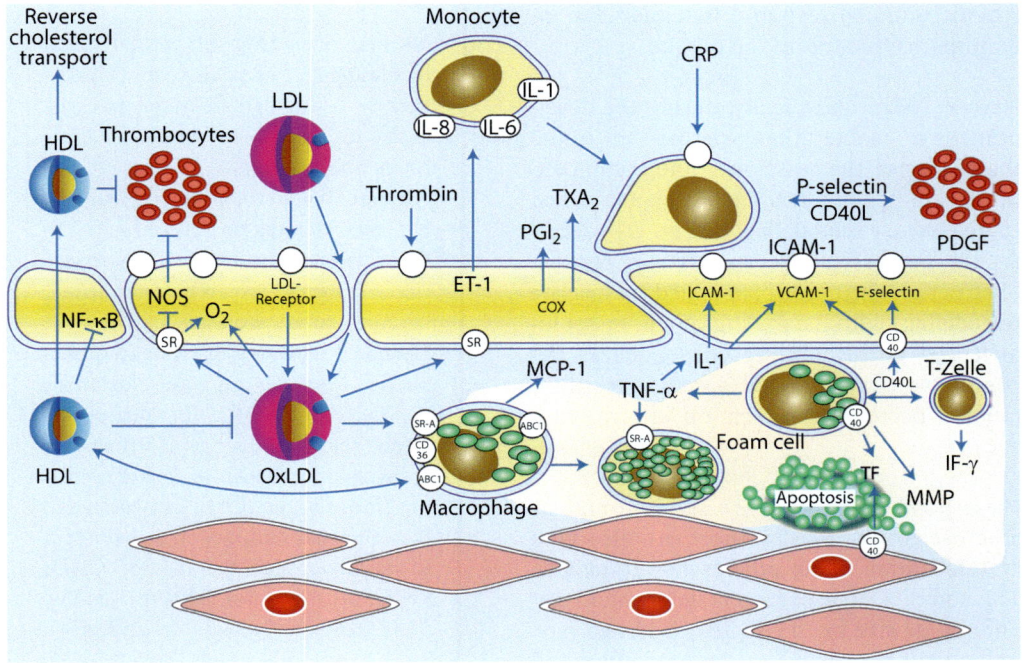

Fig. 7.2 Pathogenesis of Atherosclerosis. *HDL*: High Density Lipoprotein, *LDL:* Low Density Lipoprotein, *IL:* Interleukin, *ET:* Endothelin, *COX:* Cyclooxygenase, *TXA₂:* Thromboxane, *PGI₂:* Prostacyclin, *CRP:* C-Reactive Protein, *CD40L:* CD40-Ligand, *PDGF:* Platelet Derived Growth Factor, *NF-kB:* Nuclear Factor kB, *NOS:* NO Synthase, *oxLDL:* oxidized Low Density Lipoprotein, *ICAM:* Intercellular Adhesion Molecule, *VCAM:* Vascular Cell Adhesion Molecule, *MCP:* Monocyte Chemoattractant Protein, *TNF-a:* Tumor Necrosis Factor a, *TF:* Tissue Factor, *IF:* Interferon, *MMP:* Matrix Metalloproteinase, *SR-A:* Scavenger Receptor A

receptors leadign to inflammation and cellular dysfunction.

Phase 2 Through the **uptake of oxidized LDL**, free oxygen radicals such as O_2^- are increasingly formed locally, and NO is inactivated, leading to toxic degradation products. This and numerous other factors lead to the activation of intracellular signal transduction mechanisms, which result in an increased activation of transcription factors (including *Nuclear Factor kB, NFkB*). The resulting upregulation of the expression of adhesion molecules such as selectins (which mediate the initial "rolling" of monocytes along the endothelium) as well as the actual "docking proteins" ICAM-1 (*Intracellular Adhesion Molecule-1*) and VCAM-1 (*Vascular Cell Adhesion Molecule-1*) leads to rolling, adhesion and migration of monocytes into the intima and subsequent phagocytosis via expressed scavenger receptors of oxidized LDL-C: Foam cells are formed (Fig. 7.2).

Phase 3 **Foam cells** secrete various growth factors, including *Platelet Derived Growth Factor* (PDGF) and *Platelet Adhesion Factor* (PAF), as well as various cytokines that drive inflammation. This leads to the migration of smooth muscle cells from the media into the (neo-)intima, where they continue to proliferate ans change their phenotype. In parallel, the adaptive immune system is also activated, as antigens, particularly from the ApoB portion of the LDL complex, are presented to T cells by antigen-presenting cells, triggering a specific immune response that fuels the inflammatory process in the plaque.

Phase 4 Macroscopically, during the development of stable atherosclerosis, an initial thickening of the vessel wall and a compensatory enlargement of the vessels (so-called **compensatory remodeling;** ◘ Fig. 7.1) occur. As the process progresses, arteries become obstructed shrinking (so-called **restrictive remodeling**) with narrowing of the vessel lumen and corresponding consequences depending on the affected vascular territory (angina pectoris, claudication intermittens, etc.).

Phase 5 In addition to the stable course of atherosclerotic diseases, there can also be a **destabilization of an atherosclerotic plaque**. The stability of a plaque is determined not only by its size or the degree of lumen narrowing but above all by its composition and morphology. If the fibrous components predominate and the plaque is sealed by a robust fibrous cap, a stable plaque is present. In contrast, a high content of (oxidized) LDL leads to inflammatory changes, especially via NLRP3 and interleukin-6, and a merely thin *fibrous cap* leads to increasing instability (*vulnerable plaque*). This increases the risk of plaque erosion or rupture, with activation of platelets and coagulation, coronary occlusion, and clinically an acute coronary syndrome.

Main Risk Factors of Atherosclerosis
(► Sect. 3.3)
- **Age and Gender**: In men, the risk of atherosclerosis increases by a factor of 6 between the ages of 30 and 60, whereas in women, it increases only after menopause, probably due to the loss of protective estrogens.
- **Hypercholesterolemia/Dyslipidemia:** Main component of atherosclerotic plaque (► Sect. 3.2)
- **Nicotine**: increasing risk proportional to the number of pack-years (1 pack-year = 1 year of smoking 1 pack of cigarettes daily = 365 packs of cigarettes smoked/year)
- **Arterial Hypertension** (► Sect. 4.1)
- **Diabetes Mellitus** (► Sect. 6.1)
- **Obesity**: common cause of hypertension, diabetes, hypercholesterolemia, and metabolic syndrome
- **Genetic Predisposition**: Manifest secondary disease of atherosclerosis (CAD, CVI, PAD) in first-degree relatives before the age of 55 (men) or 65 (women) indicates a genetic predisposition. Of the genes known so far, the following chromosomal loci seem to correlate with the risk of CAD: 9p21.3 (SNP, rs1333049), 6q25.1 (rs6922269), 2q36.3 (rs2943634), 1p13.3 (rs599839), 1q41 (rs17465637), 10q11.21 (rs501120), and 15q22.33 (rs17228212)

7.2 Coronary Heart Disease (CHD)

Definition In CAD or chronic coroanry syndromes (CCS), an obstruction of one or more epicardial coronary arteries leads to reduced blood flow to the heart muscle and causes an imbalance between oxygen demand and supply in the myocardium. The most common cause of obstruction in CAD are atherosclerotic plaques. However, the clinical symptoms of CAD can also be caused by other mechanisms of myocardial blood flow disturbance, such as vasospasm, dissection, embolism, or microcirculation disorder.

Epidemiology CAD is the leading cause of death in industrialized countries. The lifetime prevalence in Europe is approximately 10% among 40- to 80-year-olds.

Etiology Atherosclerosis is the main cause of CAD (► Sect. 7.1).

Atherosclerosis and Sequelae

Clinical Findings CAD can manifest clinically in different ways.

> **Initial Clinical Manifestations of CAD are:**
> - Stable Angina Pectoris (AP) approximately 40%,
> - Acute Coronary Syndrome (ACS; Myocardial Infarction) approximately 40%,
> - Cardiac arrhythmias (mostly ventricular tachycardia or fibrillation) with or without syncope and potentially sudden death,
> - Heart failure (main symptoms: exercise intolerance, dyspnea, leg edema),
> - Sudden cardiac death (mostly ventricular fibrillation, but also asystole).

Myocardial Ischemia as a result of CAD can appear in various forms:
- **Asymptomatic CAD**: silent ischemia
- **Symptomatic CAD**: chronic coronary syndrome (CCS), acute coronary syndrome (ACS), and their consequences heart failure or sudden cardiac death

7.3 Chronic Coronary Syndrome with Stable Angina Pectoris

Definition Angina pectoris (AP, chest tightness) is the typical symptomatology of myocardial ischemia (◐ Fig. 7.3). The transient myocardial hypoperfusion, which is provoked by physical (or also psychological) stress, activates afferent nerve pathways in the myocardium, which lead to pain perception. A fundamental distinction is made between stable and unstable AP.

> Unstable angina is considered to be:
> - any first manifestation of AP,
> - an increase in the intensity or frequency of known AP,
> - AP at rest.

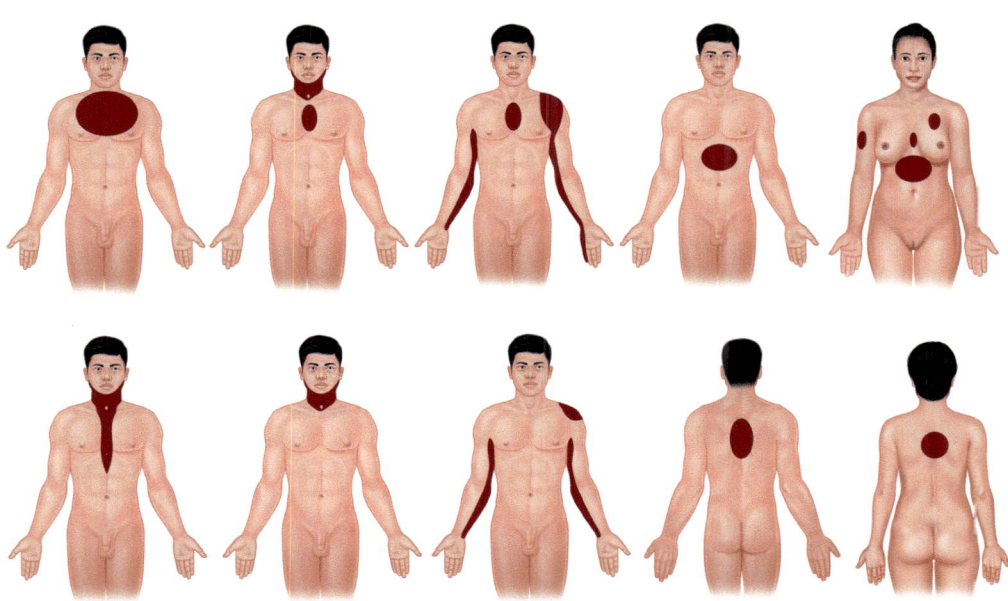

◐ **Fig. 7.3** Localization and radiation of cardiac chest pain

Clinical Findings The clinical hallmark symptom of AP is a feeling of tightness or pressure in the chest often radiating into the left arm or jaw (◘ Fig. 7.3), which occurs in stable AP upon exertion. Other triggers for AP include heavy meals, cold environmental temperatures, or psychological stress. Patients typically describe AP as a broad pressing, squeezing, or burning sensation in the chest. The symptoms usually last a few minutes and quickly improve when standing still or resting or after administration of nitroglycerin.

Classification The severity of AP is classified according to the Canadian Cardiovascular Society Score (CCS Score).

Canadian Cardiovascular Society Score (CCS Score) of Angina Pectoris
- 0: No chest pain
- I: Angina with severe exertion
- II: Angina with moderate exertion (slight impairment)
- III: Angina with mild exertion (significant impairment)
- IV: Symptoms with minimal exertion or at rest (CCS IV = unstable AP)

Differential Diagnosis Chest pain can have various causes and be due to any organ in the thorax. Musculoskeletal chest pain originating from the musculoskeletal system is more often described as stabbing or cutting, is less diffuse, often precisely localized, and usually independent of exertion. In gastroesophageal reflux, the symptoms, often described as burning, occur more frequently when lying down or at night in bed and are also not exertion-dependent. Esophageal spasms can respond to nitrates and thus be confused with AP. The symptoms of pericarditis or pleuritis are often position- (aggravation with lying) and/or breathing-dependent (aggravation with deep inspiration).

The following **conditions with chest pain** are immediately life-threatening and should be initially ruled out:
- acute Coronary Syndrome
- Pulmonary embolism
- Aortic dissection
- Tension pneumothorax
- Pericardial tamponade
- Esophageal rupture

Organ-specific differential diagnoses for chest pain
- Diseases of the **heart**: ACS (▶ Sect. 7.3), pericarditis, perimyocarditis
- Diseases of the vessels: aortic dissection (▶ Sect. 15.2)
- Diseases of the **lungs**: pulmonary embolism, pleuritis, pneumothorax, pleuritis accompanying pneumonia, empyema
- Diseases of the **musculoskeletal system**: rib fracture/contusion, musculoskeletal complaints, Tietze syndrome (chondropathy of the costal cartilage)
- Diseases of the **gastrointestinal tract**: gastroesophageal reflux, esophagitis, esophageal rupture, gastritis, pancreatitis
- Diseases of the **nerves or skin**: herpes zoster (pain may occur before the rash), disc prolapse with nerve compression, psychosomatic chest pain
- **Others**: biliary colic, splenic rupture (caution: biphasic)

Diagnostics (▶ Chap. 2) The resting ECG can be completely normal in CCS with stable angina pectoris. To provoke myocardial ischemia, a stress test can be performed in CCS. Since bicycle or treadmill ergometry has limited sensitivity (approx. 50%) and specificity (approx. 80%), especially in women, stress echocardiography, myocardial perfusion scintigraphy, or stress magnetic resonance imaging (MRI) are preferable depending on availability. In cases of low pre-test probability, coronary computed tomography can also exclude coronary artery disease with high sensitivity if the result is normal.

> **Important**
> The occurrence of ST depressions in ergometry (most frequently in V5) does not allow localization of coronary stenoses. In the rare occurrence of ST elevations, the corresponding leads indicate the anatomical ischemic area more likely.
>
> In the case of positive ischemia detection, the anatomy of the coronary arteries should be visualized using coronary CT or coronary angiography to confirm the diagnosis of coronary artery disease, perform risk stratification, and, if necessary, revascularization.

Therapy The therapy of chronic coronary syndrome aims at modifying the risk factors for atherosclerosis, preventing the progression of coronary artery disease, alleviating symptoms, and improving coronary perfusion through revascularization to improve clinical outcomes.

Fundamentals of therapy
- Non-pharmacological therapy: diet, exercise, stress reduction
- Pharmacological therapy: antithrombotics, lipid-lowering agents, antianginal drugs
- Revascularization: percutaneous coronary intervention (PCI) or coronary artery bypass grafting (CABG)

■ **Conservative Management**

Modification of **lifestyle**: weight reduction to normal weight, smoking cessation, Mediterranean diet, regular endurance exercise. The goal is optimal modification of all modifiable risk factors for coronary artery disease (▶ Sect. 3.2).

■ **Medical Therapy**
- **Antithrombotics**: Acetylsalicylic acid (75–100 mg/d) or clopidogrel (75 mg/d) alone of together are the antiplatelet agents of choice in the secondary prevention of CAD.
- **Lipid-lowering agents**: Statins are indicated in CAD regardless of LDL-C—also due to their pleiotropic effects. If lipid target levels are not achieved, ezetimibe, Bempedoic acid or PCSK9 inhibitors are available (▶ Sect. 3.3).
- **Antianginals**: During an angina attack, short-acting nitrates (1–2 sprays of nitroglycerin spray or 1 capsule sublingually) provide rapid relief. Beta-blockers are established as antianginals. Additionally, calcium antagonists (diltiazem, verapamil, long-acting dihydropyridines) are used for symptomatic therapy of angina. Second-line treatments include long-acting nitrates, nicorandil, trimetazidine, ivabradine or ranolazine.
- **ACE inhibitors**: are indicated in the secondary prophylaxis of CAD in patients with impaired left ventricular function or high-risk patients (e.g., diabetics, ▶ Chap. 6; hypertensive patients; ▶ Sect. 4.6). In case of intolerance (cough, angioedema), switching to an angiotensin II receptor blocker (ARB) is recommended. However, the simultaneous combination of ACE inhibitors and ARBs is not recommended.

❗ Always measure blood pressure before administering nitrates! Nitroglycerin is contraindicated in the presence of systolic blood pressure <100 mmHg, use of phosphodiesterase inhibitors (e.g., sildenafil, tadalafil), symptomatic severe aortic stenosis, right ventricular infarction, and hypertrophic obstructive cardiomyopathy.

■ **Revascularization**

The mechanical restoration of adequate blood flow to the myocardium is called revascularization. Essentially, either the stenosis of the coronary arteries can be resolved in an awake patient using **balloon angioplasty** and **stent implantation**, or a bypass (aortocoronary **bypass surgery**) can be created on the affected vessel distal to the stenosis during a heart operation under general anesthesia. The choice of method depends on the number of affected vessels (1-, 2-, or 3-vessel disease), the severity of atherosclerosis, the location of the narrowings, the perioperative risk, and the patient's preference. In the case of 3-vessel CAD, complex main stem stenosis, or a main stem equivalent, bypass surgery is more likely to be considered. For 1- or 2-vessel CAD or high surgical risk, percutaneous revascularization is preferred. Diabetics with 2- or 3-vessel CAD benefit more from surgery in terms of long-term survival.

Indication for Revascularization
- **Symptomatic:** Relief of angina symptoms when extensive antianginal therapy has not led to symptom relief
- **Improvement of survival** in prognostically relevant ischemia (e.g., significant main stem stenosis, 3-vessel CAD, 2-vessel CAD with proximal stenoses, proximal LAD stenosis)

■■ **Percutaneous Coronary Intervention (Percutaneous Coronary Intervention, PCI)**

The PCI (◘ Fig. 7.4) is one of the most common medical procedures overall. For the first time in 1977, Andreas Grüntzig in Zurich percutaneously dilated a coronary stenosis with a balloon catheter. In the mid-1980s, coronary stent implantation was introduced, and since the beginning of the century, drug-eluting stents (*Drug-eluting Stents*, DES) have been used to prevent restenosis. Initially, coronary anatomy is visualized by injecting contrast medium directly into the coronary arteries via diagnostic catheters (▶ Sect. 2.6). The indication for percutaneous revascularization is usually made ad hoc. After full anticoagulation (unfractionated heparin or bivalirudin), a guidewire is advanced through the narrowed vessel under fluoroscopic control via a guiding catheter. Over this wire, a still folded balloon is then placed precisely in the stenosis and inflated (6–20 bar). This dilates the stenosis. This procedure is called percutaneous transluminal coronary angioplasty (*Percutaneous Transluminal Coronary Angioplasty*, PTCA). Thereafter almost always, a durg-eluting stent crimped of another balloon is implanted with high pressure. Less commonly, a drug-coated balloon is used to prevent restenosis without a stent.

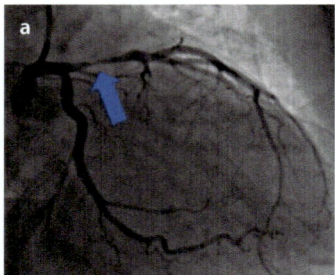 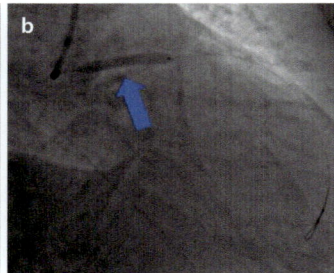 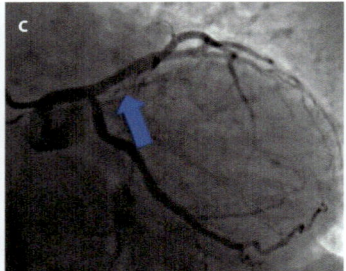

◘ **Fig. 7.4 a–c** PTCA and stenting. Patient with **a** approximately 80% stenosis of the proximal LAD and typical AP symptoms. **b** The stenosis is dilated and a stent is implanted via a guiding catheter. **c** After successful stent implantation, blood flow in the vessel is restored

Since the restenosis rate after PTCA alone is high, a stent is routinely introduced into the coronary vessel over the same guidewire following balloon dilation of the stenosis and deployed at the site of the stenosis using balloon dilation. The stent is a metal scaffold that supports the vessel wall from the inside and reduces the restenosis rate through local drug delivery. Absorbable stents (scaffolds = temporary vascular support) have not yet gained acceptance due to a higher rate of restenosis and acute occlusions.

In addition to balloon dilation and stent implantation, there are other catheter techniques to treat coronary stenoses or to prepare for stent implantation. In rotablation, a high-frequency drill is used to bore out the heavily calcified stenosis; in the cutting balloon technique (high-pressure balloon with small blades), calcified rings are broken up, and with a lithotripsy balloon, calcifications can be fragmented with shock waves.

■■ **Bypass surgery**

Since the late 1960s, an aortocoronary bypass operation (ACBP, ◘ Fig. 7.5) can be surgically created as a bypass circuit for coronary stenoses. Unlike PCI, the stenosis is not directly corrected here, but rather

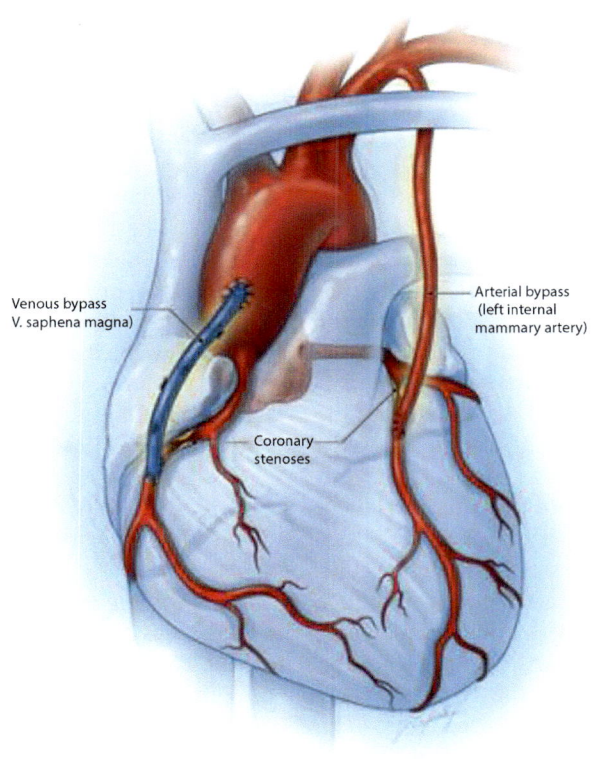

◘ **Fig. 7.5** Aortocoronary bypasses. (shown LIMA-LAD and vein-RCA). *Source*: ▶ https://www.mayoclinic.org/tests-procedures/coronary-bypass-surgery/multimedia/img-20166099

bypassed using an artery (internal thoracic artery or radial artery) or a piece of the great saphenous vein. The saphenous vein is harvested from the leg, one end is sewn into the ascending aorta, and the other end is anastomosed to the coronary artery distal to the stenosis. Similarly, the radial artery (usually from the non-dominant arm with an unremarkable Allen test) can be used as graft material. The best bypass (high patency rate over time) is considered to be the left internal mammary artery (*Left Internal Mammary Artery, LIMA*), which is used for revascularization of the left anterior descending artery (LAD). In the LIMA-LAD bypass, the origin of the artery is left in situ, but it is dissected from the thoracic wall and the distal end is anastomosed to the LAD. Strictly speaking, this is not an "aortocoronary" bypass because the blood flow runs through the subclavian artery to the LIMA, but the term is also used for these bypasses for simplicity (*Coronary Artery Bypass Grafting*, CABG).

A bypass operation can be performed on a beating heart (*Off-Pump Coronary Artery Bypass Surgery*, OPCAB) or on am arrested heart (*on-pump*). In the more common on-pump bypass operation, both the lungs and the heart are stopped and functionally replaced by the heart-lung machine. The venous blood is drawn from the right atrium through a cannula, passed through a pump and an oxygenator, and then pumped back into the aorta through an arterial cannula. The heart-lung machine takes over both the pumping function of the entire heart and the gas exchange function of the lungs. Meanwhile, the heart is perfused with a cardioplegic solution, causing asystole. Now, the bypass operation or combined heart procedures (e.g., heart valve replacement) can be performed on the arrested heart. Afterwards, the heart is rewarmed, the cardioplegic solution is washed out, and the support from the heart-lung machine is gradually reduced until the heart can independently maintain an adequate circulation.

In OPCAB, the unphysiological extracorporeal circulation is avoided. Suturing anastomoses on the beating heart is technically more demanding, requires appropriate training, a stabilizer, and is not possible with every anatomy. If no major thoracic opening (minithoracotomy; no median sternotomy) is performed, it is referred to as *Minimal Invasive Coronary Artery Bypass Surgery* (MIDCAB), which takes place *off-pump*.

Prognosis The clinical outcomes depend on:
- **Pump function** of the heart: Reduced left (LV) and/or right ventricular (RV) ejection fraction (EF) is associated with a poor prognosis.
- **Number of affected vessels**: The more coronary arteries are diseased, the worse the prognosis. In general, proximal stenoses are prognostically worse than distal ones, involvement of the LAD is less favorable than involvement of the LCX or RCA. The most unfavorable is involvement of the main stem.
- **Extent** of myocardial ischemia induced by the stenoses (▶ Sect. 2.5)
- Presence/location/extent of *hibernating myocardium*
- **Comorbidities** such as diabetes mellitus (▶ Sect. 6.3), chronic kidney disease (CKD), or chronic obstructive pulmonary disease (COPD), as well as older age, further worsen the prognosis.

The *hibernating myocardium* refers to myocardial areas that are chronically underperfused but not infarcted. This can occur in the context of CCS as well as after an ACS. The affected heart muscle cells have lost the ability to contract, as this requires a larger amount of energy and oxygen. They cannot be stimulated by catecholamines either, but they are still vital because the remaining perfusion is just sufficient to meet the basic metabolic needs (maintaining cellular integrity). These cells are, so to speak, in "hibernation" (*hibernating*), but they can recover after revascularization and thus improve the heart's pump function. The distinction between a scar and *hibernating myocardium* is achieved using ^{18}FDG-PET, which represents the metabolic activity (▶ Sect. 2.5). The detection of vitality is prognostically favorable for the patient and indicates the long-term benefit of revascularization.

7.4 Vasospastic Angina Pectoris (Prinzmetal's Angina)

Definition Angina pectoris (AP) due to temporary obstruction of the coronary arteries by vascular spasm.

Epidemiology Men and women are equally affected. They are usually younger than the average CHD patient, and smokers are more often affected as are patients of Asian ethnicity. Patients often exhibit other vascular phenomena such as migraines or Raynaud's disease. Prinzmetal's angina is significantly more common in Asians than in Caucasians.

Pathophysiology Acute structural (plaque rupture or erosion) or functional (i.e. spastic) lumen narrowing of the epicardial coronary arteries lead to persistent or transient myocardial ischemia. In patients with coronary atherosclerosis, these spasms are usually found in the area of atherosclerotic plaques und further narrow the coronary lumen therby causing ischaema. Coronary tone is ubiquitously increased, not only in the area of the focal spasm. The autonomic nervous system, which regulates vascular tone, and possibly also inflammatory mechanisms are involved in the pathogenesis.

> Frequent triggering by the intake of vasoconstrictive agents (e.g., ergotamines, cocaine) is often found, so a vasospastic genesis must be considered, especially in young patients with typical AP symptoms or myocardial infarction.

Clinical features The attacks can occur in phases. The pain location is similar to typical angina pectoris, but the pain intensity is often stronger. The attacks usually occur at night.

> In extreme cases, coronary spasms can lead to a heart attack with all consequences, including ventricular tachycardia, ventricular fibrillation, cardiogenic shock and potentially sudden death.

A typical feature is a prompt response to short-acting calcium antagonists (e.g., nifedipine) or nitroglycerin.

Diagnostics In the resting ECG, transient or reversible ST-segment elevations are found only during the attack, similar to an acute infarction. The exercise ECG is generally not very informative. Sometimes spasms with corresponding ECG changes can be provoked by hyperventilation. Conclusive diagnostics involve the demonstration of spasms during coronary angiography (provoked by intracoronary acetylcholine or ergonovine), but vasospastic angina usually remains a diagnosis of exclusion.

Therapy Therapy consists of avoiding triggering stimulants and the prophylactic administration of vasodilators (long-acting calcium antagonists, e.g., amlodipine, isosorbide mononitrate). Beta-blockers should be avoided due to their pro-spastic effect. Percutaneous revascularization of a spastic vessel segment is usually not indicated.

Prognosis The prognosis largely depends on the extent of coronary sclerosis or the presence of a systemic disease. The 5-year survival rate is 90–95%.

7.5 Acute Coronary Syndrome (ACS) and Myocardial Infarction

Definition ACS (formerly acute myocardial infarction) can present clinically in different ways.

An **ACS/acute myocardial infarction** is defined as myocardial cell death due to prolonged myocardial ischemia. Diagnostically required is an increase in cardiac biomarkers (preferably Troponin I or T) above the 99th percentile with at least one of the following factors:

- Symptoms of acute ischemia (AP, dyspnea),
- Increase in myocardial necrosis markers (primarily Troponin T/I),
- New onset of ST-segment/T-wave changes or new left bundle branch block,
- Development of pathological Q waves in the ECG, if untreated in time,
- Evidence of loss of viable myocardial cells or new onset of wall motion abnormalities in cardiac imaging after the event, commonly with delayed or no treatment (▶ Sect. 2.3 and 2.6),
- Evidence of an intracoronary thrombus in angiography or autopsy.

Symptoms and **signs of ischemia** are mandatory for the ACS diagnosis, as ECG changes and elevations of myocardial necrosis markers in the blood can also occur in other conditions such as atrial fibrillation, acutely decompensated heart failure (▶ Chap. 12), sepsis, myocarditis (▶ Sect. 8.2) and pulmonary embolism (▶ Sect. 17.3).

Manifestations According to the latest definition, different types of ACS/myocardial infarction are distinguished (◘ Tab. 7.1):
- Unstable angina pectoris (precursor of a fully developed ACS),
- NSTEMI (Non-ST-Elevation Myocardial Infarction; also NSTEMI-ACS) Commonly only subtotal coroanry occlusion with thrombus embolisation into the microcirculation
- STEMI (ST-Elevation Myocardial Infarction). Complete occlusion of a coroanry sgement.

■ **Unstable AP**
- Any newly occurring AP is referred to as **primary unstable**.
- If AP attacks occur at increasingly shorter intervals and increase in duration and pain intensity, it is referred to

◘ **Tab. 7.1** Classification of ACS/myocardial infarction according to their causes and clinical context according to ESC/ACC/AHA 2007[1]

Type 1	Spontaneous ACS due to plaque rupture or erosion
Type 2	Secondary ACS (spasm, anemia, bleeding, hypertension, tachycardic atrial fibrillation, etc.)
Type 3	Sudden cardiac death
Type 4a	Periprocedural after PCI (>3 × 99th percentile of troponin or CK levels)
Type 4b	Stent thrombosis (>3 × 99th percentile of troponin or CK levels)
Type 5	Periprocedural after CABG[1] (>5 × 99th percentile of troponin or CK levels, new left bundle branch block, new Q wave, evidence in imaging)

1 ESC = European Society of Cardiology, ACC = American College of Cardiology, AHA = American Heart Association, CABG = Coronary Artery Bypass Grafting

as **secondary unstable AP** (crescendo angina).
– If anginal symptoms occur at rest, it is referred to as **rest angina**.

In contrast to STEMI or NSTEMI, cardiac biomarkers are not elevated in unstable AP, but the clinical appearance is indistinguishable. Strictly speaking, unstable AP does not meet the criteria for acute myocardial infarction. However, since it is considered a "precursor" to it, it is part of ACS. The therapy for both forms of ACS is therefore based on the same guidelines as for non-STEMI. With the availability of highly sensitive troponin tests, the frequency of unstable angina compared to NSTEMI has significantly decreased.

▪ NSTEMI

In NSTEMI-ACS, in contrast to unstable AP with the same clinical appearance (usually AP also at rest), cardiac biomarkers (troponin T/I, myoglobin, possibly CK and CK-MB) are elevated in the serum, but the ECG does not show ST elevations. There may be ST depressions, T wave inversions (◘ Fig. 7.6), but a completely normal ECG can also be present.

▪ STEMI

In STEMI, there is typically a persistent severe AP at rest, which cannot be relieved with nitroglycerin (possibly also dyspnea, syncope, and sudden death). The ECG shows persistent ST elevations (◘ Fig. 7.7). Since the conduction system of the heart is disturbed in STEMI, malignant arrhythmias up to ventricular fibrillation are more likely to occur than in unstable AP or non-STEMI. STEMI has the highest acute mortality rate of all forms of ACS.

> ❗ STEMI is an absolute emergency and requires immediate reperfusion through prompt PCI and stenting (restoration of blood flow in the infarct vessel).

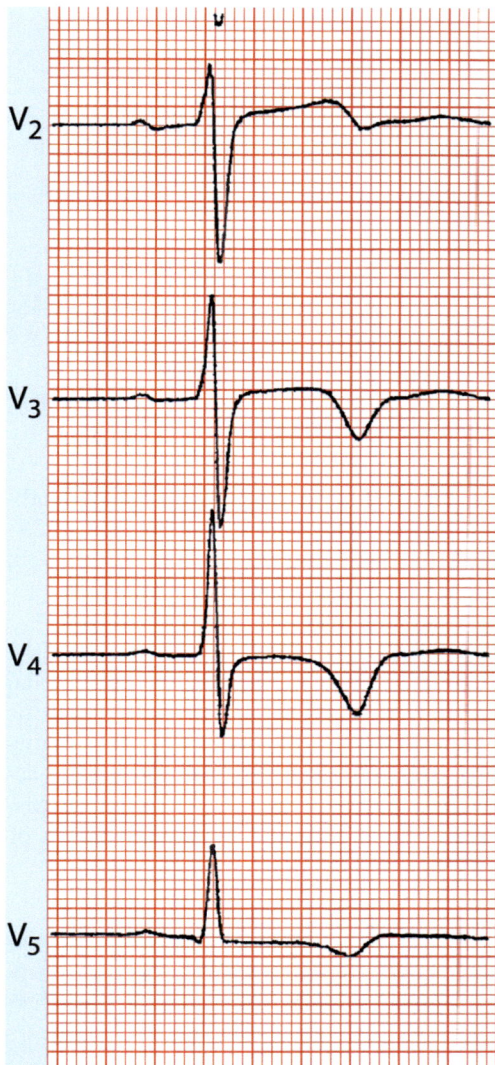

◘ **Fig. 7.6** Typical ECG changes in NSTEMI with T wave inversion over the anterior wall

Epidemiology There are significant geographical variations in the prevalence of cardiovascular diseases (▶ Sect. 3.1) and ACS. For example, the incidence of myocardial infarction in Finland or Scotland is >500/100,000 inhabitants/year and in Japan <100/100,000 inhabitants/year. In Switzerland, the incidence is relatively low at 100–200/100,000 inhabitants/year, while in

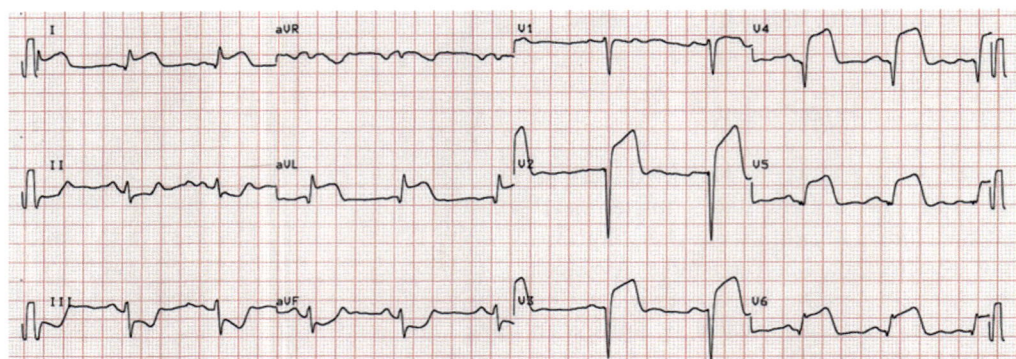

Fig. 7.7 Typical anterior wall STEMI. There are pronounced ST elevations over the entire anterior wall with reciprocal changes inferiorly (II, III, aVF)

Germany it is around 300/100,000 inhabitants/year. The lifetime prevalence is 25–30% for men and 15–18% for women in Switzerland and Germany (▶ Chap. 3).

Pathophysiology The acute myocardial ischemia in ACS is initiated by endothelial erosion or rupture of an atherosclerotic plaque (◘ Fig. 7.8), releasing the highly procoagulant content of the plaque and activating platelets and the coagulation cascade. This is followed by the formation of an intracoronary thrombus. If this thrombus completely occludes the vessel, it results in a STEMI with acute transmural ischemia and subsequent necrosis of the affected myocardial area. In NSTEMI, the thrombus is usually non-occlusive, but microembolisms occur in the microcirculation, explaining the ECG changes and elevated biomarkers.

The triggering factors for a heart attack are manifold; occasionally, a triggering factor can be identified (acute inflammation, infection, physical or psychological stress,

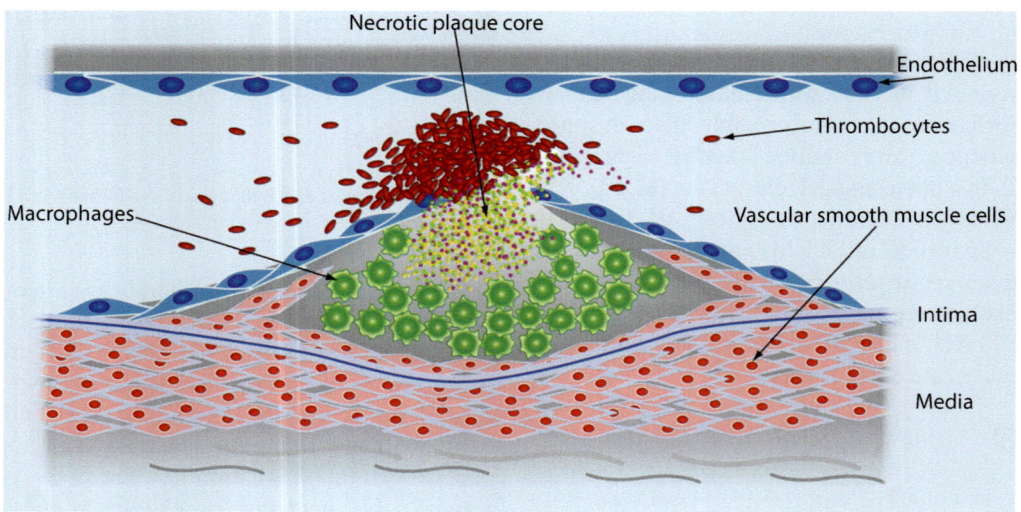

Fig. 7.8 Schematic representation of plaque rupture

accident or surgery, etc.). However, it often occurs completely "out of the blue."

❯ In almost half of all heart attack, patients had never experienced an angina episode prior to the heart attack.

The incidence of heart attacks is subject to circadian fluctuations: 40% of all heart attacks occur in the morning between 6–12 o'clock.

Regarding the **location**, the following distinctions are made:
- Anterior wall infarctions (usually occlusion of the LAD),
- lateral myocardial infarctions (usually occlusion of the LCX),
- posterior and posterior infarctions (usually occlusion of the RCA).

❯ Large anterior wall infarctions have the worst prognosis (commonly due to occlusion of the left anterior coronary artery), both acutely and in the long term, as they are associated with pronounced remodeling, ventricular dilation, aneurysm formation, and/or development of heart failure, if not timely revascularized by PCI or much less often ACBP.

Clinical Findings The main symptom is persistent retrosternal chest pain, which can radiate to the left arm, neck, and jaw (◉ Fig. 7.3). It is often accompanied by a feeling of impending doom and fear of death, which brings with it vegetative symptoms (anxiety sweat, trembling, tachycardia, nausea). The pain is not dependent on breathing and cannot be triggered by pressure on the thorax.

About 15–20% of heart attacks occur without pain, so-called **silent infarctions**, particularly in patients with diabetes mellitus (due to diabetic neuropathy) and in older patients. About half of the patients suffer from mild to severe dyspnea, which can also be the sole angina equivalent, especially in diabetics.

❯ Non-classical presentations are possible: angina can be partially or completely absent in diabetics or older patients (= "silent" myocardial infarction, see below) or manifest as dyspnea. Silent myocardial ischemia is prognostically significant, as about 50% of these patients suffer from a symptomatic form of the disease (mainly heart failure or ventricualr arrhythmias) within the next 10 years.

In posterior wall infarction, patients do not always complain of the typical pain pattern but rather of abdominal and back pain. Gastrointestinal symptoms such as vomiting, bloating, and diarrhea can also occur, complicating the diagnosis.

❗ In the acute situation, the differential diagnosis must consider aortic dissection (primary or with secondary, dissection-related myocardial infarction) and pulmonary embolism.

Patients often also show the typical signs of acute left heart failure with hypotension, tachycardia, pulmonary edema up to cardiogenic shock, or right heart failure (especially with RCA occlusion) with positive hepatojugular reflux, jugular and hepatic vein congestion.

The **complications of a myocardial infarction** can be divided into those that occur early and those that develop later.

- **Early Complications**
- Arrhythmias:
  - ventricular → extrasystole, ventricular tachycardia, ventricular fibrillation
  - atrial → sinus bradycardia, sinus arrest, extrasystole, atrial fibrillation/flutter
  - conduction disorders → AV block, left bundle branch block, right bundle branch block
- Acute left heart failure due to ischemic pump failure: pulmonary edema, blood

pressure drop up to cardiogenic shock (BP < 90 mmHg, heart rate > 100/min, lactate increase, cold extremities)
– Acute right heart failure due to right ventricular infarction

- **Late Complications**
– Ventricular rupture: free perforation with acute pericardial tamponade, covered perforation (formation of a pseudoaneurysm especially in the posterior wall area) or perforation into the right ventricle (ventricular septal defect, ◘ Figs. 7.9 and 2.7 (right))
– Papillary muscle rupture with acute severe mitral insufficiency (▶ Sect. 9.4)
– Pericarditis: early (1–2 days) or later (from 2 weeks, so-called Dressler syndrome)
– Cardiac wall aneurysm
– Cardiogenic embolism: In the case of thrombus formation in the left ventricle (especially in the context of an apical aneurysm, ◘ Fig. 7.10), it can lead to stroke and other thromboembolic complications.
– Re-infarction

Diagnostics Diagnostics are based on several pillars.

- **ECG**

The ECG is one of the basic examinations in every ACS. In the presence of an **ST elevation**, it is a STEMI. Depending on the distribution pattern of the ST elevations, conclusions can also be drawn about the location of the infarct area.

> An ST elevation is defined as an elevation of the ST segment by >1 mm in at least 2 contiguous limb leads or by >2 mm in the chest leads, which is typically accompanied by ST depression in the reciprocal leads.

In the case of ST elevation infarction, the indication for immediate reperfusion therapy by means of PCI and stenting of the occluded coronary segment is given.

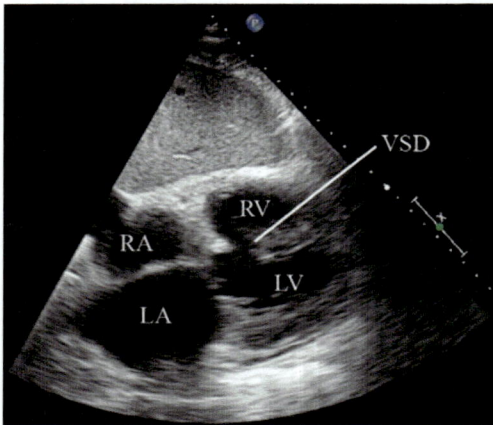

◘ **Fig. 7.9** Ventricular septal defect (VSD) as a result of a myocardial infarction. Subcostal view. *LA*: left atrium, *LV*: left ventricle, *RA*: right atrium, *RV*: right ventricle. (Echocardiography, subcostal view; see ◘ Fig. 2.8)

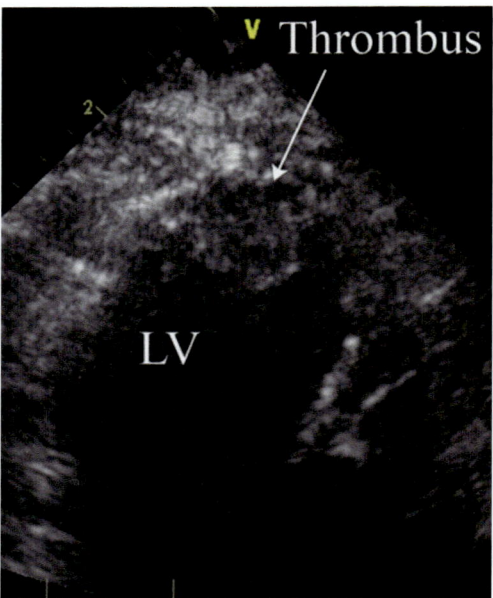

◘ **Fig. 7.10** Apical left ventricular (LV) thrombus 3 days after a myocardial infarction. (Echocardiography, enlarged view from apical 3-chamber view; see ◘ Fig. 2.7)

▶ Serum markers have no significance in the acute diagnosis of STEMI: on the one hand, because they are not yet elevated due to their kinetics in those with early presentation, and on the other hand, because the diagnosis is made based on the typical ECG changes and clinical presentation (acute chest pain), which does not justify waiting for laboratory results.

The extent of ST elevations in the different ECG leads allows for an approximate **infarct localization**:
- anteroseptal: V2, V3
- anterior: V2–V4
- lateral: aVL, I, (V5, V6)
- inferior: II, III, aVF
- posterior: reciprocal (ST depression) in V1, V2, possibly elevations in V7–9
- right ventricular infarction: possibly elevations in the right-sided leads rV1–4

The **Pardee Q** is a pathological Q wave that is either longer than 0.04 s or at least ¼ the amplitude of the following R wave. In the appropriate clinical context, it indicates a past myocardial infarction.

■ Laboratory

Specific laboratory parameters are of great use in the diagnosis of ACS. They also allow for an approximate assessment of the severity of an infarction and the patient's risk of complications. Of particular importance are:
- Troponin T or I,
- Myoglobin,
- CK-MB,
- Total creatine kinase (CK),
- Aspartate aminotransferase (AST), and
- Lactate dehydrogenase (LDH),

which show different kinetics after infarction (◘ Fig. 7.11). Due to the ongoing ischemia, necrosis of the myocardial cells occurs, during which these intracellular enzymes are released into the blood.

The **myoglobin** plasma levels can be easily and quickly measured. It reaches a very high test sensitivity after just 2 hours, and after 4 hours it is almost always elevated, but it is not specific for the myocardium as troponins are.

▶ However, myoglobin is not heart-specific (e.g., skeletal muscle injuries also lead to an increase in serum), so it is mainly suitable for ruling out a heart attack.

The determination of **troponin T** (hsTNT) or hsTNI using high-sensitivity (hs) assays is now the gold standard in the laboratory

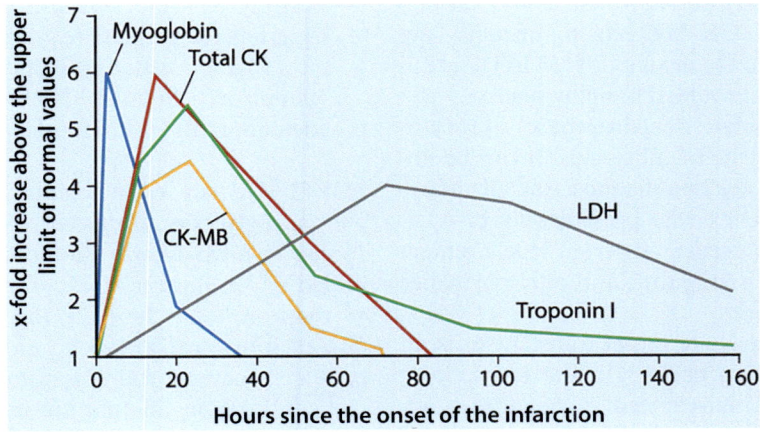

◘ Fig. 7.11 **Enzyme progression after myocardial infarction.** Abbreviations see text. (Modified from Braunwald's Heart Disease, 8th edition)

diagnosis of heart attack. Troponins are heart-specific and detectable in serum after just 1 hour, reaching their maximum after about 20 hours. The values normalize again within about a week. With the 0/1 hour algorithm, a heart attack can be ruled out if the high-sensitivity troponin assay shows very low values and/or no increase in the necrosis marker within one hour.

> However, hsTn can also be elevated in other conditions associated with ventricular stress (e.g., hypertensive crisis, prolonged tachycardia, acute heart failure or pulmonary embolism). For the diagnosis of myocardial infarction, the clinical presentation (see above) and the enzyme progression are crucial.

The **total CK**, the creatine kinase concentration in serum, is a marker for heart and skeletal muscle damage.

> The serum level of total CK also allows for an approximate estimation of the infarct size and thus has prognostic value.

The **CK-MB** is an isoenzyme of creatine kinase that is predominantly found in the heart. The CK-MB fractions in an infarction event range between 6–20% of the total CK. More sensitive than the CK-MB mass is the CK-MB activity, which is determined using an enzymatic assay. The significance of CK-MB has significantly decreased since the availability of hsTn and is no longer determined in many places.

LDH (lactate dehydrogenase) is a cytoplasmic enzyme of all tissues. It can be important for the late diagnosis of an infarction (in patients who present only days after the pain event), as serum levels remain elevated for a long time and only normalize after 1–2 weeks.

AST (aspartate aminotransferase) is an enzyme that is present in the heart, liver, and skeletal muscle and is therefore a relatively nonspecific marker. Both AST and LDH were integral parts of infarction diagnostics before the introduction of CK (and later troponin), but they no longer have any significance today.

Therapy Every patient with an ACS is initially treated according to a basic scheme. Depending on whether they are primarily treated by emergency services or in the clinic, different approaches are taken:

- **Emergency Services**
- If necessary, resuscitation (sudden cardiac death in 20% of first manifestations of CHD!)
- ECG monitoring
- 2–6 l oxygen/min (only with reduced oxygen saturation)
- Initially 0.8 mg nitroglycerin spray or capsules, provided the sBP >100 mmHg and no right heart infarction is present (contraindication for nitroglycerin!). Also beware: intake of phosphodiesterase inhibitors (sildenafil, etc.) in the last 24–48 h
- Analgesia (morphine 3–5 mg i.v.), possibly parallel antiemesis, possibly sedation (e.g., diazepam 1–5 mg)
- Immediately 250–500 mg aspirin i.v.
- Unfractionated heparin: bolus of 60–70 IU/kg, followed by infusion of 12–15 IU/kg/h. Alternatively, low molecular weight heparin can be given.
- Possibly beta-blockers i.v., especially in hypertensive patients (e.g., metoprolol 5 mg i.v. fractionated), except with HR < 50/min or > 90/min, shock, pulmonary edema, or sBP < 100 mmHg

In STEMI, pain relief cannot be achieved with **nitroglycerin**. In this case, a lack of response to nitroglycerin should not be interpreted as "exclusion of a coronary origin" of the symptoms. In ACS, the administration of nitroglycerin has no prognostic impact, i.e., acute mortality is not reduced. On the contrary, in an inferior infarction involving the right heart, nitroglycerin can induce hypotension up to circulatory arrest.

Atherosclerosis and Sequelae

Therefore, careful and prudent use of nitroglycerin in acute infarction!

❗ In STEMI, the most important measure is the rapid transport of the patient to a cardiac catheterization center for revascularzation by immediate PCI and stenting of the occluded coronary artery. Time is crucial, as with each passing minute more heart muscle cells are irreversibly damaged ("*Time is muscle!*").

▪ **Emergency Department**
- ECG Monitoring: 12-lead ECG
- Laboratory: Cardiac enzymes
- Analgesia (Morphine 3–5 mg i.v.), possibly parallel antiemesis, possibly sedation (e.g., Diazepam 1-5 mg)
- If not already done (see above): Aspirin i.v., O_2 (in case of reduced saturation), Heparin, possibly Nitroglycerin
- ADP receptor antagonist (either one together with Aspirin = Dual Antiplatelet Therapy or DAPT):
  - Prasugrel (Efient®): Loading dose 60 mg
  - Ticagrelor (Brilique®): Loading dose 180 mg
  - Clopidogrel (Plavix®): Loading dose 300–600 mg
  - Ticagrelor and especially Prasugrel have higher efficacy in ACS (reduced reinfarction and mortality rates) than Clopidogrel, but are each associated with an increased tendency to bleed.
- Unfractionated Heparin: initially as a bolus with 60–70 IU/kg, then as an infusion 12–15 IU/kg/h. Alternatively, low molecular weight Heparin can be administered.
- Statin: high dose, e.g., Atorvastatin 80 mg or Rosuvastatin 20–40 mg.
- Additionally, if there are no contraindications (AV block, inferior infarction, blood pressure instability), a beta-blocker should be administered within 12 hours.

- ACE inhibitor administration within the first 24 hours, if there are no contraindications. The benefit of this therapy is particularly pronounced in high-risk patients (reduced pump function, initial presentation with heart failure).

▶ Acronym for the most important elements of basic therapy: MONAS BH (Morphine, Oxygen, Nitrate, Aspirin, Statin, Beta-blocker, Heparin)

The therapy of unstable angina pectoris and non-STEMI is based on specific risk stratification (◐ Fig. 7.12). In cases of high and medium risk (according to GRACE Score), rapid reperfusion via PCI and stenting within 24–48 hours is to be aimed for

▶ In the case of STEMI, the earliest possible reperfusion should be sought under all circumstances.

▪ **Acute Therapy for STEMI**
Two different reperfusion strategies are available: Primary PCI and systemic thrombolysis.

▪▪ **Catheter Intervention**
Whenever possible, immediate reperfusion is performed by **PCI** (percutaneous coronary intervention, ◐ Fig. 7.13) with **stent implantation**. However, in rare cases, an emergency **bypass surgery** may be necessary. With optimal therapy, a hospital mortality rate of less than 10% is generally possible.

▶ In the acute situation, PCI and stent implantation are the therapy of choice whenever and as quickly as possible.

Advantages of catheter intervention:
- No absolute contraindications to PCI/stenting in acute myocardial infarction (in contrast to thrombolysis due to risk of cerebral and systemic bleeding).

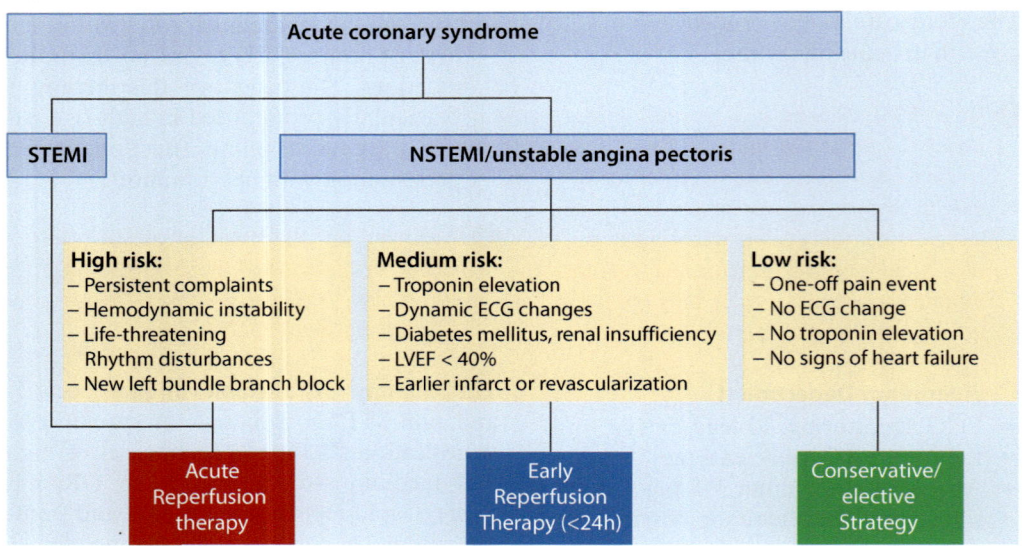

Fig. 7.12 Risk stratification of acute coronary syndrome (ACS)

- Complete reopening of the stenosed vessel is achieved with PTCA in over 95%, with thrombolysis only in 60–70%.
- A risk of any reperfusion technique is the development of a stroke, which, however, is only half as large with PCI as with thrombolysis.

■■ **Pharmacological systemic thrombolysis**
Thrombolysis Thrombolysis (also: Fibrinolysis, ◻ Fig. 7.14) is rarely used today in the Western world for the treatment of STEMI. If a catheter intervention cannot be performed within 2 hours of symptom onset, e.g., in rural areas without a rapidly accessible PCI center, systemic thrombolysis may be used, but it should be performed within 6 hours of infarction onset: the earlier, the higher the chances of success and the lower the morbidity/mortality. Three different fibrinolytics are considered:
- Streptokinase,
- Urokinase,
- recombinant tissue plasminogen activator (preferred fibrinolytic).

Absolute contraindications for a thrombolysis are:
- Stroke within the past 6 months (but not within the last 3 hours, ▶ Sect. 7.5),
- known central nervous system lesions, e.g., tumor, etc.,
- head trauma or neurosurgical operation in the last 6 months,
- gastrointestinal bleeding in the past month,
- aortic dissection (▶ Sect. 15.2),
- hemorrhagic diathesis.

■ **Early invasive approach in moderate risk**
In patients with unstable angina or non-STEMI and certain risk factors, an early invasive approach is indicated. Coronary angiography (and possibly PCI/stenting) should be performed within 24 hours of pain onset. As concomitant therapy, either unfractionated heparin, low molecular weight heparin, e.g., enoxaparin, dalteparin, or nadroparin, or fondaparinux is administered. Treatment with a Gp IIb/IIIa antagonist is rarely indicated except with large coroanry thrombi.

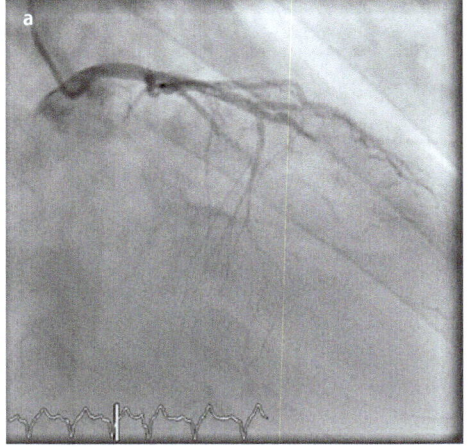
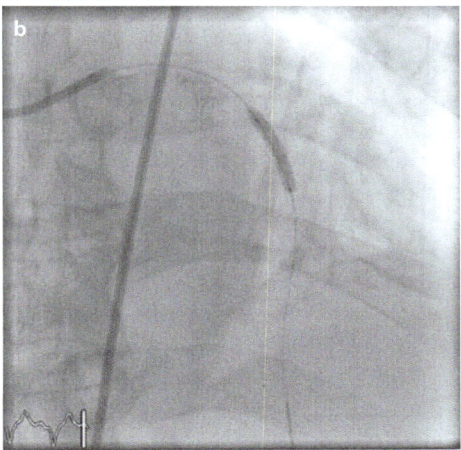
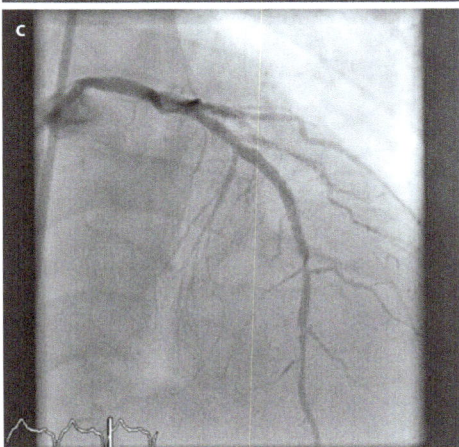

Fig. 7.13 a–c Acute PCI a in thrombotic LAD occlusion, b after guide wire placement, balloon dilation, and stent implantation, c LAD with restored perfusion

- **Conservative therapy/elective further evaluation in low risk**

In low-risk cases, coronary angiography does not necessarily have to be performed in the acute situation. Instead, optimal drug therapy is administered, which includes the following medications:
- Aspirin: 100 mg/day for life,
- Clopidogrel: 75 mg/day for 12 months, Prasugrel 10mg/day or ticagrelor 90 mg/2 × daily for 12 months,
- therapeutic unfractionated heparin, low molecular weight heparin, or fondaparinux until hospital discharge,
- expansion of antianginal therapy (nitrate, molsidomine, nicorandil, beta-blockers; possibly calcium antagonists, especially in suspected vasospastic genesis).

A formal ischemia test using a stress test and/or imaging should be performed as soon as possible, followed by (elective) coronary angiography depending on the findings.

▶ Regardless of acute therapy, optimal secondary prophylaxis is a cornerstone of therapy in any ACS in the further course.

Optimal therapy of cardiovascular **risk factors** according to secondary preventive goals is sought:

Secondary preventive target values of cardiovascular risk factors (▶ Sect. 3.3; ◘ Fig. 3.5)
- LDL cholesterol in CAD < 1.4 mmol/l (or < 55 mg/dl)
- Blood pressure < 130/80 mmHg (<65 years) or < 140/90 mmHg (older patients; ▶ Sect. 4.3)
- Fasting glucose < 6 mmol/l, HbA1c < 7.0% (▶ Sect. 6.3)
- BMI < 25 kg/m^2 (▶ Sect. 3.3)
- Waist circumference men < 102 cm, women < 88 cm (▶ Sect. 3.3)

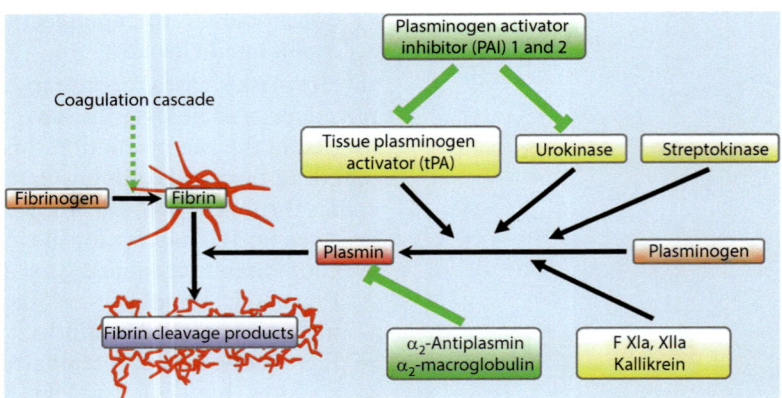

Fig. 7.14 Schematic representation of fibrinolysis

Especially after stent implantation, a **dual antiplatelet therapy** with aspirin and a P_2Y_{12} antagonist (clopidogrel, ticagrelor, or prasugrel) is mandatory, as it protects against the dreaded **stent thrombosis** (Fig. 7.15), an acute stent occlusion with a mortality rate of up to 50%! A stent thrombosis presents like a STEMI and must be treated accordingly. The duration of therapy with an ADP receptor antagonist after an acute coronary syndrome is generally 12 months, regardless of the type of acute treatment. If there is a high ischemic and low bleeding risk, the therapy can also be continued. Therapy with aspirin (alternatively clopidogrel 75 mg) is carried out for life. In patients with hgh bleeding riks, DAPT duration can be shortened.

Statins for **cholesterol reduction** have a firm place in secondary prevention after myocardial infarction (e.g., atorvastatin 80 mg or rosuvastatin 20–40 mg). Patients treated accordingly have a lower risk of recurrent events. LDL target values can now be routinely achieved, especially through the combination with other lipid-lowering agents such as ezetimibe, bempedoic acid, and PCSK9-targeted therapies.

Finally, lifestyle-modifying measures are also crucial for optimal secondary prevention, including the initiation and expansion of physical activity and sports, a Mediterranean diet (fish, fruits, and vegetables), and weight normalization. Nicotine abstinence (▶ Sect. 3.2) is crucial, which also reduces the risk of peripheral arterial occlusive disease, stroke, dementia, impotence, malignancies, and others. Both specialized counseling and pharmacological therapies are used for this purpose.

Prognosis A heart attack is a life-threatening emergency.

❗ Almost half of all acute heart attacks do not reach the hospital but die before a doctor can be alerted (sudden cardiac death).

Among the patients who can be brought to the clinic, up to 10% still die during the hospital stay (mainly those with cardigenic shock) even under optimal conditions (Fig. 7.16). For hemodynamically stable patients, it is 3–4%, but for patients with cardiogenic shock, it is up to 40%. The 1-year mortality rate for survivors after a heart attack is 7–10%.

Atherosclerosis and Sequelae

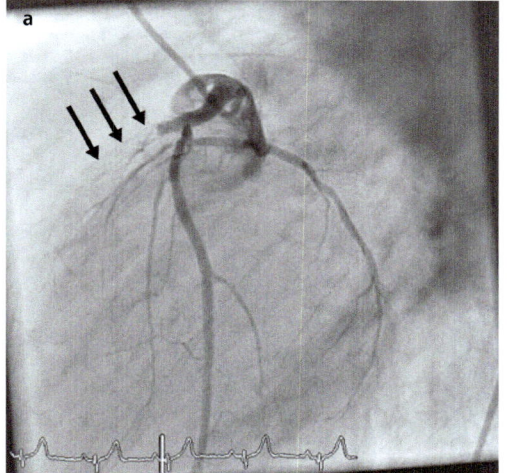

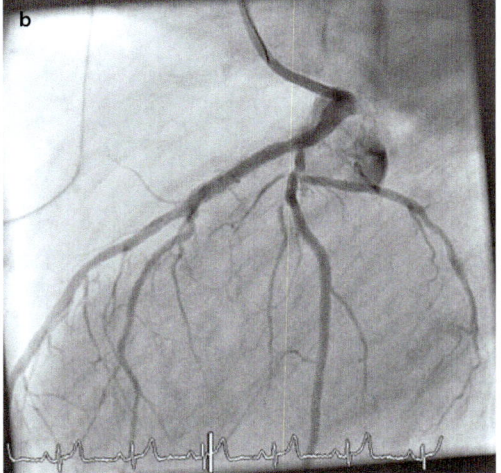

Fig. 7.15 a, b Acute stent thrombosis a of the LAD with interruption of contrast flow and occluded stent (arrows). b After emergency PCI, the thrombosis can be resolved and flow in the LAD restored

7.6 Peripheral Arterial Occlusive Disease (PAOD)

Definition In PAOD, there is hypoperfusion of one or more extremities due to mostly atherosclerotic stenoses or occlusions of the peripheral artery. The ischemia can be asymptomatic or lead to functional impairment (claudication), rest pain, wound healing disorders, or in extreme cases, gangrene of the extremity with an indication for amputation. In 90% of cases, the legs are affected, less frequently the upper extremity.

Epidemiology The prevalence increases with age and is 2–3% for men and 1–2% for women over 60 years old. The clinically silent form of PAOD is much more common and is 21% in men and 17% in women over 60 years old.

> **Coincidence of CAD and PAOD**
> - 70% of patients with PAOD have atherosclerotic changes in the carotids with an increased risk of stroke.
> - 70% of patients with PAOD also have CAD.

The most important causes of death in patients with PAOD are myocardial infarction and cerebrovascular stroke. The prognosis correlates with the extent of peripheral blood flow restriction.

Etiology In over 80% of cases, the cause of PAOD is atherosclerosis based on classic risk factors (especially nicotine; "smoker's leg").

Rarer causes are
- Embolisms, e.g., in atrial fibrillation, arterio-arterial embolisms mainly from aortic and iliac aneurysms,
- Thrombosis of a popliteal aneurysm,
- Aortic dissections with malperfusion of the lower extremity,
- Entrapment syndrome (entrapment of the popliteal artery by the gastrocnemius muscle),
- Cystic adventitial degeneration,

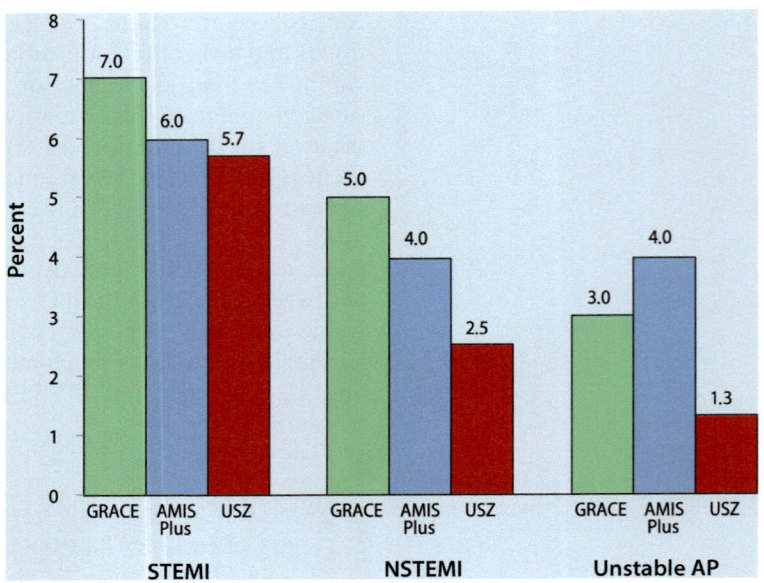

Fig. 7.16 Hospital mortality in the GRACE registry (Global Registry of Acute Coronary Events, 1999–2000), in the AMIS (Acute Myocardial Infarction in Switzerland)-Plus registry (2007–2009), and at the University Hospital Zurich (2007–2010)

- Inflammatory vascular diseases such as thromboangiitis obliterans (Buerger's disease in smokers) or Takayasu arteritis,
- Autoimmune vasculitis.

Clinical Findings Most PAOD patients are asymptomatic. Some patients report foot/calf/thigh or buttock claudication when walking, which is due to exercise-induced ischemia and typically disappears at rest (standing still) after a few minutes (window shopping disease). The location of the symptoms is usually distal to the expected location of the stenosis (e.g., thigh pain when walking with stenosis of the pelvic arteries). In severe blood flow restrictions (critical limb ischemia), there is rest pain and wound healing disorders up to tissue necrosis.

If PAOD is of atherosclerotic origin, the symptoms increase with increasing obstruction. In the case of acute occlusion of the extremity arteries (e.g., embolic or arterial in-situ thrombosis), rest pain suddenly occurs accompanied by several symptoms: "The 6 P's" *P*ain, *P*ulslessness, *P*aresthesia, *P*aralysis, *P*aleness, *P*rostration. If the origin is not atherosclerotic but due to an inflammatory or systemic disease, the symptoms of the underlying disease or general symptoms (fever, fatigue, etc.) may also be present.

Clinical Stages of Chronic PAD (according to Fontaine)
- I Asymptomatic
- II Symptoms only under exertion (claudication, exertional insufficiency)
  - Pain-free walking distance over 200 m: IIa
  - Pain-free walking distance under 200 m: IIb
- III Rest pain (often at night/while lying down)
- IV Ischemia-induced trophic disorders (necrosis, gangrene)

Atherosclerosis and Sequelae

> In stage III/IV, the vitality of the extremity is at risk (critical ischemia).

Diagnostics Diagnostics are based on several pillars.

- **Clinical Examination**
- Inspection:
  - Skin: pale (acute), reddish (chronic), blue (peripheral cyanosis)
  - disturbed trophic: hair growth, nail growth
- Palpation:
  - along thigh/lower leg to the foot: asymmetric temperature difference
  - test sensitivity and motor function: present/restricted/not present
  - Pulse status femoral/popliteal as well as foot pulses present/not present
  - capillary refill time delayed
- Auscultation:
  - flow noise in the stenosis area

- **Diagnostics tests for PAD**
- Calculation of the Ankle-Brachial Index (ABI): ABI < 0.9 or > 1.3 = pathological, ABI 0.91–1.0 = borderline (further clarification indicated)
- Measurement of blood pressure at the ankle using a Doppler probe and calculation of the ratio to systemic systolic blood pressure
- Oscillography (pulse wave curves): used for segment diagnostics/localization of the obstruction as well as semi-quantitative blood flow restriction
- Color-coded Doppler sonography: as non-invasive, radiation-free imaging diagnostics for detection, localization, and severity assessment of an obstruction (Fig. 7.17)
- MRI/CT angiography (Fig. 7.18)
- Digital subtraction angiography

Therapy The management of PAD is based on several pillars.

- **Medication Therapy and Risk Factor Modification**
- Antiplatelet agents (Aspirin, 100 mg/day or Clopidogrel 75 mg/day); after stenting in combination as dual antiplatelet therapy
- Lipid-lowering agents (initially statin, if necessary Ezetimibe, Bempedoic acid and/or PCSK9 inhibitors (▶ Sect. 3.3)
- Optimal therapy of diabetes (▶ Sect. 6.3), arterial hypertension (▶ Sect. 4.3), dyslipidemia (▶ Sect. 3.2)
- Walking training (at least 3–5 times/week for 30–60 min) promotes blood circulation and the formation of collaterals. While one should not provoke angina pectoris, in PAD one can exercise to the pain threshold.
- Smoking cessation
- Vasodilators in stages II and IV (e.g., iloprost)

- **Revascularization**

Similar to PCI in CAD, symptomatic stenoses/occlusions can be dilated and also stented using balloon catheters with or without stents (percutaneous transluminal angioplasty, PTA, Fig. 7.19). Surgical methods are used depending on the anatomical location and extent of an obstruction. These include thrombendarterectomy ("excision" of the stenosis with the vascular intima) and bypass surgery with an autologous graft (usually saphenous veina) or synthetic material (Dacron, polytetrafluoroethylene). When percutaneous and surgical techniques are combined, it is referred to as a "hybrid procedure".

> Revascularization is indicated to improve symptoms (severely limited walking dis-

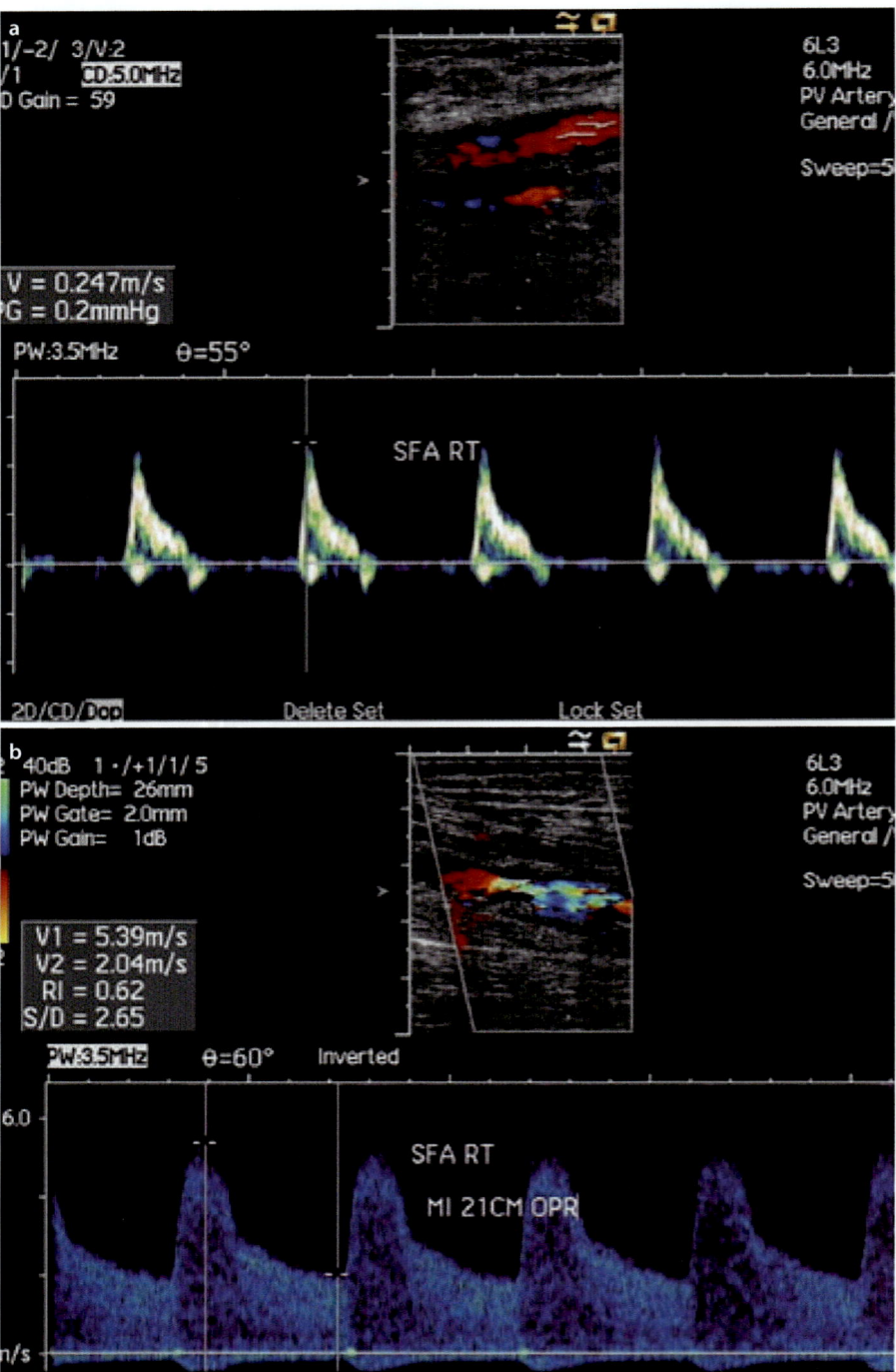

Fig. 7.17 a, b Doppler sonography. Lower extremity before **a** and in **b** a significant stenosis. The flow acceleration in the color duplex (turbulent flow) as well as in the Doppler measurement (0.247 m/s and 5.39 m/s) is clearly visible. (Courtesy of Mark Husmann, Angiology, University Hospital Zurich)

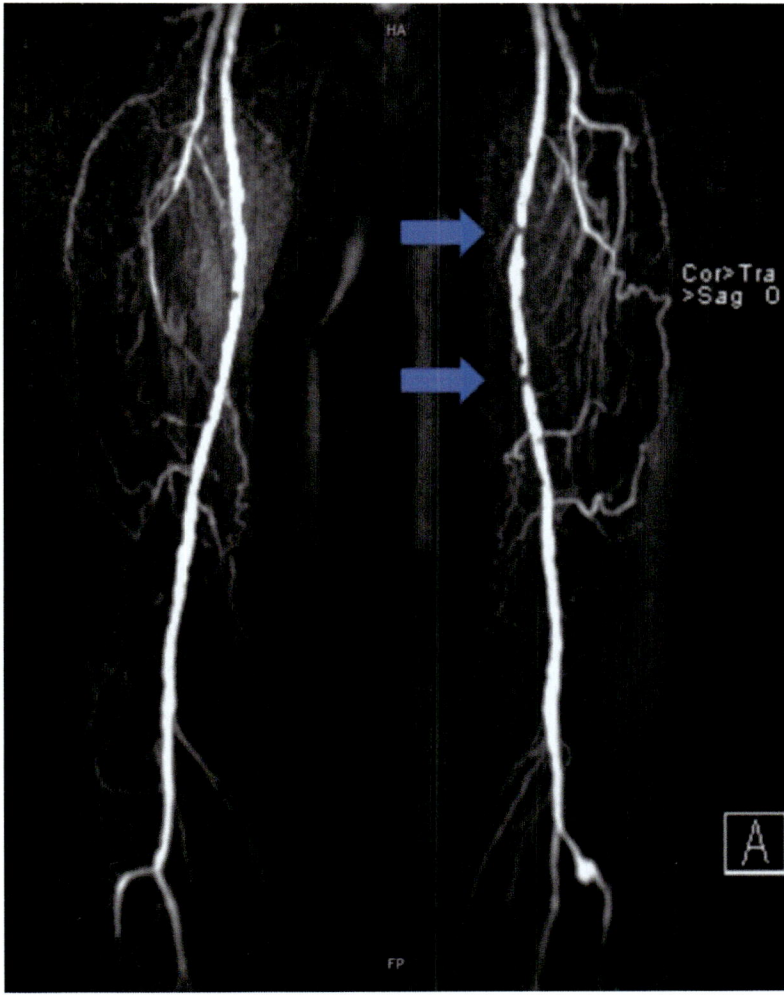

Fig. 7.18 **MR angiography of the thighs with stenoses in the superficial femoral artery.** (Courtesy of René Müller-Wille, Klinikum Wels)

tance <200 m or persistent limitation in daily life despite walking training at distances >200 m) or to save the limb in critical ischemia (rest pain/wound/gangrene).

7.7 Cerebrovascular Accident (CVA)

Definition A sudden cerebrovascular ischemia in a brain region leads either to transient neurological deficits (transient ischemic attack; TIA) or to subsequent death of brain tissue (cerebrovascular accident; CVA). The CVA, along with intracerebral hemorrhage, is a form of stroke.

Epidemiology Ischemic strokes (70–80%) are significantly more common than hemorrhagic strokes, but they can bleed secondarily, i.e., "hemorrhagic transformation". The following will only address ischemic brain infarction; for further information on hemorrhagic stroke, refer to neurology textbooks.

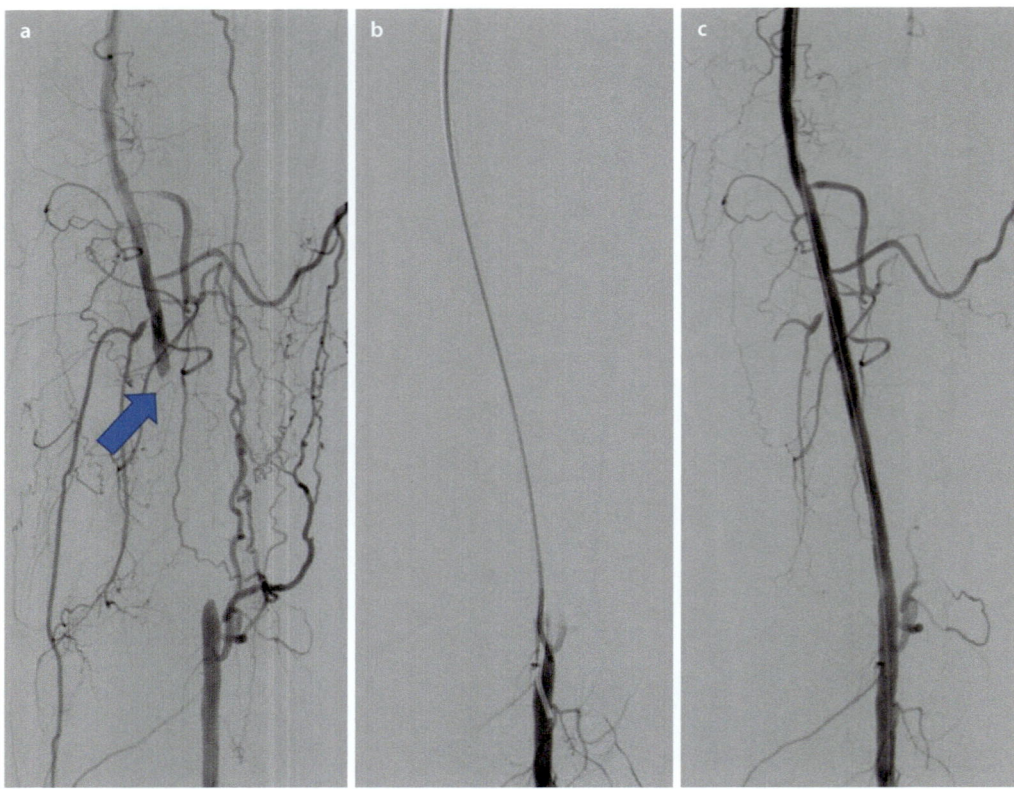

Fig. 7.19 a–c PTA and stent implantation in occlusion of the superficial femoral artery. a The obstruction is **b** treated by PTA and stenting. **c** After the intervention, a good result with restored flow is shown. (Courtesy of René Müller-Wille, Klinikum Wels)

> In Europe, CVA is the third leading cause of death after myocardial infarction and malignancies, accounting for 15% of all deaths.

It is also the most common cause of acquired disabilities in adulthood. The incidence of CVA in Central Europe is about 2 per thousand per year, and in those over 85 years old, it is 1% per year.

Pathogenesis CVI usually occurs as a secondary disease of atherosclerosis in atherosclerotically altered cerebral arteries. A distinction is made between a macrovascular genesis (approx. 25% thromboembolism from an atherosclerotic wall change in a large cerebral artery, e.g., the carotid artery) and a microvascular genesis (approx. 25%, changes in the small vessels in the brain, especially the perforators to the basal ganglia). Pathophysiologically, a common endpoint results in a circulatory disorder in the brain, which usually cannot be compensated for, as the cerebral arteries are functional end arteries.

Furthermore, there can be a cardioembolic occlusion of the cerebral vessels (approx. 25%). Embolism sources include the left atrium (in the context of atrial fibrillation, 90% of all thrombi originate from the left atrial appendage; ▶ Chap. 11) and the left ventricle (subacute in anterior wall infarction or anterior wall aneurysm). The remaining 25% of CVIs are distributed among a variety of rare disease patterns or remain etiologically unclear (cryptogenic stroke).

> Most commonly, circulatory disorders occur in the area of the middle cerebral artery (Fig. 7.20) and the basilar artery. These are associated with the highest morbidity and mortality.

Clinical Findings As with ACS, different degrees of severity are also distinguished in cerebral ischemia.

Transient Ischemic Attack (TIA)

In TIA, the symptoms typically regress within a few minutes to hours. The earlier definition of TIA (arbitrarily) required a complete remission of symptoms within 24 hours. According to the current definition, a TIA is defined as a transient neurological deficit without evidence of an infarction on cerebral imaging (e.g., in diffusion-weighted MRI). However, this does not make TIA a harmless event, as it is a strong predictor of a subsequent cerebral infarction.

> 40% of patients with TIA suffer an ischemic insult within 4 years, half of them within 3 months.

Cerebrovascular Insult (CVI)

In contrast to TIA, a stroke leaves a neurological deficit of varying severity, and an ischemic area is found in cerebral computed tomography. In the acute phase, imaging may still be inconspicuous until the infarction demarcates over time. MRI is more sensitive in the acute event.

In the early phase after an insult (hours to days), a distinction is made in CVI between the **infarct core**, where the cells are already dead, and the surrounding **penumbra**, where the cells are still structurally intact but functionally impaired and at risk of survival due to insufficient supply. In the penumbra, the reduced oxygen supply is still sufficient to maintain the basic metabo-

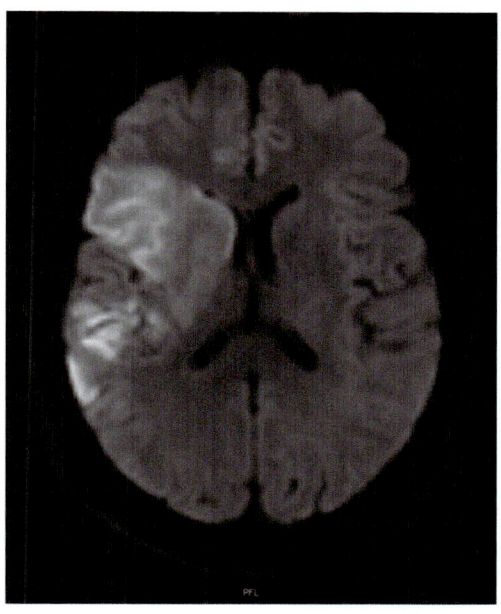

Fig. 7.20 MRI after ischemic cerebral infarction due to occlusion of the right middle cerebral artery (diffusion weighting). (Courtesy of René Müller-Wille, Klinikum Wels)

lism of the nerve cells but no longer for the working metabolism.

The symptomatology of cerebral infarction is determined by the location of the occlusion. Common symptoms include (hemi-)paresis with or without a sensory component, speech and language disorders (motor, sensory, or global aphasia), dizziness, and visual disturbances. In the case of a middle cerebral artery infarction, there is a typical sensorimotor hemiparesis contralateral to the occluded vessel. For detailed symptomatology and clinical examination in occlusion of specific cerebral arteries (anterior cerebral artery, middle cerebral artery, posterior cerebral artery, basilar artery, vertebral artery, etc.), see neurology textbooks.

Diagnostics After the neurological examination, the most important measure is the differentiation between cerebral ischemia and intracranial hemorrhage. The standard procedure is contrast-enhanced computed tomography, which can easily detect hemorrhages but cannot reliably identify ischemias in the early phase. The latter is achieved with diffusion-weighted MRI of the brain (◘ Fig. 7.20). The vascular occlusion can be localized using CT or MR angiography (◘ Fig. 7.21).

Therapy In the case of CVA, the timing of the start of therapy is of utmost importance.

> The general rule is: The sooner the therapy begins, the better the long-term prognosis. *"Time is brain!"*

▪ Peracute Therapy

Within the first 4–5 hours after the onset of symptoms, the ischemic brain area can be reopened using systemic thrombolysis, with rt-PA (recombinant plasminogen activator) being the drug of choice.

> ❗ Thrombolysis should only be performed if a brain hemorrhage has been ruled out by CT.

Thrombolysis can be performed either intravenously or intra-arterially using catheter angiography. Mechanical thrombectomy can also be performed via the intra-arterial route. These procedures can also extend the time window. Thrombectomy is offered in stroke centers and should be coordinated within a "stroke network" with peripheral hospitals.

The most important (partly only relative) **contraindications** for systemic thrombolysis are:
- Brian tumor, cerebral metastases,
- intracranial hemorrhage (absolute contraindication),
- therapy-resistant hypertension,
- active bleeding (e.g., gastric ulcer),
- status post facial or skull trauma <3 months,

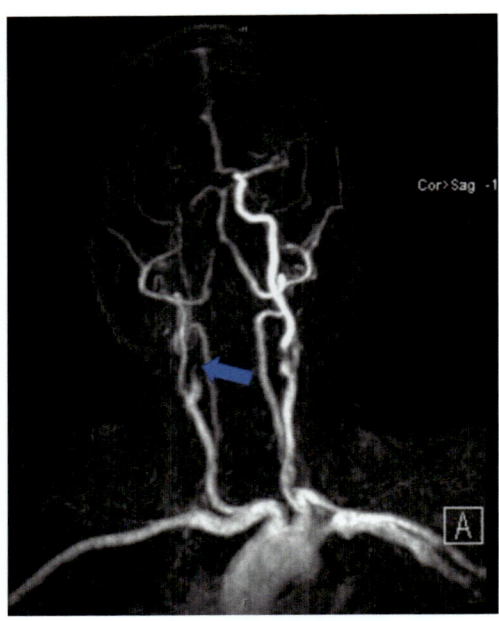

◘ Fig. 7.21 MRI after ischemic stroke with occlusion of the right internal carotid artery (blue arrow). (Courtesy of René Müller-Wille, Klinikum Wels)

- INR > 1.7,
- oral anticoagulation with a NOAC (if necessary, administer NOAC antidote before thrombolysis, e.g., idarucizumab for dabigatran, andexanet-a for apixaban and rivaroxaban),
- major surgical procedure <3 weeks (relative contraindication),
- pregnancy.

All contraindications must be individually and carefully weighed against the expected neurological disability in each case.

▪ Acute Therapy

Purpose: Maintenance of vital functions, providing the best possible "survival conditions" for brain tissue.

Acute therapy is usually carried out in a specialized unit (stroke unit) that includes a specially trained team of medical, therapeutic, and nursing staff. After the completion of acute treatment, inpatient or outpatient neurorehabilitation is connected depending on the course and neurological deficits.

Components of acute therapy are:
- O_2 administration; in case of respiratory insufficiency, non-invasive or invasive ventilation,
- maintenance of normal glucose levels,
- optimal secondary prevention (aspirin, if necessary, anticoagulation),
- thrombosis prophylaxis,
- prevention of aspiration,
- reduction of any elevated body temperature,
- treatment of increased intracranial pressure,
- early rehabilitation, especially early mobilization.

❗ Careful blood pressure lowering in case of severely elevated blood pressure (risk of secondary hemorrhage)—generally not <160 mmHg, to avoid local hypoperfusion due to infarct-related dysregulation of cerebral vessels.

▪ Secondary Prevention

Secondary prevention must be initiated both after a CVI and after a TIA and is determined by the cause of the brain infarction. In the case of high-grade carotid stenosis, this is surgically corrected by endarterectomy or interventionally by stenting (◘ Fig. 7.22). In the case of atheroembolic origin, usually originating from an aortic plaque (◘ Fig. 7.23), the therapy consists of optimal secondary prophylaxis of atherosclerotic risk factors (▶ Sect. 3.2). If the CVI is of cardioembolic origin, oral anticoagulation with NOACs is indicated. If a crossed embolism is suspected in the presence of a persistent foramen ovale (PFO)

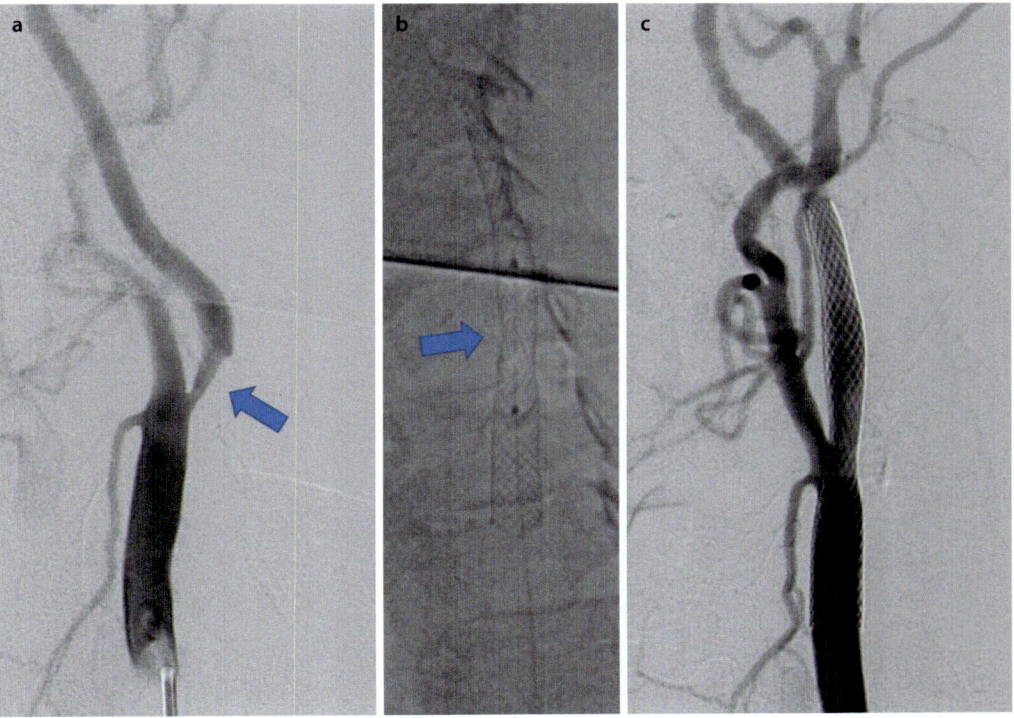

◘ **Fig. 7.22** a, b Stenting of a high-grade internal carotid artery stenosis (arrow) with very good angiographic result c

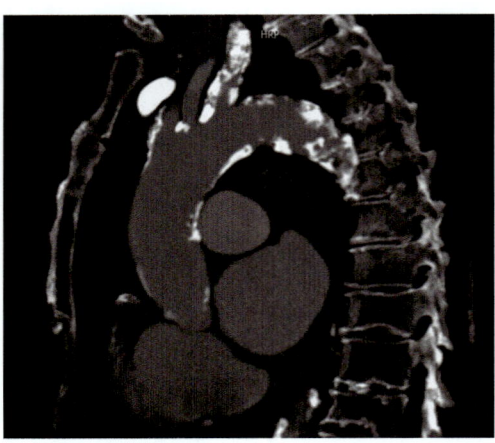

Fig. 7.23 Computed tomography of the aorta with severe atherosclerosis of the entire aorta and the origins of the brain-supplying vessels

with/without atrial septal aneurysm, a percutaneous closure of the PFO should be performed.

Secondary prevention in atherosclerotic CVI includes (▶ Sect. 3.2):
- ASA, clopidogrel, or ASA + dipyridamole for platelet aggregation inhibition,
- Statin; target: LDL cholesterol <1.4 mmol/l,
- Blood pressure control (<130/80 mmHg <65 years, <140/90 mmHg older patients),
- Lifestyle modification (smoking cessation, Mediterranean diet, regular endurance exercise),
- Oral anticoagulation with NOAC after cardioembolic insult (atrial fibrillation).

Prognosis Morbidity and mortality after CVI are high: 25% of patients die within a year, and another 30–50% remain more or less severely disabled. Within 5 years, 20–30% of patients suffer a second insult.

Myocardial Diseases

Benjamin Meder and Urs Eriksson

Contents

8.1 Cardiomyopathies – 122
8.1.1 Introduction and Systematics – 122
8.1.2 Dilated Cardiomyopathy (DCM) – 123
8.1.3 Hypertrophic Cardiomyopathy (HCM) – 126
8.1.4 Restrictive Cardiomyopathy (RCM) – 130
8.1.5 Cardiac Amyloidosis – 131
8.1.6 Arrhythmogenic (Right Ventricular) Cardiomyopathy (ARVC, ACM) – 133
8.1.7 Left Ventricular Non-compaction Cardiomyopathy (LVNC) – 136

8.2 Myocarditis – 138

Earlier versions with contributions from U. Eriksson, D. Hürlimann, C. Gruner, U. Eriksson, J. Steffel, T. F. Lüscher

© The Author(s), under exclusive license to Springer-Verlag GmbH, DE, part of Springer Nature 2025
T. F. Lüscher and U. Landmesser (eds.), *Cardiovascular System*,
https://doi.org/10.1007/978-3-662-70152-2_8

Trailer

Cardiomyopathies are heart muscle diseases that are usually genetically determined or lead to mechanical and/or electrical dysfunction of the heart muscle as part of a secondary cause. Myocarditis is an infectious or non-infectious inflammation of the heart muscle that can be acute or chronic leading to similar dysfunction of the heart muscle.

Both disease entities can cause severe limitations for the patient in terms of dyspnea due to heart failure, arrhythmias up to sudden cardiac death, and stroke. Diagnostics today are multimodal and include molecular genetic markers, biomarkers, and modern imaging techniques. The so-called red-flag principle uses conspicuous clinical and apparatus findings to infer specific causes of the respective cardiomyopathy, thereby enabling a rational use of diagnostic possibilities and identifying specifically treatable causes.

8.1 Cardiomyopathies

8.1.1 Background

- **Frequency and Causes**

Cardiomyopathies are overall common and affect 1:200 people in the general population. Alongside ischemic heart disease, they are the main causes of heart failure, sudden cardiac death, and heart transplantation. A distinction is made between primary and secondary forms, with transitions being fluid, as in the same patient, a genetic predisposition can interact with an external noxa, leading eventually to a clinical manifestation *(Multiple Hit)*. The classification of cardiomyopathies can be based either on morphological grounds (World Health Organization; WHO 1995) or based on etiology (American Heart Association; AHA).

Classification according to AHA 2006

Predominantly genetic
- Hypertrophic cardiomyopathy (*Hypertrophic Cardiomyopathy*; HCM)
- Arrhythmogenic cardiomyopathy (*Arrhythmogenic Right Ventricular Cardiomyopathy*; ARVC or *Arrhythmogenic Right Ventricular Dysplasia*; ARVD)
- Left ventricular non-compaction cardiomyopathy (LVNC)
- Glycogen storage diseases
- Conduction disorder
- Mitochondrial cardiomyopathies
- Ion channel diseases

Mixed
- Dilated cardiomyopathy (*Dilated Cardiomyopathy*; DCM)
- Restrictive cardiomyopathy (*Restrictive Cardiomyopathy*; RCM)

Acquired
- Inflammatory cardiomyopathy
- Myocarditis (▶ Sect. 8.2).
- Takotsubo syndrome (▶ Sect. 7.3).
- Peripartum cardiomyopathy
- Tachycardiomyopathy
- Children of insulin-dependent diabetic mothers

Other acquired (secondary) cardiomyopathies include:
- Ischemic cardiomyopathy (▶ Chap. 7),
- Valvular cardiomyopathy (▶ Chap. 9)
- Hypertensive heart disease (▶ Chap. 4),
- Cardiomyopathy as a result of a systemic disease (e.g., sarcoidosis, mitochondrial cytopathy, cardiac transthyretin [TTR] and light chain (AL) amyloidosis, Fabry disease),
- Metabolic-toxic cardiomyopathy (alcohol, cocaine, radiation, chemotherapy, etc.),
- Pacemaker-induced cardiomyopathy (▶ Sect. 12.4).

Criteria of Classification

Cardiac TTRmt amyloidosis is a genetic disease and leads to a restrictive filling pattern, but it is a secondary disease of the heart muscle and formally does not count as restrictive cardiomyopathy (RCM) because it results in a thickening of the heart walls and valves—which by definition is not the case with RCM. This example clearly shows that the massive increase in knowledge over the past decades has not simultaneously led to a generally accepted new classification of these diseases. The clinical approach to patients with cardiomyopathy, should therefore be conceptually guided and aim to ensure that:

- Disease triggers and predisposing factors should be identified (e.g., causal gene variant),
- Patients should be risk-stratified according to the latest findings (e.g., risk scores for sudden cardiac death),
- Therapies should target causal factors, i.e. heart failure and arrhythmias, as well as the prevention of sudden cardiac death,
- Due to the often genetic nature of cardiomyopathies, the family should be included in the considerations and diagnostics.

8.1.2 Dilated Cardiomyopathy (DCM)

Definition DCM is characterized by an enlargement of all heart chambers, which are usually most pronounced in the left ventricle. These structural changes of DCM can also be the common macro- and microscopic phenotype of the end stage of primary and secondary cardiomyopathies. In newer classifications, DCM is therefore seen as a continuum from the establishment of a risk to the full picture of the disease. Arrhythmias can precede the functional impairment of the left ventricle (e.g., paroxysmal or persistant tachycardic atrial fibrillation); (▶ Sect. 12.5). Likewise, there are hypocontractile subtypes without significant dilation of the left ventricle (Non-Dilated Left Ventricular Cardiomyopathy, NDLVC).

Epidemiology The incidence of DCM is approximately 6:100,000 poeple/year, the prevalence is about 1:250. Men are twice as likely to be affected as women. In about 25–40% of all patients with heart failure, DCM is the underlying cause. Monogenetic forms of DCM account for about 20–30% of cases.

Etiology and Pathophysiology The causes of DCM are heterogeneous, and only after excluding all causal factors can it be referred to as idiopathic DCM. In >30% of cases, a familial clustering is notable, indicating a genetic cause. In 20–30% of cases, a causal gene variant with predominantly autosomal dominant inheritance can be found using new sequencing methods (panel sequencing). There are forms that lead to isolated DCM, while others, as part of a syndrome, affect multiple organ systems and often include peripheral myopathy.

Further, **inflammatory causes** are not uncommon in DCM and can be triggered by exogenous factors (pathogens such as cardiotropic viruses) or autoimmune mechanisms. The checkpoint inhibitor-induced inflammatory cascades belong tocardio-oncological conditions. Virus-induced cardiomyopathies, and acute myocarditis are discussed in ▶ Sect. 8.2. Other secondary causes are excessive alcohol consumption, malnutrition (protein deficiency, carnitine deficiency), thyroid dysfunction, or pregnancy.

In the course of the disease, a progressive enlargement of the left ventricle occurs (◘ Fig. 8.1, cf. normal finding, ◘ Fig. 2.5). The enlargement of the left ventricle corresponds to a passive physiological compen-

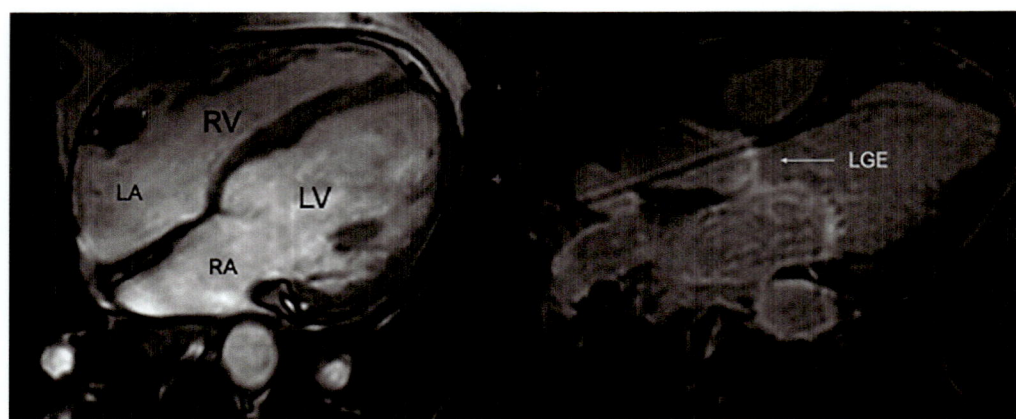

◘ **Fig. 8.1 Dilated cardiomyopathy in MRI.** Left: 4-chamber view with dilated left ventricle (LVEDD = 72 mm) and still normal-sized atria. Right: Late-Gadolinium Enhancement with a pronounced "Mid-Wall Sign," i.e., contrast agent deposition in the area of replacement fibrosis in the muscular septum

sation mechanism, i.e. as the stroke volume decreases in the diseased heart, the end-diastolic volume and finally the filling pressure increase. The dilatation and in turn the increase in end-diastolic volume of the left ventricle allows the ejected stroke volume to be temporarily kept constant via the Frank-Starling law. However, with the dilation of the left ventricle, the myocardial wall tension necessary to generate a certain transmural pressure and the myocardial O_2 consumption increase (Laplace's law). This eventuallyoverloads the heart: A vicious cycle ensues with a progressive decrease in contractility and reduction in ejection fraction, leading to demand tachycardia and eventually to chronic underperfusion of the organs. In the course of the disease, all heart chambers may become enlarged.

Complications In a severely dilated left ventricle with reduced ejection fraction (*Left Ventricular Ejection Fraction*; LVEF), thrombi can form, which can lead to systemic embolisms with the corresponding clinical consequences (cerebrovascular insult, CVI, ▶ Sect. 7.7; acute peripheral occlusion, ▶ Sect. 7.6; etc.). Another source of systemic embolisms in these patients is concomitant atrial fibrillation present in about a quarter of cases, whose development is favored by dilation of the atria (especially the left atrium). Finally, ventricular dilation and the associated intramyocardial remodeling processes also favor the development of malignant ventricular arrhythmias, which in the worst case can result in sudden cardiac death (▶ Sect. 12.5). In syndromic forms of DCM, complications such a left vdentricualr thromus formation due to heart failure (▶ Chap. 13) and respiratory failure due to pneumonia are more common.

Clinical Findings DCM usually leads to the clinical picture of left heart failure with typical symptoms such as exercise intolerance, dyspnea (initially only on exertion, later also at rest), orthopnea, nocturia, peripheral edema, jugular venous distention among others. (▶ Sect. 13.2). Palpitations due to tachycardic arrhythmias are also frequently reported, as is episodes of dizzines up to syncope. Increasingly important is the consideration of preclinical stages, which often have no or few symptoms, but can be associated with a risk of cardiac arrhythmias. Even an asymptomatic stage with left ventricular dysfunction is today an indication for initiating therapy, among other reasons.

Diagnostics The medical history should always include a detailed family history. The creation of a 3-generation pedigree is generally advisable for cardiomyopathies. In laboratory chemistry, high-sensitivity troponins (i.e. inflammation) and NT-proBNP (increased left ventricular strain) play a central rolediagnostistically and in the monitoring of disease progression. To confirm the diagnosis and for monitoring, echocardiography (▶ Sect. 2.5) is the method of choice as it allows to assess the size and contractility of heart chambers, to calculate the LVEF, and the assessment of other accompanying changes such as secondary mitral regurgitation, ▶ Sect. 9.4, diastolic dysfunction, intracardiac thrombi, hypertrabeculation, pulmonary hypertension, among others. Cardiac magnetic resonance imaging (Cardio-MRI; ◘ Fig. 8.1) is now an integral part of the diagnostic algorhith, with approximately 50% of all Cardio-MRIs being conducted with the question of cardiomyopathy. In addition to a precise quantitative assessment of the heart's morphology and function, tissue characterization using mapping techniques (T1, T2 times) and contrast agent accumulation (Late-Gadolinium Enhancement, LGE; ▶ Sect. 2.5) can also be achieved. The latter is an independent predictor of ventricular arrhythmias and sudden cardiac death (▶ Sect. 12.5) regardless of the LVEF. Especially in cases of suspected storage diseases or inflammatory processes, a myocardial biopsy should be considered. Nowadays, myocardial specimens can also be processed using molecular techniques allowing for therapy-altering decisions in 5–10% of cases. Genetic diagnostics are indicated for all DCM patients with a positive family history or in the presence of certain features (AV block as a sign of an LMNA/C variant among others).

> Important for the diagnosis of primary DCM is the exclusion of possible secondary causes (especially CAD), as many cardiomyopathies show the picture of DCM as a "common final pathway" in the end stage of the disease.

Therapy If a specific secondary cause of DCM is found (especially CAD, ▶ Sect. 7.2; enzyme defects, hemochromatosis, etc.), specitif therapeutic measures take priority. For example, if myocardial perfusion in CAD can be successfully improved through revascularization (PTCA/stenting or bypass surgery; ▶ Sect. 7.1), it may lead to a regression of ventricular dilation and an increase in pump function (i.e. reverse remodeling). In smaller studies, improvement through immunomodulation/suppression has also been shown effective in inflammatory forms of DCM (inflammatory virus-negative DCM, cardiac sarcoidosis, eosinophilic myocarditis, etc.; ▶ Sect. 8.2).

Otherwise, the treatment of DCM is based on the pharmacotherapy used for heart failure (▶ Sect. 13.4). In advanced stages, heart transplantation or the implantation of bi- or leftventricular support devices (*Left/Bi-Ventricular Assist Device*, LVAD or BIVAD) may represent the last therapeutic option either as bridge-to-transplant or destination therapy.

> In the presence of a severely reduced LVEF (<35%), there is an indication for the implantation of an ICD (Implantable Cardioverter-Defibrillator) in symptomatic patients due to the increased risk of malignant ventricular arrhythmias, possibly in combination with cardiac resynchronization therapy (CRT, ▶ Sect. 13.4). Recent studies highlight the value of risk scores, which also emphasize the particular importance of Late Gadolinium Enhancement; LGE) on MRI. Indeed, the presence of LGE can lead to a significantly increased risk of sudden cardiac death even with an LVEF >35%. Corresponding randomized studies in this patient population are currently underway.

Clinical Outcomes The prognosis of DCM is very variable and primarily dependent on the etiology. The 10-year survival rate is currently 50–80%; if LVEF falls below 30%, the 5-year survival probability is less than 50%.

8.1.3 Hypertrophic Cardiomyopathy (HCM)

Definition HCM is characterized by hypertrophy of the left ventricle muscle of at least ≥15 mm wall thicknes at its thickest point, if other causes that can also lead to hypertrophy or wall thickening (e.g. hypertension; ▶ Chap. 4) have been excluded. Typically, the hypertrophy is asymmetrical and particulalry dominant in the basal interventricular septum. However, the apex and the lateral wall can also be affected on certain forms of HCM.

Epidemiology The prevalence of HCM in the western world is about 0.2%, i.e., 200:100,000 inhabitants.

Etiology The disease is usually genetically determined with an autosomal dominant inheritance pattern. In about 50% of cases, a mutation in sarcomeric proteins can be found. Most frequently (>70%), genetic variants are found in myosin heavy chains (MYH7) as well as myosin binding proteins (MYBPC3). somewhat less common are mutations in the troponin genes (◘ Table 8.1). Meanwhile, >1000 mutations in >10 gene loci are known; however, since no mutation can be detected in 50% of cases, it must be assumed that both environmental factors and more complex genetic backgrounds (*polygenetic causes*) must play an important role (◘ Fig. 8.2).

Pathophysiology Most commonly, the hypertrophic process involves mainly the interventricular septum. About 10% of cases

◘ **Table 8.1** Disease genes of isolated DCM

DCM disease genes according to Clingen	Other disease genes of DCM
ACTC1, ACTN2, BAG3, DES, DSP, FLNC, JPH2, LMNA, MYH7, NEXN, RBM20, SCN5A, TNNC1, TNNI3, TNNT2, TPM1, TTN, VCL	PLN, ILK, MYBPC3, LDB3, mtDNA, ACTN1, CHD2

present as apical hypertrophic cardiomyopathy, whose prevalence is twice as high in Japan than, for instance, in Germany. In this case, the left ventricular apex is particularly hypertrophix and electrocardiographically, there are typically pronounced T-wave inversions ("giant negative T-wave"; ◘ Fig. 8.3 right). The right ventricle is very rarely involved. Other forms and causes of left ventricular hypertrophy must be differentiated from hypertrophic cardiomyopathy (◘ Table 8.2 and also ▶ Chap. 4).

Histologically, a disturbed alignment of the cardiomyocytes (so-called disarray) is characteristic, in which their normal parallel arrangement is disrupted and the structure appears chaotic. This disarray, together with interstitial fibrosis, can represent the morphological substrate for the development of a reentrant electrical excitation, which can result in ventricular arrhythmias (up to ventricular fibrillation; ▶ Sect. 12.5). Furthermore, there is involvement of the arterioles with hyperplasia of the intima and media, resulting in microvascular dysfunction.

> If the ventricular septum is involved, the left ventricular outflow tract can be narrowed. This is referred to as the obstructive form of HCM (hypertrophic obstructive cardiomyopathy, HOCM or oHCM). The obstructive form of HCM is present in about 30–50% of patients at rest and in up to 60% at rest and/or

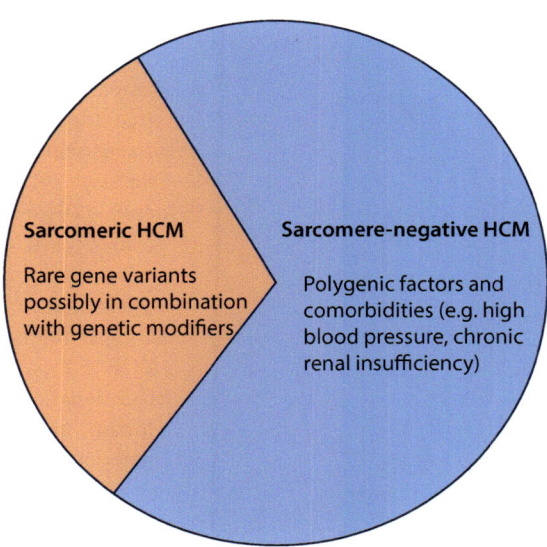

Fig. 8.2 Sarcomeric HCM with detectable genetic variants in known disease genes (orange). The proportion without detection of known highly penetrant gene variants is most likely determined by comorbidities (diastolic hypertension), environmental factors, and complex genetic backgrounds. (From Hugh Watkins, Circulation 2021;143:2415–2417)

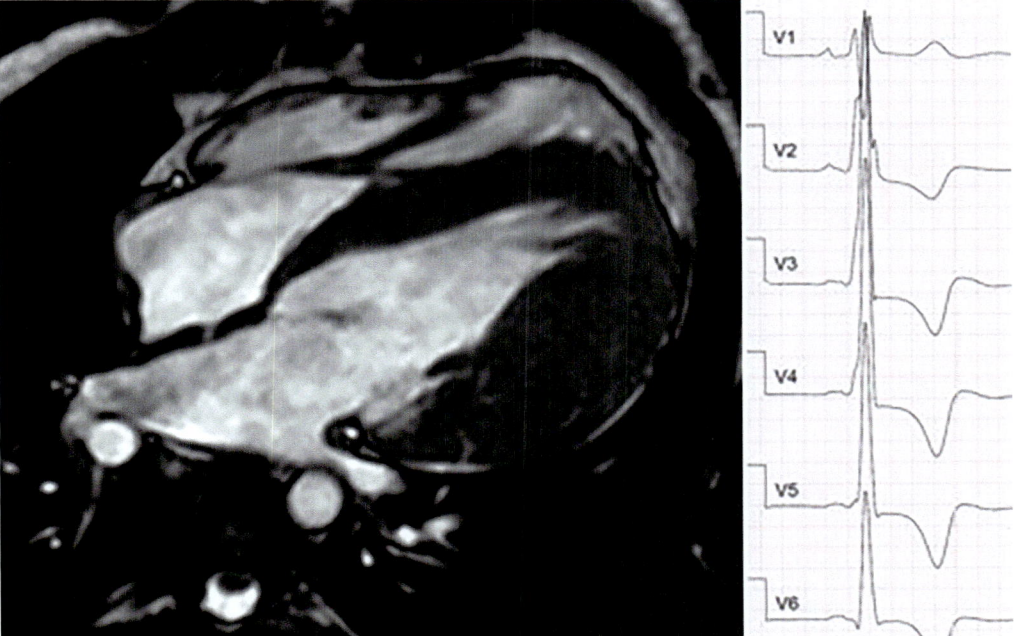

Fig. 8.3 Hypertrophic cardiomyopathy in cMRI. Shown is the 4-chamber view with massive hypertrophy, particularly of the lateral wall. This atypical hypertrophic pattern is much less common than septal hypertrophy. Right: Chest wall leads V1–V6 of the same patient with incomplete right bundle branch block, positive Sokolow-Lyon index, and typical end-stage changes

Table 8.2 Disease genes in syndromes with DCM manifestation

Syndrome with DCM phenotype	Disease gene
Barth syndrome	TAZ
Carvajal syndrome	DSP
Laminopathy, Emery-Dreifuss muscular dystrophy	LMNA
Duchenne muscular dystrophy	DMD
Myofibrillar myopathies	BAG3, DES, DMPK, FLNC, CRYAB, FHL1, MYPN, DNAJB6, LDB3

under stress. For this form, there are effective therapies available (i.e. interventional, surgical, medical, ◘ Table 8.2).

Differential Diagnoses of Myocardial Thickening:
- **Hypertensive Heart Disease** (▶ Chap. 4), **Athlete's Heart** (▶ Sect. 3.5)
- **Storage Diseases**
  - Fabry Disease (lysosomal storage disease)
  - Glycogen storage diseases (e.g., Cori disease = glycogen storage disease type III, Danon disease, glycogen storage disease type IIb)
  - PRKAG2 cardiomyopathy (associated with WPW syndrome, glycogen storage disease confined to the myocardium)
  - Mucopolysaccharidoses
  - Oxalosis
  - Obesity
  - Hypothyroidism
  - Mitochondrial cytopathies
- **Infiltrative Diseases**
  - Amyloidosis
  - Hemochromatosis
  - Sarcoidosis
- **Neuromuscular Diseases**
  - Friedreich's Ataxia
- **Syndromic Diseases**
  - Noonan syndrome (short stature, hypertelorism, pterygium colli, cryptorchidism, pulmonary stenosis, hypertrophic cardiomyopathy)
  - LEOPARD syndrome (lentiginosis, ECG: bundle branch block, hypertelorism, pulmonary stenosis, hypertrophic cardiomyopathy, cryptorchidism, skeletal anomalies, deafness)

Clinical Findings The clinical manifestation of HCM is very variable and ranges from completely absent to very mild symptoms up to sudden cardiac death. Typical symptoms are exertional dyspnea, angina-like symptoms, palpitations, dizziness, or syncope. As regards syncope, it is important to distinguish between hemodynamically induced syncope due to severe obstruction with an increasing pressure gradient across the left ventricular outflow tract (LVOT) under stress and in turn reduced stroke volume during exertion and consequently reduced cerebral perfusion, and arrhythmogenic or vasovagal syncope. Here, a detailed history is particularly informative.

Due to the redistribution of blood pools, many patients experience increased obstruction gradients postprandially, leading to increased symptoms.

Angina pectoris in HCM is usually multifactorial, caused by microvascular dysfunction, increased filling pressures, and an imbalance between the sheer number of capillaries and increased muscle mass.

The feared malignant ventricular arrhythmias occur in 50% of cases during sympathetic stimulation, e.g., during exertion, and the remaining ones during low-stress activities or sleep.

> Undiagnosed HCM is one of the most common causes of sudden death in young athletes. Competitive athletes should regularly undergo cardiac screening.

Diagnostic Work-up The diagnosis of HCM, as with all cardiomyopathies, is always made considering various modalities. Important are the medical history as well as the family history and the clinical examination (systolic murmur in case of obstruction, provokable by Valsalva maneuver). Indications of a systemic disease should be noted (skin, neurology, peripheral muscle strength). Since in well over 90% of HCM patients a pathological ECG with signs of left ventricular hypertrophy, T-wave inversions, and septal Q waves is present, the ECG (▶ Sect. 2.2) plays a crucial role in screening. Ultimately, imaging plays a key role, with Doppler echocardiography as a first step (▶ Sect. 2.5). Doppler echocardiography allows for determination of the maximal wall thickness and of the presence of left ventricular outflow tract obstruction. The obstruction can be accentuated by provocation maneuvers such as the Valsalva maneuver leading to a reduction in venous return. Further provocation maneuvers should be particularly used, if the patient complains of exertional symptoms and no gradient can be provoked by the Valsalva maneuver, i.e. handgrip test, postprandial measurements, stair climbing, or stress echocardiography (▶ Sect. 2.5).

Nowadays, a cardiac MRI (◉ Fig. 8.3) with detection of LGE (after intravenous administration of gadolinium as a contrast agent; ▶ Sect. 2.5) is also routinely performed to determine the extent of hypertrophy and to evaluate the presence of myocardial fibrosis. A myocardial biopsy should be performed especially in cases of storage disease/infiltration and can be done with low risk in the left ventricle. Since the disease is predominantly genetic in nature, it is a guideline recommendation to genetically test HCM patients after appropriate counseling.

Therapy The management of HCM is primarily symptomatic in nature. The obstruction of the left ventricular outflow tract can be primarily reduced with beta-blockers (negative chronotropic and negative inotropic effects), disopyramide (class IA antiarrhythmic, negative inotropic sodium channel blocker; not available in many countries), and central, non-vasodilating calcium channel blockers. Such medications primarily serve to reduce contractility and thus reduce the obstruction in the left ventricular outflow tract. A newly introduced drugs (Mavacamten, Aficamptem) are potent inhibitors of the contractile myosin proteins, which leads to a significant reduction in the gradient in the left ventricular outflow tract and is symptomatically very effective. The drugs are now available in many countries and are recommended in the European guidelines as a therapeutic options after the administration of beta-blockers. If such medications are not effective, invasive options such as catheter-based alcohol septal ablation and surgical myectomy are available.

> In the case of hypertension and the presence of HOCM, afterload-reducing antihypertensives such as ACE inhibitors, ATII blockers, or nitrates are contraindicated, as they can further increase the gradient across the left ventricular outflow tract. Effective management of the obstruction is often challenging and can sometimes only be achieved after interventional or surgical septum reduction.

Patients with a non-obstructive form who suffer from dyspnea and angina pectoris respond best to calcium channel blockers of the verapamil type and as second choice to beta-blockers. The cause of their symptoms is usually coronary microvascular dysfunction.

In the case of survived sudden cardiac death, the indication for secondary prophylactic implantation of an implantable cardioverter-defibrillator (ICD, ▶ Sect. 12.5) is given. In addition, primary prophylactic ICD implantation is generally recommended for patients who have an increased risk of sudden cardiac death. Risk scores are used to assess the risk of sudden cardiac death (*ESC HCM Risk Score*). The statistical risk should be explained to the patient, and a balanced decision considering arrhythmic risk, ICD protection, and possible ICD complications should be made.

The identification of potential HCM-mimicking diseases often has therapeutic consequences, which is why the response to therapy in presumed HCM should be closely observed.

Clinical Outcomes In principle, the prognosis for HCM is good, and patients have an almost normal life expectancy. The general population has a sudden cardiac death rate of 0.4% per year, and HCM patients have an average of 1% per year, although there are patients with significantly higher risk. About 10% of patients develop significant heart failure (▶ Chap. 13) and only a small fraction of these patients ultimately undergo heart transplantation.

8.1.4 Restrictive Cardiomyopathy (RCM)

Definition RCM refers to heart muscle diseases with (severe) diastolic dysfunction with preserved systolic LVEF and normal wall thicknesses.

Etiology Half of the cases are idiopathic. Genetic forms are found through variants in the genes *ACTC1, MYH7, TNNI3, TNNT2, TTN, FLNC*. Here, overlap with other forms of cardiomyopathy within the same family is common. A secondary cause is **endomyocardial fibrosis**, which involves eosinophilic infiltration of the endocardium and myocardium. There is an endemic and a sporadic form. *Endemic* endomyocardial fibrosis occurs more frequently in the tropical belt. It is thougt that genetic factors, diet (cassava in indigenous people in South America), parasitic infections, and cerium play a role. In Central Europe, the *sporadic form* is more common, where the hypereosinophilia syndrome (formerly called Löffler endocarditis) must be distinguished from secondary eosinophilias. Secondary forms can occur in the context of infections, drug side effects or allergies, malignancies, amyloidosis (▶ Sect. 8.1.5), autoimmune diseases (Churg-Strauss, scleroderma, sarcoidosis, etc.), or acute leukemias.

Pathophysiology Pathognomonic for RCM is a severely restricted diastolic function with largely preserved systolic ventricular function. The underlying cause is a change in the mechanical properties of the myocardium. The consequences are similar to those of cardiac amyloidosis: due to increased left ventricular filling pressures there is a backlog of blood in the left and/or right atrium with corresponding clinical consequences (pulmonary hypertension, dyspnea, pulmonary edema, or jugular vein distention, peripheral edema, pleural effusions, ascites).

Clinical Findings Patients present with more or less pronounced signs of heart failure (▶ Sect. 13.3). Additionally, other signs of an underlying disease (see above) may be detectable. Edema and jugular vein distention can be very pronounced and lead to hepatosplenomegaly up to liver cirrhosis (*cirrhose cardiaque*).

Diagnostics Doppler echocardiography (▶ Sect. 2.5) of RCM typically shows pronounced diastolic dysfunction with significant restriction of ventricular filling (restrictive filling pattern). The atria are often very large and can exceed the volume of the ventricles. NT-proBNP is usually significantly elevated. Further diagnostics, particularly invasive hemodynamic measurement, CT, MRI (◘ Fig. 8.4), and possibly a myocardial biopsy, may be required depending on the suspected cause (see above). In particular, hypereosinophilia should be sought and consequently systemic diseases associated with it.

Therapy Therapy is directed on the one hand (symptomatically) according to the severity of heart failure, and on the other hand (causally) according to an underlying systemic disease. Diuretics are often the central therapeutic agent for symptom relieve. The efficacy of SGLT-2 inhibitors has not yet been systematically studied. If the underlying disease cannot be treated or can only be inadequately treated, surgical decortication (removal of the fibrosed endocardium) is a possibility in endomyocardial fibrosis, which can improve both symptoms and survival. In advanced stages, heart transplantation may be necessary as a last resort.

8.1.5 Cardiac Amyloidosis

Definition In cardiac amyloidosis, the myocardium is primarily infiltrated in the interstitium with deposits of abnormally altered insoluble protein deposits (= amyloid fibrils). The detection of amyloid is achieved histologically in biopsy tissue stained with Congo red. Under polarized light, a characteristic green birefringence can be observed.

The amyloid deposits impair the mechanical function of the heart and can also lead to severe conduction delays and arrhythmias. Classically, patients present with a picture similar to restrictive cardiomyopathy (RCM; ▶ Sect. 8.1.4), but in advanced disease, there is often also a restriction of systolic function.

Epidemiology Depending on the type of amyloid, there are different forms of the disease. Light chain Amyloidosis (AL) is a systemic hematological disease (plasmacytoma) in which the heart is involved in 70% of cases. The incidence is about 5–12 patients/1 million inhabitants.

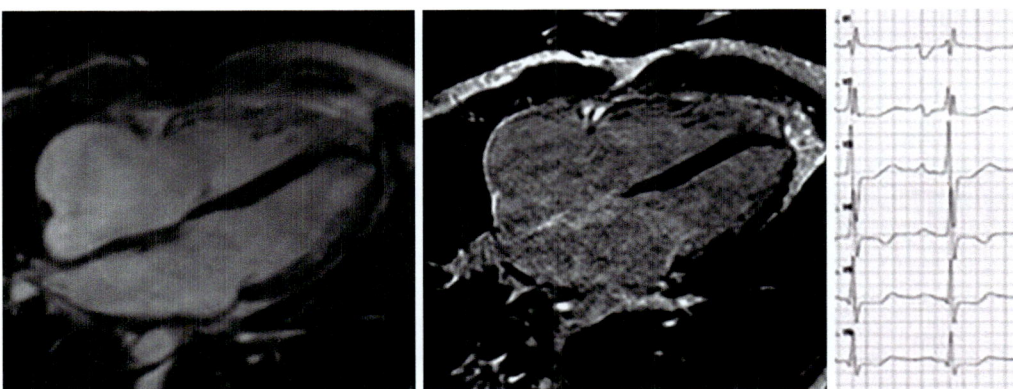

◘ **Fig. 8.4 Restrictive Cardiomyopathy.** cMRI in the 4-chamber view (left) with normal wall thickness and normal LV diameters. Atria and the right ventricle are significantly (secondarily) dilated. Middle: negative late gadolinium enhancement, amyloidosis can therefore be excluded. Right: chest wall leads with signs of right heart strain, P-mitrale and P-dextroatriale, end-stage changes

Hereditary, hereditary ATTRv (also ATTRmt) amyloidosis is very rare. It affects only a few thousand patients worldwide.

In contrast, acquired, age-related wild-type transthyretin amyloidosis (ATTRwt) is being diagnosed more and more frequently. In certain populations (e.g., aortic stenosis, TAVI population), up to 20% of those over 80 years old are affected (men > women).

> Cardiac amyloidosis is an increasingly frequently diagnosed disease in older people.

Pathogenesis In amyloidosis, endogenous proteins undergo a conformational change, leading to the formation of insoluble fibrils that deposit in tissues. Over 30 proteins can form amyloid fibrils, but only 9 of them show relevant deposits in the heart, most commonly AL and TTR. Cardiac amyloid deposits as a result of chronic inflammation (so-called AA amyloidoses) are very rare.

More than 98% of diagnosed cardiac amyloidosis can be classified as AL amyloidoses or transthyretin amyloidosis (ATTR). AL amyloidosis is the result of monoclonal light chain deposition. The light chains are the result of a plasma cell dyscrasia, most often a monoclonal gammopathy, or an asymptomatic multiple myeloma, in 10% of cases a symptomatic myeloma or a B-cell lymphoma.

Hereditary ATTRv amyloidosis results from a transthyretin mutation, while acquired ATTRwt amyloidosis is the result of a not yet fully understood aging process.

Clinical Findings The cardiac symptoms are nonspecific, variable, and include signs of heart failure (▶ Sect. 13.3) as well as syncope and dizziness as expressions of bradycardic arrhythmias (▶ Sect. 12.4), autonomic dysfunction, and/or atrial fibrillation (▶ Sect. 12.5).

However, there are clinical findings that significantly increase the pretest probability of the presence of cardiac amyloidosis.

On the one hand, in AL the presence of a known monoclonal gammopathy or an asymptomatic myeloma or as regards ATTRwt amyloidosis, bilateral carpal tunnel syndromes, spinal canal stenoses, and biceps tendon ruptures are often found. In addition, ATTRwt amyloidosis is frequently observed in older patients with degenerative aortic stenosis.

Diagnostics The medical history and clinical findings often reveal heart failure with typically preserved LVEF or preserved radial systolic function (HFpEF; ▶ Sect. 13.2), "unclear" right heart failure, the presence of pericardial effusions, as well as bradyarrhythmias with AV block patterns, typically in older patients.

In the ECG, apart from bradyarrhythmias and "pseudo" Q-waves, a relative "low-voltage" pattern is typically seen, which contrasts with marled left ventricualr wallthickening as detected by echocardiography (◘ Fig. 8.5).

Echocardiographically, in addition to left ventricular wall thickening, signs of advanced diastolic dysfunction, increases in pulmonary systolic pressure, and a typically apex-sparing restriction of the longitudinal strain rate ("strain"; ◘ Fig. 8.5) are found.

If cardiac amyloidosis is suspected based on the medical history, free light chains in the serum and a clonal gammopathy are sought using immunofixation in serum and urine. Additionally, a ^{99m}Tc-DPD (diphosphono-1,2-propanedicarboxylic acid) bone scintigraphy is usually performed. The latter confirms, after excluding a monoclonal gammopathy, with almost 100% specificity the presence of ATTR amyloidosis through tracer accumulation in the cardiac wall. Depending on the scintigraphic findings and whether a monoclonal gammopathy is present or not, the diagnosis can be further confirmed or ruled out by a cardiac MRI examination. In case of

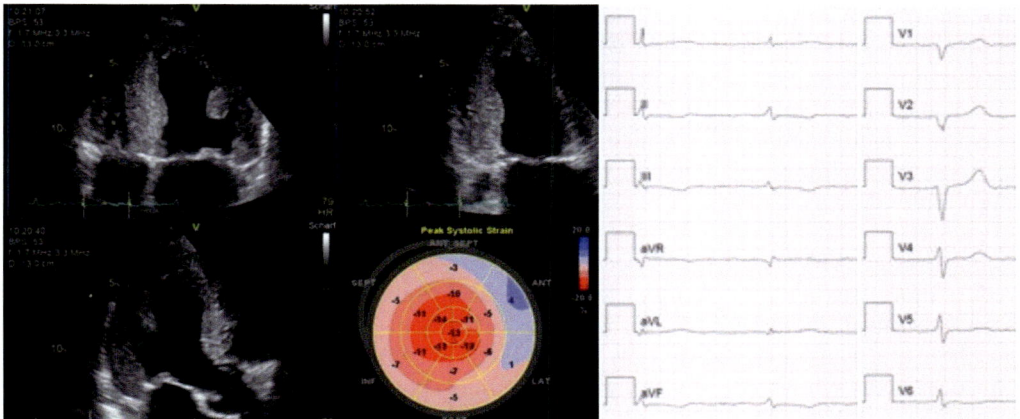

Fig. 8.5 Echocardiography and ECG as basic diagnostics in TTR amyloidosis. Shown is a 4-, 3-, and 2-chamber view with massive thickening of the heart walls (RV, LV, atrial septum). In the strain analysis, a preserved deformation of the apex can be seen with reduced strain in the basal segments. Right: In the ECG of the same patient, low voltage, ST-segment depressions in II, III, aVF with terminal T-wave inversion are apparent. (Courtesy of Dr. A. Amr)

doubt, myocardial biopsy is the diagnostic gold standard.

> The ^{99m}Tc-DPD bone scintigraphy plays a central role in the diagnosis of cardiac ATTR amyloidosis alongside cMRI. Cardiac AL amyloidosis can be suspected through the detection of clonal light chain production and a suggestive MRI finding—however, AL amyloid must be immunohistologically proven for diagnostic confirmation.

Therapy In addition to symptomatic therapy with diuretics, arrhythmias must be managed properly, e.g. patients with atrial fibrillation must be anticoagulated independent of their CHA_2DS_2-VASc score. ICD therapy (▶ Sect. 12.5) is usually not indicated due to the lack of evidence for an improvement in clinical outcomes.

The specific treatment of AL amyloidosis is carried out individually by a multidisciplinary team and includes cytostatic medication as well as autologous stem cell transplantation.

For the treatment of patients with ATTRwt and ATTRv, the transthyretin stabilizer tafamidis is currently available, which can delay the progression of the disease and reduces mortality. siRNA therapies are approved for ATTR polyneuropathy and soon for cardiac TTR. Finally, gene therapy using CRISPR-Cas9 is currently in clinical trials with encouraging early results.

Clinical Outcomes The prognosis varies depending on the type of amyloid, comorbidity, and treatment approach. Most series report 5-year survival rates between 50 and 70%.

8.1.6 Arrhythmogenic (Right Ventricular) Cardiomyopathy (ARVC, ACM)

Definition In ARVC, the myocardium of typically the right ventricle is replaced by fat and connective tissue, leading to the formation of right ventricular aneurysms and in turn dilation, reduction of right ventricular pump function, and the development of ventricular arrhythmias. Left ventricular involvement is not uncommon, which is why the term "Arrhythmogenic Cardiomyopathy (AC)" should be used today.

Epidemiology ARVC is a rare disease that occurs more frequently in families and has been described in syndromic forms, primarily in the Veneto region of Italy and in Greece (Naxos syndrome). It usually occurs in young and physically active people, with diagnosis typically made between the ages of 10 and 40. The prevalence is estimated to be between 1:2000–1:5000.

Pathogenesis ARVC is usually inherited in an autosomal-dominant manner. Mutations are mostly found in genes that code for proteins of the intercalated disc and desmosomes. This has consequences for the excitation process, cellular signaling pathways, and mechanics. Morphologically, there is a remodeling of the right ventricle, i.e. myocardial tissue is successively replaced by fat and connective tissue. Due to the remodeling processes, both the conduction of excitation and the contractility of the right ventricle are severely impaired. Additionally, the remodeled areas provide a substrate for ventricular tachycardias up to ventricular fibrillation. The involvement of the left ventricle can be explained by similar mechanisms, but also affects genes and secondary causes of DCM/HCM (Laminin LMNA/C variant, sarcoidosis, etc.).

Clinical Findings Commonly, a long asymptomatic course is followed by rhythm disturbances and signs of right or biventricular heart failure. Sudden cardiac death can be the first manifestation of AC, which is why autopsy including molecular genetic analysis is useful for further family clarification in people with sudden cardiac death.

> It is not uncommon that patients who suffer sudden cardiac death in the context of AC have previously experienced (pre-)syncope. An autopsy including molecular genetic analysis should be performed, but it is not yet well established in many countries.

Diagnostics Symptoms of cardiac rhythm disturbance (palpitations, syncope) are common. The family history often includes cases of sudden cardiac death. The ECG may show an epsilon wave at the end of the QRS complex (V1–V3), which corresponds to a late potential, as well as typical T-wave inversions in V1–V3 (◘ Fig. 8.6 below). Echocardiography (◘ Fig. 8.6 top right, cf. normal finding ◘ Fig. 2.5) may reveal typical signs, but may also be inconspicuous in the early stages. Fat deposits can be detected by MRI (currently probably the best diagnostic modality; ► Sect. 2.5) or using endomyocardial biopsy, However, endomyocardial biopsy is prone by a high rate of false-negative results due to *sampling errors* due to the uneven distribution of the changes). Similar to HCM, the diagnosis is based on various factors, and the so-called revised Task Force criteria should be applied (◘ Fig. 8.7).

Therapy The therapy consists of treating any existing heart failure as well as arrhythmias (primarily using beta-blockers, if necessary, amiodarone). In cases of survived sudden cardiac death and in the presence of risk factors such as a history of syncope, evidence of ventricular tachycardia in the 24-hour ECG, or during an electrophysiological study, an ICD implantation is indicated (► Sect. 12.5). In these patients, a subcutaneous ICD without a shock electrode in the often sufficient. Heart failure therapy is indicated in left or biventricular AC (► Sect. 13.3). As a last resort, especially in refractory heart failure, a heart transplant may be necessary.

Myocardial Diseases

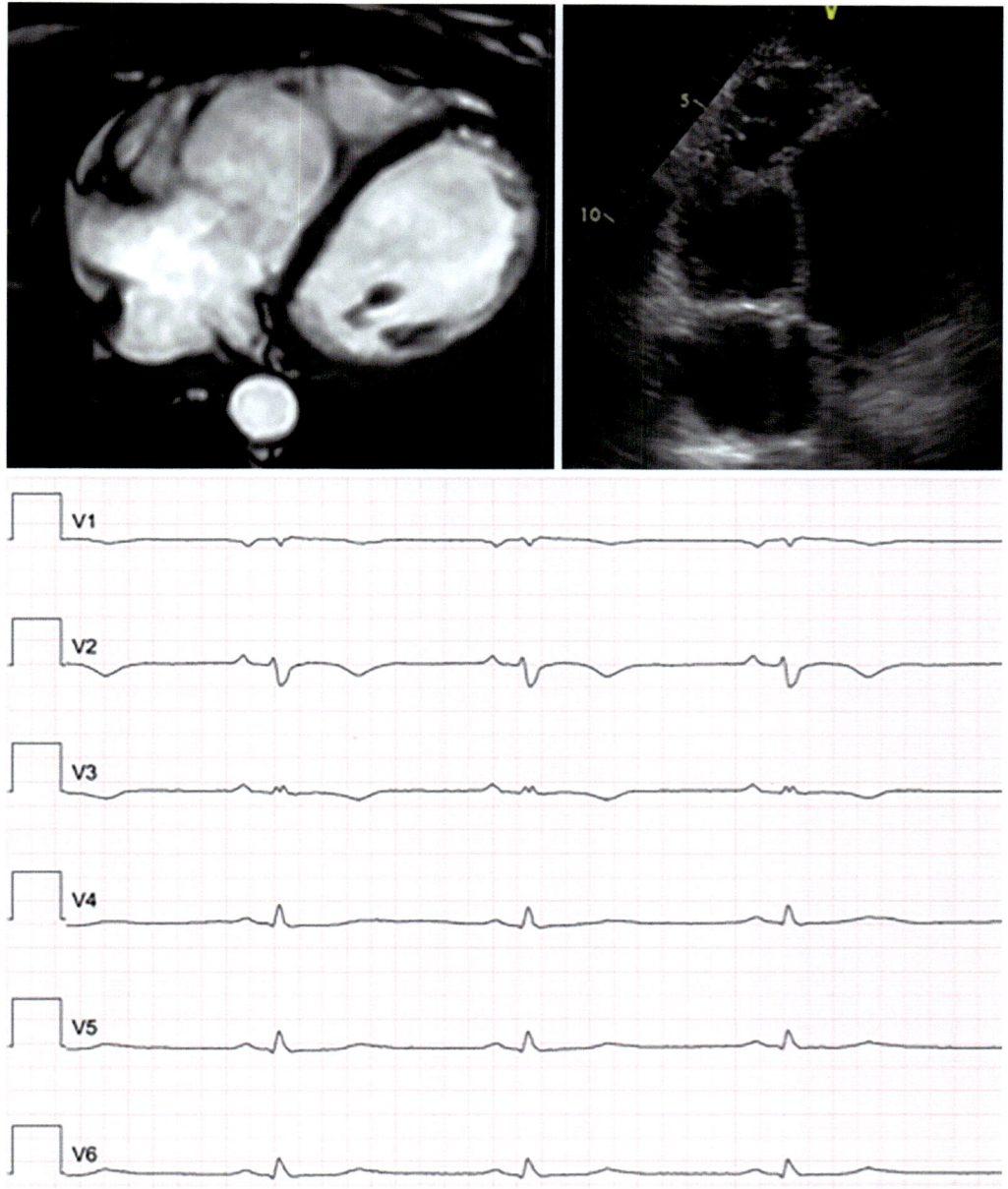

Fig. 8.6 **Arrhythmogenic right ventricular cardiomyopathy (ARVC)** with significantly enlarged right ventricle (top left: MRI; top right: echocardiography) with aneurysmal bulges. This leads to corresponding changes in the surface resting ECG (bottom) with right precordial T-wave inversions in V1–V3. Indicated epsilon potential (V1, V3)

Since competitive sports are particularly associated with an increased manifestation and progression of AC, such activities should be discouraged. Light physical activity, on the other hand, seems unproblematic.

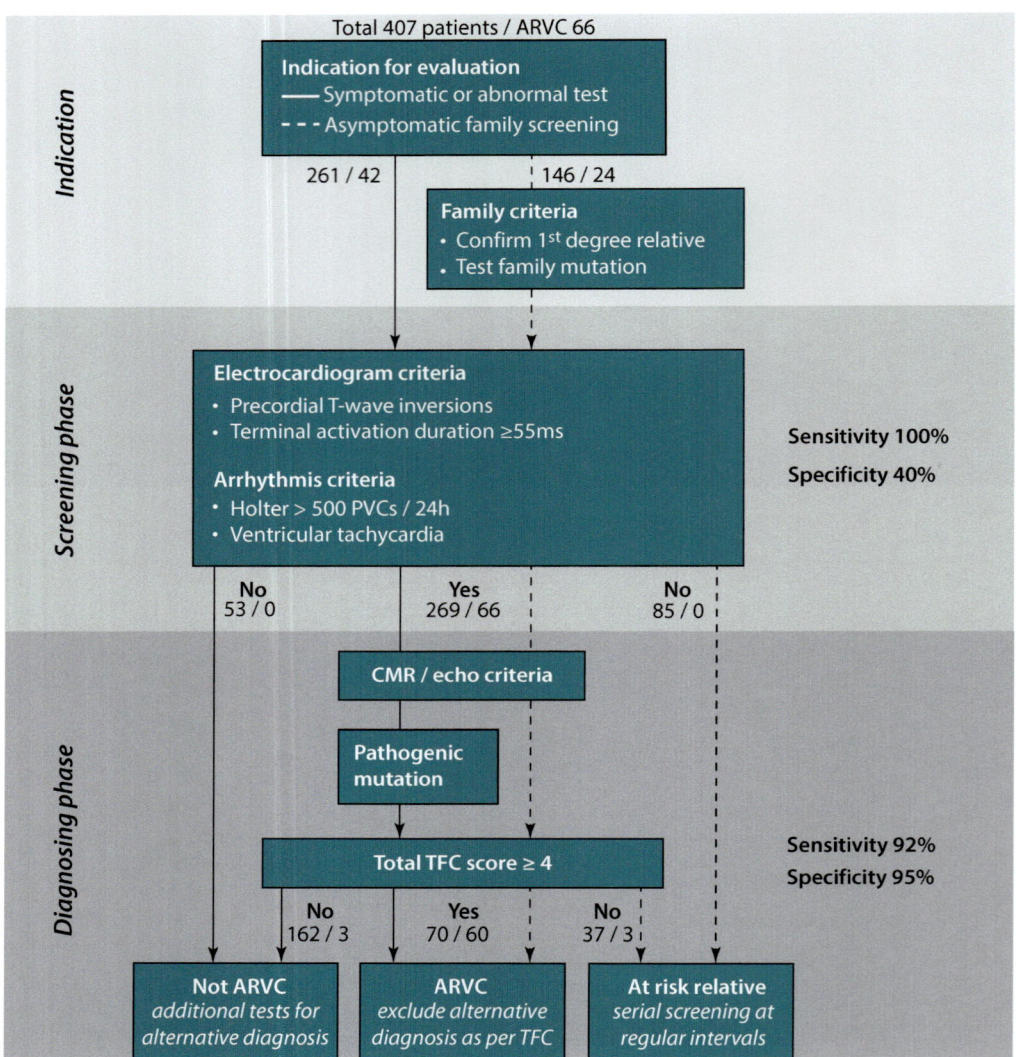

☐ **Fig. 8.7** Simplified practical procedure for applying the Task Force criteria. (From Bosman et al. EP Europace, Volume 22, Issue 5, May 2020, Pages 787–796)

8.1.7 Left Ventricular Non-compaction Cardiomyopathy (LVNC)

Definition In LVNC, the myocardium is loosened and interspersed with trabeculae. The disease can also occur biventricularly. The transition to the other described forms of cardiomyopathies is fluid, and it is debated whether LVNC is truly an independent cardiomyopathy or a special phenotype of various forms of cardiomyopathies. Indeed, the disease can be congenital, genetic, or acquired. Distinguishing it from a physiologically benign phenotype, which occurs more frequently in different ethnicities and has no disease value, is sometimes difficult. Thus, te 2023 ESC Guidelines on cardiomyopathies therefore recommend 'hypertrabeculation', rather than LVNC.

Epidemiology Exact prevalence figures are not available, but criteria for LVNC are found in approximately 0.5–1% of performed echocardiographic studies. Overall, it is the most common cardiomyopathy phenotype after DCM and HCM.

Pathogenesis In congenital LVNC, genetic mechanism disturbances during embryonic development lead to a disrupted process of myocardial compaction. This normally progresses in the ventricle from basal to apical, resulting in the greatest effects being apically located. A cardiomyopathy should only be considered, if the phenotype leads to functional or clinical signs of heart failure, arrhythmias, cardiac embolisms, or elevated cardiac biomarkers. Overdiagnosis must be avoided. In LVNC occurring later in life, it is likely an adaptive response to stressors, such as aortic regurgitation, DCM, pregnancy, or sports. Here too, signs of heart muscle disease must be present to identify the relevant risk groups.

Clinical Findings It is often an incidental finding in asymptomatic individuals. The prevalence of stroke and thromboembolism is increased in LVNC, and signs of heart failure only appear with accompanying systolic heart failure. Registries have shown an increased rate of arrhythmias in LVNC with systolic dysfunction.

> Recent Guidelines do not consider non-compaction to be an independent cardiomyopathy. To avoid overdiagnosis, other pathological signs of myocardial disease must be considered (based on ECG, biomarkers, LV dysfunction, arrhythmias, cardioembolic stroke).

Diagnostics The family history is indicative of a genetic LVNC. In imaging, there are various criteria for echocardiography (Jenni Criteria; J Am Soc Echo 2005;18:865; Fig. 8.8) and cardiac MRI (Fig. 8.8; Petersen Criteria; J Am Coll Cardiol 2005;46:101; Fig. 8.9). Here, the ratio of compacted to non-compacted myocardium plays a crucial role. Elevated troponin or natriuretic peptides are signs of pathological non-compaction. The ECG is often uneventful except in end-stages. A myocardial biopsy is rarely indicated; molecular genetic testing should be performed in familial cases. The disease genes overlap particularly with those of DCM.

Therapy In LVNC with systolic heart failure, appropriate heart failure therapy should be initiated (▶ Sect. 13.4). A causal therapy is not established. Anticoagulation in the case of pronounced hypertrabecula-

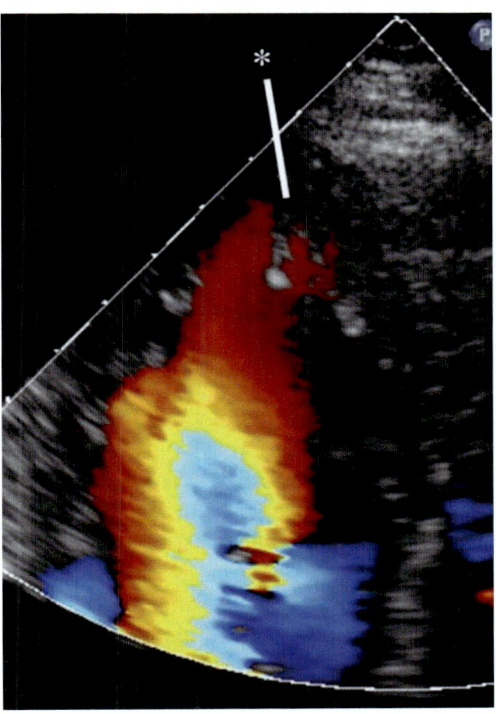

Fig. 8.8 LVNC in echocardiography and cardiac MRI. Here, the criteria according to Jenni and Petersen are positive. The LVEF in this patient is 45%, the ECG is essentially unremarkable

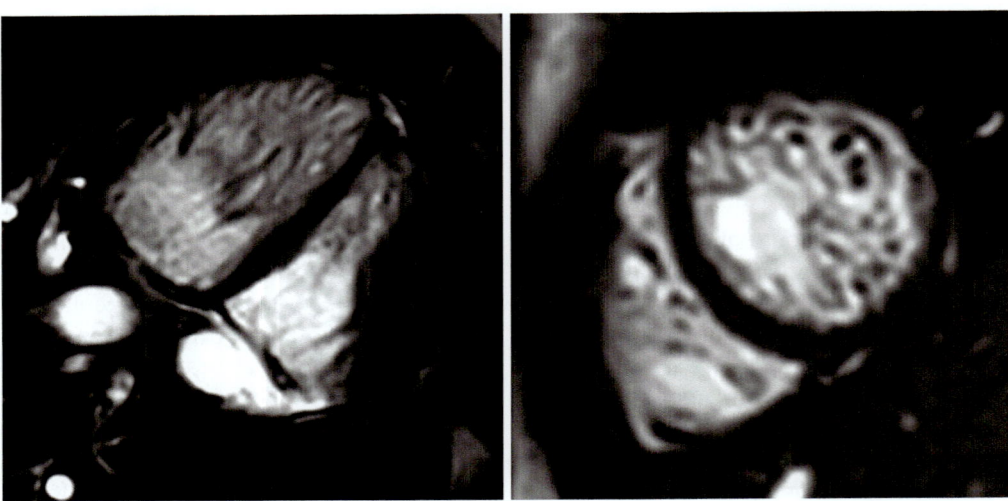

Fig. 8.9 cMRI findings in non-compaction cardiomyopathy. Shown are a shortened 4-chamber view (left) and the short axis (SAX; right). The spongy structure of the left and partially right ventricular myocardium can be seen

tion (in particular with detectable thrombi) or an embolic stroke is a case-by-case decision and should be based on echocardiographic findings, the presence of atrial fibrillation (▶ Sect. 12.5) and bleeding risk.

8.2 Myocarditis

Definition The term "myocarditis" essentially refers to any inflammation of the heart muscle and is strictly speaking a histological term that presupposes both the conventionally histologically detectable presence of inflammatory cells and the detection of apoptotic or necrotic cardiomyocytes. In the literature, the terms "inflammatory cardiomyopathy" and "inflammatory dilated cardiomyopathy" have become established. The latter terms refer to cardiac dysfunction ("cardiomyopathy"), a dilated heart ("dilated"; ▶ Sect. 8.1.2) and an immunohistochemically proven inflammation. Immunohistochemical criteria for cardiac inflammation are the detection of more than 14 leukocytes, more than 7 CD3-expressing T-cells, and/or more than 4 CD14-expressing monocytes per view field.

Clinically, depending on the course and severity of the disease, myocarditis is referred to as fulminant, acute, chronic, or subclinical form. However, these terms are not clearly defined in terms of time. Most authors refer to acute myocarditis when less than 4 weeks have passed between the onset of symptoms and the first medical contact. Fulminant myocarditis is present when a patient with acute myocarditis requires additional pharmacological or mechanical circulatory support (▶ Sect. 13.4).

Epidemiology The annual prevalence of myocarditis in Europe is reported to be 130 cases/1 million inhabitants. However, the true prevalence is likely to be significantly higher, as many myocarditis cases pass subclinically. It is important to note that up to 40% of idiopathic dilated cardiomyopathies (DCM; ▶ Sect. 8.1.2) are late consequences of subclinical myocarditis. In addition, myocarditis is an important cause of sudden cardiac death in young people.

Myocardial Diseases

> Symptomatic and subclinical myocarditis can develop into inflammatory dilated cardiomyopathies, with inflammatory changes often no longer detectable in the late course.

> Myocarditis is a common cause of sudden cardiac death in young patients (<40 years).

Etiology Myocarditis can fundamentally be triggered by any heart muscle hazard. Infections are the most common cause, with the parasite *Trypanosoma cruzi* playing a central role in South America. In developed countries, myocarditis is most frequently associated with viruses, primarily enteroviruses such as *Coxsackie B3* (◘ Table 8.3). However, certain bacteria or even fungi can also lead to myocarditis. Finally, myocarditis can occur due to toxin and drug exposure, in the context of sepsis, in autoimmune diseases such as systemic lupus erythematosus or collagen diseases, and sometimes as an expression of a hypersensitivity reaction. Giant cell myocarditis represents an etiologically unexplained primary myocarditis with a poor prognosis. The histological detection of multinucleated giant cells without granuloma formation is specific to this condition.

Pathophysiology The current understanding of the pathophysiological processes of myocarditis largely stems from mouse models and observational studies. In principle, any heart muscle hazard, depending on the genetic and immunological predisposition of the affected patient and the properties of the infecting or hazardous agent, can trigger a persistent cardiac inflammation.

The process of virus-induced myocarditis is the best investigated. It can be divided into 3 phases:
1. Viral or infectious phase
2. Immunological reaction
3. Inflammatory triggered remodeling

In the 1st phase, the virus infects the cardiomyocytes. This leads to tissue damage and activation of the immune response. Certain viruses can also directly impair the contractile apparatus of the cardiomyocates.

In the 2nd phase, the immune system attempts to eliminate the virus. Ideally, the pathogen is eliminated, and the inflammation heals without consequences. However, the immune response often remains inadequate. Either the elimination of the virus does not succeed, leading to chronic inflammation, or the immune response loses its pathogen specificity and targets the heart muscle tissue itself (autoimmune response). The underlying mechanisms are the subject of ongoing research. In certain cases, molecular mimicry or cross-reactivity between specific viral antigens and myocardial structural proteins could result in continuous immune activation and cardiomyocyte damage. More relevant is the finding that practically after every myocate damage, cardiac proteins are taken up by antigen-presenting cells. If the extent of the accompanying nonspecific inflammatory response exceeds a genetically determined threshold, an autoimmune response directed against the heart muscle can develop. Indeed, numerous cardiac-specific autoantibodies have been identified, especially in patients with (idiopathic) dilated cardiomyopathy (DCM; ▶ Sect. 8.1.2). Pathophysiologically, the activation of cardiac-specific T-lymphocytes and humoral immune defense mechanisms leads to the production and secretion of a variety of inflammatory cytokines and mediators, further recruitment of inflammatory cells, and ultimately the destruction of cardiomyocytes. In parallel, the inflammatory response leads to the formation of fibrotic, non-functional scar tissue. The entire process ultimately results in the typical phenotype of dilated cardiomyopathy.

Clinical Findings Patients often, but not always, report previous flu-like general symp-

Table 8.3 Causes of Myocarditis

Viruses (most common)	Coxsackie virus	
	Adenovirus	
	Parvovirus B19	
	Human herpesvirus type 6	
	Epstein-Barr virus	
	Cytomegalovirus	
	Echovirus	
	Mumps virus	
	Influenza viruses A, B	
	Flavivirus	
	HIV (Human Immunodeficiency Virus)	
	Measles virus	
	Poliovirus	
	Hepatitis C virus	
	Rabies virus	
	Rubella virus	
	Varicella-zoster virus	
Parasites	Schistosomes	
	Trypanosoma cruzi	
	Larva migrans	
Bacteria	Streptococci	
	Chlamydia pneumoniae	
	Mycoplasma pneumoniae	
	Treponema pallidum	
	Mycobacteria	
Fungi	Candida	
	Histoplasma	
	Aspergillus	
	Coccidioides species	
	Cryptococci	

(continued)

Table 8.3 (continued)

Toxins	Cocaine, Alcohol
	Anthracyclines
Hypersensitivity Reactions	Penicillins
	Tricyclic antidepressants
	Clozapine
	Sulfonamides
	Cephalosporins
Autoimmune Reactions/Diseases	Giant cell myocarditis
	Churg-Strauss syndrome
	Systemic lupus erythematosus (SLE)
	Wegener's granulomatosis
	Sjögren's syndrome
	Takayasu arteritis
	Sarcoidosis
	Inflammatory bowel diseases
Histologically specific idiopathic forms	Giant cell myocarditis
	Eosinophilic necrotizing myocarditis

toms such as a runny nose, headaches, body aches, abdominal discomfort, or diarrhea. However, such symptoms are nonspecific and are often also reported by patients with new onset symptomatic heart failure or coronary artery disease. Myocarditis often progresses subclinically. It is not clear what percentage of patients with subclinically progressing myocarditis ultimately develop dilated cardiomyopathy.

If myocarditis becomes clinically manifest, various forms of presentation can be distinguished:

− **Acute non-fulminant Myocarditis** (time span between symptom onset and doctor contact <4 weeks): In acute non-fulminant myocarditis, signs of heart failure (▶ Sect. 13.2) and arrhythmias (▶ Chap. 12) are usually predominant. Sometimes patients have angina-like symptoms that must be differentiated from acute coronary syndrome. The differential diagnosis of acute coronary syndrome (▶ Sect. 7.5) is complicated by the fact that, in addition to the symptoms, EKG changes (ST elevations) and an increase in cardiac enzymes (CK-MB, troponin) can also be detected. To definitively rule out an acute coronary syndrome, coronary angiography is often unavoidable. In the case of myocarditis, the latter shows no (or at least no disease-explaining) stenoses.

- **Acute fulminant Myocarditis:** If patients with acute myocarditis require intensive medical care or even the use of an left ventricularassist device (▶ Sect. 13.4), it is referred to as fulminant myocarditis. Echocardiographically, the LVEF is usually severely impaired with a still normal dimensions of the left and/or right ventricle. The fulminant course is rare, and the prognosis for patients is serious. However, if the acute phase is overcome, the long-term prognosis is commonly good.

▶ Acute fulminant myocarditis is a life-threatening condition with high mortality, requiring etensive therapeutic measures involving the full spectrum of heart failure and intensive care medications and potentially left ventricualr assist devices.

- **Chronic Myocarditis** (time span between symptom onset and doctor contact >4 weeks): Often, the onset of symptoms is difficult to determine, or the insidious onset of symptoms occurred more than 4 weeks ago. In these cases, heart failure symptoms (▶ Sect. 13.2) or arrhythmias (▶ Sect. 12.5) are often predominant. Echocardiographically, a dilation of the heart chambers is often already evident. The affected patients usually show a progressive course and often develop the phenotype of dilated cardiomyopathy with signs of heart failure.

Diagnostics The detailed medical history (including recent infections and assessment of the cardiovascular risk profile), clinical examination (signs of heart failure; ▶ Sect. 13.3), ECG, echocardiography, and cardiac MRI may suggest the diagnosis of myocarditis. However, the findings obtained from the ECG and echocardiography are neither specific nor sensitive for myocarditis. The MRI provides a fairly high sensitivity, but the specificity is controversial and currently under investigation. In the ECG, both ST-segment changes and conduction disturbances (e.g. AV block, bundle branch block) and higher-grade arrhythmias (ve.g. entricular tachycardia to ventricular fibrillation; ▶ Sect. 12.5) can be observed. Echocardiography may show wall thickening due to edema, wall motion abnormalities, and impaired pumping function in the acute phase. In the subacute to chronic phase, the findings of DCM (▶ Sect. 8.1.2 and ◘ Fig. 8.1) with enlarged and poorly contracting cardiac chambers are usually seen.

Traditionally, the diagnosis of myocarditis required the detection of inflammatory infiltrates with necrosis/apoptosis of cardiomyocytes (Dallas criteria, ◘ Fig. 7.8a, b). Recently, staining of infiltrating T-cells and monocytes using immunohistochemistry has been used more commonly. In principle, a myocardial biopsy should be performed to definitively prove the presence of a myocarditis. However, in clinical practice, this is often avoided due to the lack of therapeutic consequences and potential complications (e.g. cardiac tamponade, tissue embolism, damage to the tricuspide valve). The diagnosis is then made

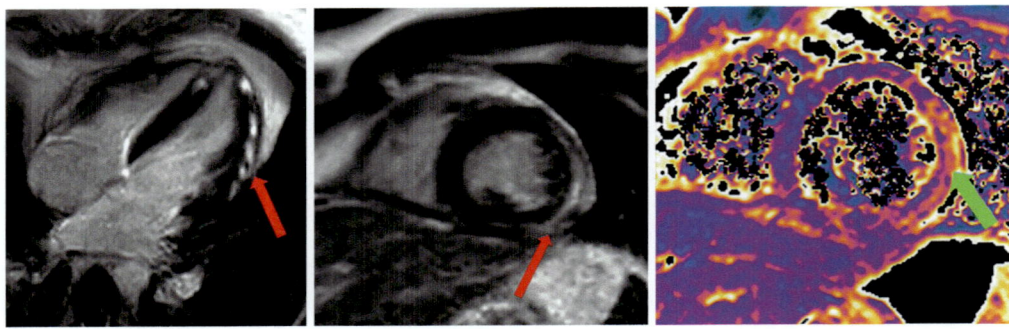

Fig. 8.10 MRI in acute myocarditis. It shows the typical "late enhancement" after gadolinium (red arrows), apical lateral wall, and significant edema formation (green arrow) in T2 mapping at the same site. (courtesy of Prof. Urs Eriksson)

by excluding other differential diagnoses and combining clinical findings with newer imaging techniques (MRI; ◘ Fig. 8.10).

Only with a prolonged course and progressive decrease in LVEF should a biopsy be routinely performed to identify the subgroup of patients with virus-negative myocarditis who might respond to immunosuppression. In patients with fulminant myocarditis, the risk of intervention must be weighed against the potential therapeutically usefulness of the obtained information. Some experts pursue a more aggressive diagnostic strategy here to avoid missing the rare giant cell myocarditis, which would also respond to immunosuppression in the highly acute phase (◘ Fig. 8.11).

Therapy The focus is on treating symptoms, heart failure, and arrhythmias. In fulminant myocarditis, the entire repertoire of intensive carem ust be used. Heart failure patients are treated with ACE inhibitors, AT receptor blockers/neprilysin inhibitors, beta-blockers, diuretics, SGLT2-inhibitors and aldosterone antagonists. In selected cases with left bundle branch block and severyl reduce LVEF, cardiac resynchronization therapy may be considered (▶ Sect. 13.4). In therapy-refractory cases, endomyocardial biopsy can be used to select patients in whom the infecting virus has been eliminated at the cost of a heart-specific autoimmuneresponse. For these latter patients, there are not yet sufficiently

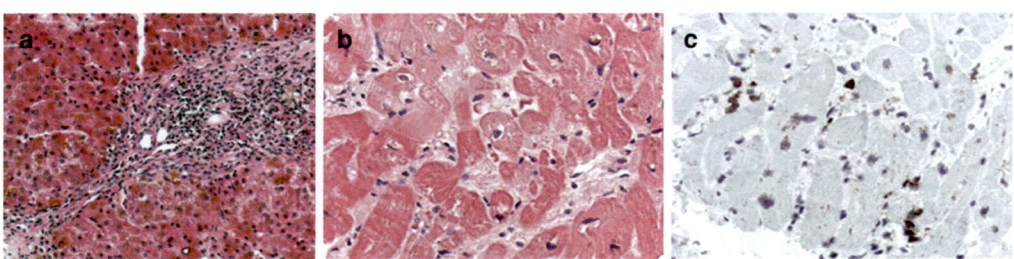

Fig. 8.11 a–c Different manifestations of cardiac inflammation. **a** Lymphocytic myocarditis: inflammatory infiltrate and apoptotic cardiomyocytes in hematoxylin-eosin preparation, **b** minimal inflammation in "inflammatory dilated cardiomyopathy": hematoxylin-eosin staining without relevant inflammatory cells, **c** after immunohistochemistry for CD3, significant T-cells can be stained brown in the sample of the same patient. (Prof. U. Eriksson)

validated immunomodulatory and immunosuppressive treatment options available. Whether antiviral therapy with interferons is beneficial is currently being investigated.

Prognosis The prognosis depends on the genetic predisposition: This determines whether the disease becomes symptomatic at all, whether spontaneous healing occurs, or whether the disease becomes chronic in nature. Furthermore, the prognosis is determined by the clinical findings (fulminant vs. non-fulminant).

Chronically progressing myocarditis has a rather unfavorable prognosis. In prospective studies, the progression to heart failure and the occurrence of arrhythmias are relatively common, with the 10-year survival rate being around 45%.

Valvular Heart Diseases

Christian Hengstenberg, Thomas Pilgrim, Philipp Bartko, Fabien Praz, Georg Goliasch and Stephan Windecker

Contents

9.1 Aortic Valve Stenosis – 146

9.2 Aortic Valve Insufficiency – 152

9.3 Mitral Valve Stenosis – 157

9.4 Mitral Valve Insufficiency – 160

9.5 Mitral Valve Prolapse – 164

9.6 Tricuspid Valve Insufficiency – 165

© The Author(s), under exclusive license to Springer-Verlag GmbH, DE, part of Springer Nature 2025
T. Lüscher and U. Landmesser (eds.), *Cardiovascular System*,
https://doi.org/10.1007/978-3-662-70152-2_9

Heart valve diseases can affect all four valves, such as the aortic, mitral, tricuspid, and pulmonary valves. Heart valves can either become narrow (stenosis) or leaky (regurgitation). The most common are aortic stenosis, especially in older patients, and mitral regurgitation. They typically cause shortness of breath and eventually cause cardiac dysfunction. Severe aortic stenosis is treated with an aortic valve replacement, either surgically or catheter-based. Mitral regurgitation is initally treated conservatively and medically, and at later stages surgically, or with percutaneous mitral valve clipping, depending on anatomy and severity.

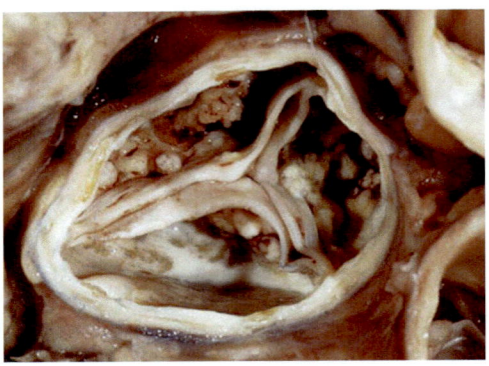

Fig. 9.1 Severely calcified aortic valve. View from the aorta. (Courtesy of Paul Vogt, Institute of Clinical Pathology, University Hospital Zurich)

9.1 Aortic Valve Stenosis

Definition An aortic valve stenosis is caused by restricted opening and in turn narrowing of the native aortic valve. A reduction in the aortic valve opening area results in a pressure load on the left ventricle, which, due to structural changes (remodeling), leads to heart failure and premature death in the long run.

Epidemiology Aortic valve stenosis is the second most common degenerative heart valve disease after mitral regurgitation and the most common heart valve disease leading to percutaneous or surgical interventions. It is responsible for more than two-thirds of all deaths due to non-rheumatic heart valve disease. The prevalence of aortic valve stenosis increases exponentially with advancing age (> 70 years).

Etiology The most common causes of aortic valve stenosis can be distinguished as follows.
- **Degenerative/calcifying (Fig. 9.1):** Lipid deposits (especially elevated lipoprotein(a) levels; ▶ Sect. 3.3), oxidative stress, and inflammatory processes play a central role in the pathogenesis of degenerative aortic valve stenosis and lead to increasing calcifications and consequently reduced mobility of the valve leaflets. This most common form of aortic valve stenosis typically manifests in individuals > 70 years.
- **Rheumatic:** Untreated streptococcal infections in childhood can sustain a chronic inflammatory reaction through an autoimmune response, leading to fibrotic fusion of the valve leaflets with partial secondary calcification. Rheumatic aortic valve stenosis rarely occurs in isolation and is often accompanied by aortic valve regurgitation or concommitent characteristic changes of the mitral valve. Rheumatic heart valve defects typically manifest in middle age. While the prevalence in highly developed countries is significantly declining, in fact today quite rare, rheumatic fever remains endemic in socio-economically disadvantaged regions.
- **Congenital:** In 2% of the normal population, the aortic valve is not tricuspid but unicuspid, bicuspid, or quadricuspid. The most common congenital malformation is the bicuspid aortic valve, which is classified according to the number and location of the raphe (fusion of the commissures of the valve leaflets). The bicuspid aortic valve is associated with an enlargement of the aorta

(with or without involvement of the aortic root) and occasionally with aortic coarctation in about half of the affected individuals. Increased shear forces lead to early degeneration, necessitating aortic valve replacement in about a quarter of the affected individuals (mostly under the age of 50).

Classification The severity of aortic valve stenosis is defined by the valve opening area (normal 4 cm^2). Severe aortic valve stenosis is present when the aortic valve opening area is ≤ 1 cm^2. Valvular aortic valve stenosis can be classified into four groups considering the transvalvular gradient, systolic left ventricular function, and stroke volume (◘ Table 9.1)

In addition to aortic valve stenosis, there are subvalvular and supravalvular aortic stenoses; these are rare and most commonly occur in combination with congenital malformations.

Pathophysiology A narrowing of the aortic valve leads to an increased transvalvular gradient between the left ventricle and the ascending aorta, which is indirectly documented by the flow acceleration in Doppler echocardiography (Vmax in m/sec.). The increase in afterload results in a pressure rise in the left ventricle. According to the Laplace law, the increased wall tension leads to concentric hypertrophy of the left ventricle as a compensatory mechanism. An increase in myocardial mass results, on the one hand, in reduced compliance of the left ventricle and thus in diastolic dysfunction. On the other hand, it leads to increased oxygen consumption and reduced coronary flow reserve potentially associated with ischaemia and angina.

Cardiac sequelae of chronic pressure overload are not limited to the left ventricle (hypertrophy, diastolic dysfunction) but can also lead to secondary mitral regurgitation and enlargement of the left atrium as an expression of congestion in the long run, and eventually affect the pulmonary circulation (i.e. pulmonary hypertension, right ventricular dysfunction and tricuspid regurgitation). These complications can be used to delineate different stages of the disease and are of prognostic relevance. Degenerative aortic valve stenosis can further lead to atrioventricular conduction disturbances

◘ **Table 9.1** Types of aortic stenosis and their hemodynamic characteristics

Types of aortic valve stenosis	Mean transvalvular pressure gradient	LVEF	Indexed stroke volume	Remarks
High-gradient aortic valve stenosis	≥ 40 mmHg	–	–	Classic form of aortic valve stenosis
Low-flow/low-gradient aortic valve stenosis with impaired LV function	< 40 mmHg	< 50 %	≤ 35 ml/m^2	Low-dose dobutamine stress echocardiography recommended to exclude pseudo-severe aortic valve stenosis and to demonstrate contractile reserve
Low-flow/low-gradient aortic valve stenosis with preserved LV function	< 40 mmHg	≥ 50 %	≤ 35 ml/m^2	Diagnosis is supported by evidence of LV hypertrophy and advanced calcification
Normal-flow/low-gradient aortic valve stenosis	< 40 mmHg	≥ 50 %	> 35 ml/m^2	In the majority of cases, moderate aortic valve stenosis is present

due to the anatomical proximity to the conduction system.

Clinic Aortic valve stenosis often remains asymptomatic for a long time and manifests with a heart murmur during a routine clinical examination. The slow progression of the disease can mask a gradually increasing exercise intolerance and allow for a symptom-free daily life at a reduced activity level. At last, when clinical symptoms appear, action is required. Early detection of left ventricular dysfunction and/or clinical symptoms are therefore crucial.

Exertional dyspnea (NYHA I-IV; ▶ Sect. 13.2) is the most common symptom of aortic valve stenosis and can be attributed to increased left ventricular filling pressures and diastolic dysfunction. The combination of increased left ventricular filling pressure and increased myocardial oxygen consumption, together with shortened diastolic filling time can also lead to exertion-induced chest pain even in the absence of coronary artery disease. Additionally, a limited coronary flow reserve may unmask mild concomitant coronary artery disease, which is present in 20–50% of patients with aortic valve stenosis. Dizziness and (pre-)syncope during physical exertion occur less frequently and are indicative of cardiac arrhythmias or reduced left ventricular output.

Prognosis If left untreated, the prognosis of aortic valve stenosis is poor; although there is a long asymptomatic phase (◘ Fig. 9.2), remodeling of the left ventricle already occurs (Sects. 4.2 and 13.3) with clinical complications such as HFpEF or even HfrEF, arrhythmias and sudden cardiac death. With the onset of symptoms, life expectancy decreases rapidly (◘ Fig. 9.2).

Diagnostic Work-up Auscultation is at the forefront of the physical examination. Echocardiography is the method of choice to confirm the diagnosis and to grade the severity of aortic valve stenosis. An exercise test can be performed in asymptomatic patients to unmask hidden exercise intolerance. However, caution is advised in patients with advanced aortic stenosis. Cardiac catheterization and computed tomography are primarily used prior to a percutaneous or surgical intervention.

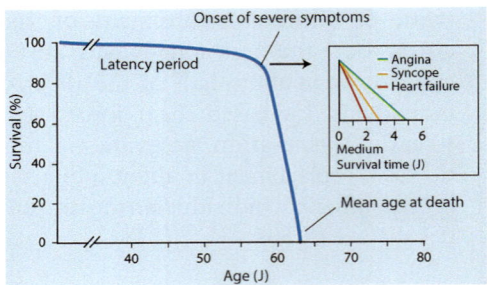

◘ **Fig. 9.2** Natural course of untreated aortic valve stenosis with a long asymptomatic latency period and rapid deterioration upon symptom onset

▪ **Physical Examination**

Auscultation is helpful in the diagnosis, but is not specific nor suitable for assessing the severity of aortic valve stenosis. As a correlate to the turbulent flow over the aortic valve, a spindle-shaped (crescendo-decrescendo), rough, low-frequency ejection murmur with a point of maximum intensity in the second intercostal space on the right or over Erb's point can typically be heard. Occasionally, the maximum intensity of the murmur is in the area of the apex. Radiation into the carotids can help differentiate the murmur from mitral valve regurgitation. A shift of the murmur to late systole and a weakening of the second heart sound may indicate an advanced degree of stenosis.

Palpation reveals a weak pulse with a delayed rise in blood pressure amplitude ("pulsus parvus et tardus"). At the same time, left ventricular hypertrophy may cause a lateral displacement of the apex beat.

▪ **Echocardiography** (◘ Fig. 9.3)

Transthoracic echocardiography allows for the differentiation of etiology, quantifica-

Valvular Heart Diseases

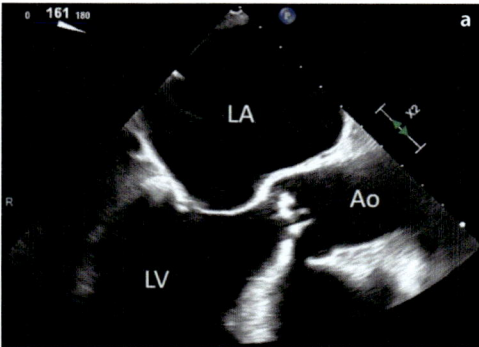

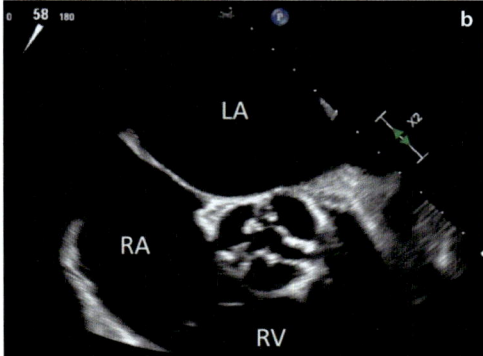

Fig. 9.3 a, b Echocardiographic findings in aortic valve stenosis. Transesophageal echocardiography of a degenerative tricuspid aortic valve stenosis in the long axis (**a**) and in the short axis (**b**). *Ao:* Aorta; *LA:* left atrium; *LV:* left ventricle; *RA:* right atrium; *RV:* right ventricle

tion of severity, and assessment of hemodynamic consequences of aortic valve stenosis as well as the dimensions of the ascending aorta. A definitive morphological assessment of the aortic valve is often only possible with transesophageal echocardiography. Using Doppler echocardiography, the maximum transaortic flow velocity can be measured and the mean gradient can be derived using the Bernoulli equation. With a flow velocity of > 4 m/s, a mean gradient of ≥ 40 mmHg severe aortic valve stenosis is present. The aortic valve opening area can be calculated using the continuity equation. A planimetric determination of the aortic valve opening area is often only relia-

bly possible with 3D-transesophageal echocardiography. At the same time, systolic LV function and stroke volume can be obtained with echocardiography, which allows classification of aortic valve stenosis into one of the types listed in ◘ Table 9.1.

- **Cardiac Catheterization**

Using left ventricular catheterization, the transvalvular gradient across the aortic valve can be invasively determined. At the same time, the coronary arteries are selectively visualized to detect any accompanying coronary artery disease. The valve opening area is calculated using the Gorlin formula. The cardiac output required for this formula is determined by thermodilution or calculated using the Fick principle. In right heart catheterization, the pulmonary arterial oxygen saturation value required for the latter is measured. At the same time, pulmonary, right ventricular, and right atrial pressure values, which have prognostic relevance, can be recorded (◘ Fig. 9.4).

- **Computed Tomography**

Computed tomography is helpful for confirming low-flow/low-gradient aortic stenosis with preserved LV function (◘ Table 9.1). Using the Agatston score, the degree of calcification of the aortic valve can be determined, and thus the likelihood of severe stenosis estimated (◘ Fig. 9.5). Furthermore, computed tomography is crucial for planning a transcatheter aortic valve implantation (TAVI-CT) in patients with aortic valve stenosis requiring treatment.

Therapy Currently, there are no medications that have been proven to delay the progression of degenerative aortic valve stenosis. However, a first possibility might soon open up for patients with elevated lipoprotein(a) levels (e.g. PCSK9 inhibitors, antisense oligonucleotides and siRNAs).

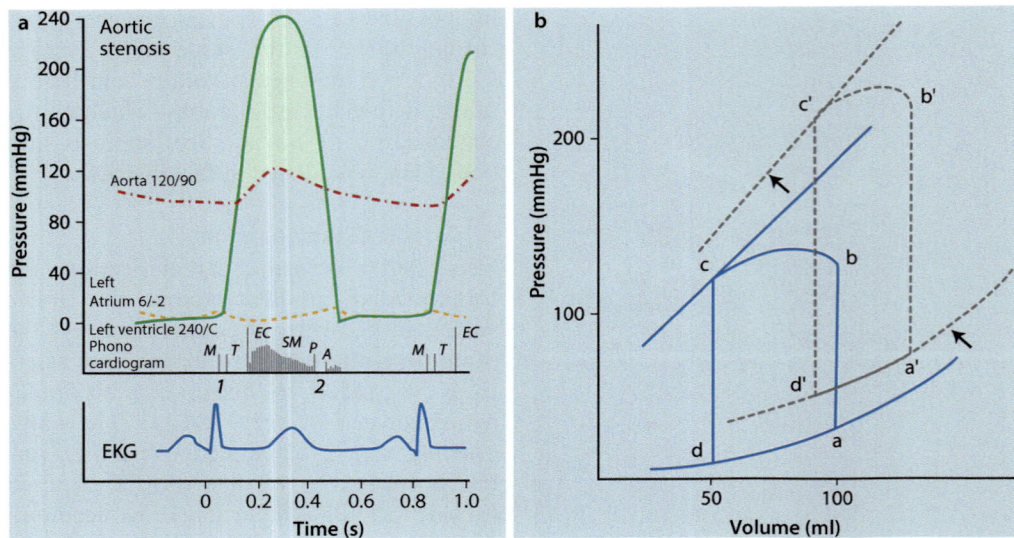

Fig. 9.4 a, b a Hemodynamic conditions in the aorta, left ventricle, and left atrium in relation to the ECG and phonocardiogram in aortic stenosis, **b** pressure-volume curve in the left ventricle in normal condition (solid line) and in aortic stenosis (dashed line)

Since patients with aortic valve stenosis often have cardiac comorbidities, cardiovascular secondary prevention is recommended. The treatment of severe aortic valve stenosis consists of valve replacement using a mechanical or biological prosthesis. The optimal timing of aortic valve replacement is determined by the severity of the stenosis, now even with or without the occurrence of clinical symptoms or the presence of comorbidities (e.g. coronary artery disease) requiring intervention and ideally occurs before the onset of long-term side effects such as a decrease in left ventricular ejection fraction, evidence of pulmonary arterial hypertension, or the occurrence of atrial fibrillation.

Depending on life expectancy, comorbidities, and morphology, different aortic valve replacement procedures are used.

Mechanical Aortic Valve Replacement

Mechanical aortic valve replacement is a permanent solution for the treatment of aortic valve stenosis in patients < 50–60 years. However, mechanical aortic valve replacement requires lifelong oral anticoagulation with vitamin K antagonists to prevent thrombus formation in the valve leaflets.

Autograft/Ross Procedure

A Ross Procedure is an alternative to mechanical aortic valve replacement in adolescents and young adults (< 45 years) who wish to avoid long-term oral anticoagulation (e.g., young women with a desire to have children). In this procedure, the aortic valve is replaced with the patient's pulmonary valve (autograft). The removed pulmonary valve is replaced with a homograft or a xenograft. However, the procedure is only performed in experienced centers.

Biological Aortic Valve Replacement

Bioprostheses do not require oral anticoagulation, but have limited durability (with increasing durability with increasing age), which may necessitate a repeat aortic valve

Valvular Heart Diseases

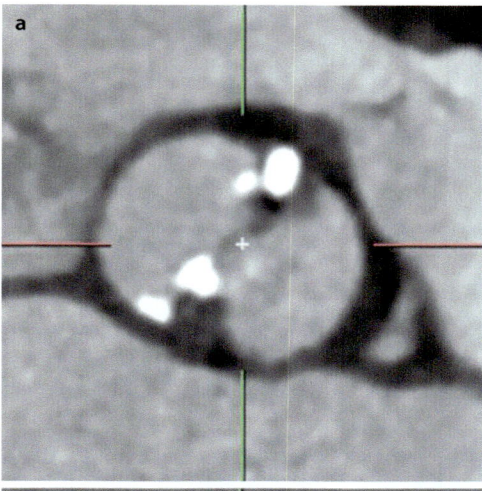

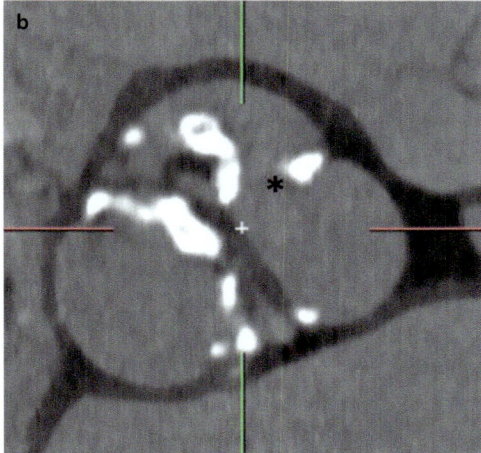

Fig. 9.5 a, b Computed tomographic image of a bicuspid aortic valve in the short axis. a Bicuspid aortic valve without raphe; b bicuspid aortic valve with raphe (*) between the right coronary and left coronary cusps

replacement after 10–20 years. For this reason, bioprostheses are suitable for patients who cannot tolerate or do not wish oral anticoagulation, those whose life expectancy is shorter than the durability of the bioprosthesis, and individuals > 65 years. Aortic valve bioprostheses can be implanted conventionally surgically via a sternotomy requiring cardioplegia and a heart-lung machine.

■ **Transcatheter Aortic Valve Implantation**
Transcatheter aortic valve implantation (TAVI; ◘ Fig. 9.6) represents a newer therapeutic alternative, which is now most frequently performed. In this procedure, a stented aortic valve bioprosthesis is implanted under local anesthesia, usually retrogradely via the femoral artery (> 95%) in a beating heart. Unlike the surgical procedure, the native aortic valve leaflets are not removed, but are pressed against the aortic wall in a permanently open position. TAVI aortic valve prostheses are differentiated into balloon-expandable and self-expanding prostheses according to the release mechanism. The latter can be repositionable during the procedure. TAVI significantly shortens the recovery time and restoration of quality of life compared to surgical aortic valve replacement. The TAVI procedure is the method of choice for older patients (> 70–75 years) and those with increased perioperative risk. With increasing experience and improvement of materials, TAVI procedures are also considered in selected patients < 70 years and those with low surgical risk.

▶ **Practical Decision Making**

TAVI vs. Surgical Aortic Valve Replacement
The two treatment modalities for the treatment of aortic valve stenosis in older patients showed comparable results in several randomized studies regarding mortality and the occurrence of a stroke over a follow-up period of up to 5 years. In TAVI, compared to surgical aortic valve replacement, there is an increased risk of paravalvular aortic valve regurgutation and atrioventricular conduction disorder requiring a pacemaker. In contrast, patients with surgical aortic valve replacement more frequently experience bleeding complications, renal failure, and atrial fibrillation.
The choice of the appropriate treatment strategy in individual cases depends on the

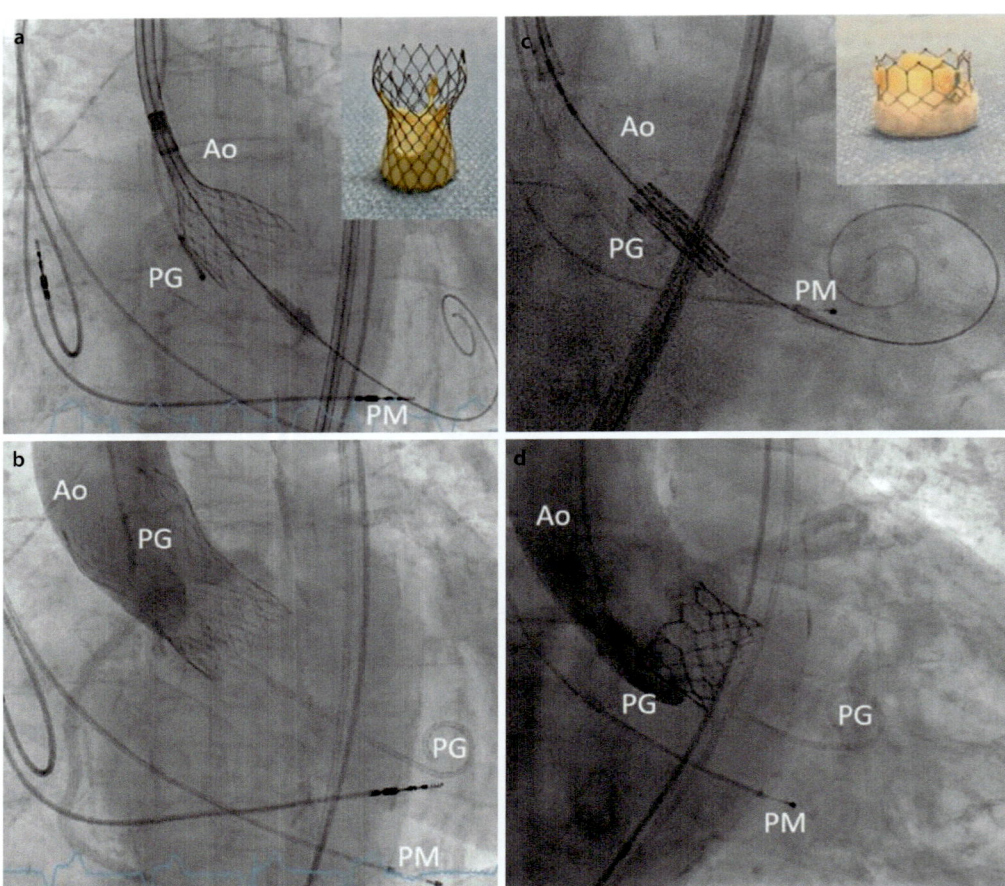

Fig. 9.6 **a–d** Fluoroscopy of a transcatheter aortic valve implantation with a self-expanding biopro-sthesis (**a, b**) and a balloon-expandable bioprosthesis (**c, d**). *Ao:* Aorta, *PG* Pigtail catheter, *PM:* temporary pacemaker in the right ventricle

presence of comorbidities (coronary heart disease, combined valve defects), life expectancy, and the anatomical conditions in the area of the aortic valve complex (cuspidity, extent and distribution of calcification, distance to coronary ostium) and the peripheral access vessels (diameter, tortuosity, degree of calcification of femoral and iliac arteries).

Degenerated bioprostheses can be treated using transcatheter aortic valve implantation (*Valve-in-Valve*). This facilitates the decision for a bioprosthesis in younger patients and has far-reaching consequences for planning a long-term strategy in patients with aortic valve stenosis. ◄

9.2 Aortic Valve Insufficiency

Definition Aortic valve regurgitation is characterized by an inadequate closure of the aortic valve with diastolic backflow into the left ventricle. The regurgitant volume leads to a volume overload on the left ventricle.

Epidemiology Aortic valve regurgitation is markedly less common than aortic valve stenosis and occurs in isolation or in combination with other valve defects or diseases of the aortic root and ascending aorta. Aortic valve regurgitation is more

Valvular Heart Diseases

common in men and typically manifests itself between the ages of 50 and 70 years.

Etiology The causes of aortic valve regurgitation are diverse (◨ Table 9.2) and are etiologically divided into primary diseases of the aortic valve leaflets and secondary aortic valve regurgitation due to diseases of the aortic root and ascending aorta. Additionally, a distinction is made between acute and chronic aortic valve regurgitation. Infective endocarditis is the most common cause of acute primary aortic valve regurgitation, while the degeneration of a bicuspid or tricuspid aortic valve is the most common form of chronic primary aortic valve regurgitation in the Western world. Secondary aortic valve regurgitation due to disease of the aortic root or ascending aorta is now the most common cause of aortic valve regurgitation. In the acute setting, severe aortic regurgitation occurs often in the context of aortic dissection (see ► Chap. 15.2)

Classification The classification of aortic valve regurgitation is based on etiology and type of clinical presentation (acute vs. chronic) (◨ Table 9.2). The severity of aortic valve regurgitation is primarily determined by echocardiography (◨ Table 9.3). In the presence of severe aortic valve regurgitation, it is important to watch for early signs of left ventricular dilation and dysfunction in asymptomatic patients to prevent irreversible myocardial damage.

Pathophysiology Aortic valve regurgitation primarily caused by a pathology of the aortic leaflets is based on reduced mobility and thus on a diastolic coaptation disorder of the degeneratively calcified or destructed valve leaflets (the latter typical due to infective endocarditis). Secondary aortic valve regurgitation due to diseases of the aortic root or ascending aorta is commonly due to annular dilation, leading to a coaptation disorder or a geometric distortion of the annular plane. Aortic dissection can also lead to annular dilation or cause aortic regurgitation due to intimal intussusception during diastole (◨ Fig. 9.7).

An inadequate closure of the aortic valve leads, regardless of the underlying etiology, to diastolic backflow of blood into the left ventricle. This results in a regurgitant volume and a volume overload on the left ventricle. In chronic aortic regurgitation, the backflow is initially compensated via the Frank-Starling mechanism with an increase in stroke volume. This leads to long-term eccentric hypertrophy with enlargement of the left ventricle (in extreme cases *Cor bovinum*).

◨ **Table 9.2** Causes of Aortic Valve Regurgitationy

Anatomical Involvement	Acute	Chronic
Aortic Valve Leaflets	Infective Endocarditis	Rheumatic Heart Disease Degeneration of the Native Aortic Valve (due to calcification or myxomatous changes) Degeneration of an Aortic Valve Bioprosthesis
Aortic Root/Ascending Aorta	Aortic Dissection	Aortic Aneurysm as a Result of Long-standing Uncontrolled Hypertension or Marfan Syndrome, Ehlers-Danlos Syndrome, or Osteogenesis Imperfecta Aortitis (Takayasu Arteritis, Syphilis, Lupus Erythematosus)
Combined Valve Defects	Aortic Stenosis and Regurgitation	Bicuspid Aortic Valve Ankylosing Spondylitis

Table 9.3 Classification of the severity of aortic regurgitation

Criterion	Light	Moderate	Heavy
Qualitative			
Color Doppler jet width*	Central; width <25% of the LVOT*	Between light and heavy	Central; width >25% of LVOT*
Doppler Vena contracta (= narrowest diameter of the flow stream in cm)	<0.3	0.3-0.6	>0.6
Qualitative (catheter or echo)			
Regurgitation volume (ml/beat)*	<30	30-59	>60
Regurgitation fracture (%)*			
Regurgitation opening (cm²)*	<0.10	0.10-0.29	>0.30

*LVOT: left ventricular outflow tract; color Doppler jet width: width of the aortic regurgitation jet in color Doppler (◘ Fig. 9.8); regurgitation volume and fraction can be calculated using various echocardiographic or invasive measurements

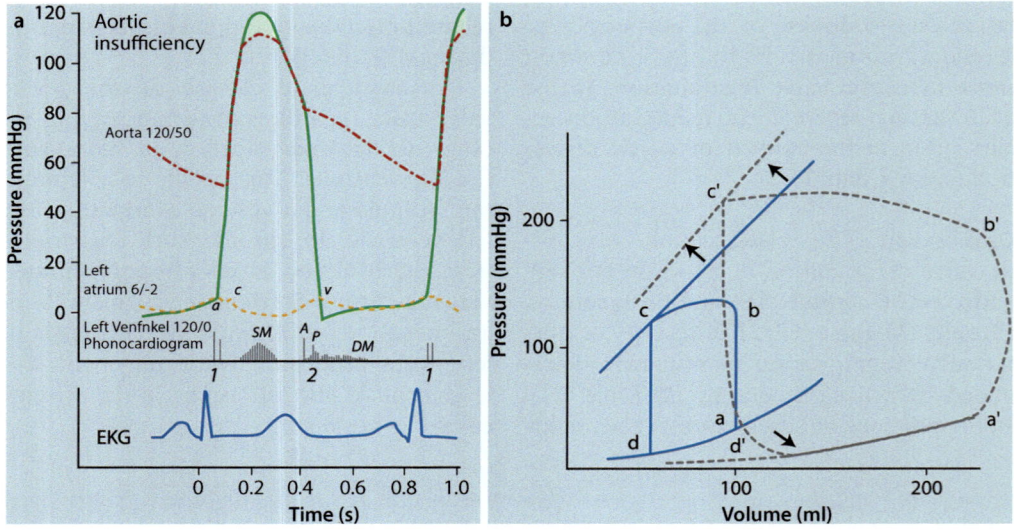

◘ **Fig. 9.7** a, b a **Hemodynamic conditions** in the aorta, left ventricle, and left atrium in relation to the ECG and phonocardiogram in aortic valve regurgitation, b **Pressure-volume loops** in the left ventricle under normal conditions (solid line) and in aortic valve regurgitation (dashed line)

In acute aortic regurgitation, there is no compensatory enlargement of the left ventricle as under chronic conditions. In contrast, the sudden backflow of blood leads to a significant increase in end-diastolic pressure in the left ventricle and to a pressure equalization with diastolic aortic pressure. A reduced forward flow results in compensatory tachycardia. Left untreated, severe acute aortic insufficiency will lead to cardiogenic shock due to insufficient compensatory mechanisms.

Clinical Presentation Aortic valve regurgitation often remains asymptomatic for a long time. Exertional dyspnea is, along with insidious exercise intolerance, the most common symptom. In the advanced stage, aortic regurgitation manifests as left ventricular dysfunction with signs of left heart failure. Simultaneously, due to increased myocardial oxygen consumption and low myocardial perfusion pressure, angina pectoris may occur.

Acute aortic valve regurgitation manifests with acute left heart decompensation with pulmonary edema, orthopnea, and resting dyspnea up to cardiogenic shock and sudden death.

Diagnostics Echocardiography is the primary imaging modality for assessing aortic valve regurgitation. Cardiac magnetic resonance imaging and computed tomography are supplementary modalities for grading the severity of aortic valve regurgitation and for precise measurement of aortic dimensions.

- **Physical Examination**

Chronic aortic valve regurgitation typically presents with a high-frequency diastolic murmur with a decrescendo character, with the point of maximum intensity parasternal in the 3rd or 4th intercostal space. Due to the increased stroke volume, a systolic ejection murmur may also be present in severe regurgitation. A mid-diastolic low-frequency murmur may be heard over the apex correlating with an echocardiographically detectable jet-induced vibration of the anterior mitral leaflet and mimicing mitral valve stenosis (Austin Flint murmur). In acute aortic valve regurgitation, a rough low-frequency murmur can be heard, which is limited to early diastole due to the rapid pressure equalization between the aorta and the left ventricle and is difficult to detect.

Tachycardia and a wide pulse pressure are other features of chronic aortic valve regurgitation ("*pulsus celer et altus*"). The latter can manifest with a "water hammer pulse" (*Corrigan Pulse*) and visible systolic pulsation of the nail bed with slight pressure (Quincke's sign). The regurgitant volume can lead to a systolic and diastolic murmur over the femoral arteries (Duroziez's sign). Very severe aortic valve regurgitation can result in head bobbing synchronous with the pulse (Musset's sign).

- **Echocardiography**

Transthoracic echocardiography allows for quantification of the severity of aortic valve regurgitation (◘ Table 9.3) and an assessment of the size and function of the left ventricle as well as the size of the aortic root and ascending aorta. Using Doppler ultrasound, a holodiastolic flow reversal in the descending aorta (◘ Fig. 9.8) (end-diastolic flow velocity > 20 cm/s) and the abdominal aorta can be documented in severe aortic valve regurgitation. In acute aortic valve regurgitation, transesophageal echocardiography can visualize a destruction of the aortic valve leaflets due to infectious endocarditis or detect dissection of the ascending aorta.

- **Cardiac Magnetic Resonance Imaging (MRI)**

Cardiac MRI allows for an accurate determination of the regurgitant volume and regurgitant fraction in patients with echocardiographically borderline severe aortic valve regurgitation, as well as an exact determination of left ventricular dimensions and mass. At the same time, cardiac MRI allows for the early detection of subclinical myocardial damage in individuals with asymptomatic aortic valve regurgitation.

- **Computed Tomography**

Computed tomography can quantify aortic valve regurgitation and accurately determine the diameter of the aortic root and ascending aorta in patients with aortic aneurysm. At the same time, in younger patients with a low-risk profile, the coronary arteries can be preoperatively assessed (as an alternative to coronary angiography). Computed tomography is also the gold standard for detecting aortic dissection.

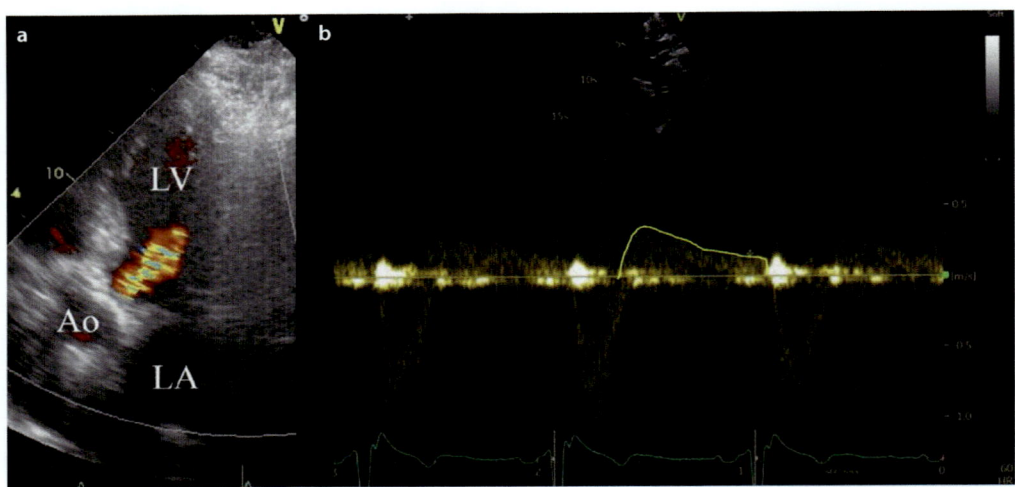

Fig. 9.8 a, b a Color Doppler findings in aortic valve regurgitation (*Ao:* Aorta, *LA:* left atrium, LV: left ventricle). **b** Doppler echocardiography shows a holodiastolic flow reversal in the descending aorta with an end-diastolic flow velocity of 16 cm/s, corresponding to moderate aortic valve regurgitation

Therapy Symptomatic medical therapy of chronic aortic valve insufficiency consists of afterload reduction using ACE inhibitors or calcium antagonists (dihydropyridines). In patients with Marfan syndrome, beta-blockers are also used to reduce wall tension in the area of the aortic aneurysm to prevent dissection. However, prolongation of diastole due to betablocker-induced bradycardia can functionally exacerbate aortic regurgitation. Conversely, patients with acute aortic valve can benefit from an increase in heart rate using a temporary pacemaker, as the regurgitant volume decreases under these conditions.

Aortic valve regurgitation should be surgically treated before the onset of clinical symptoms when there are signs of myocardial strain (e.g. increaes in natriuretic peptides), early signs of left ventricualr dilation or a decrease in systolic left ventricular function. Often, left ventricular damage occurs in asymptomatic patients, which must be prevented. Close monitoring using echocardiography is therefore crucial. In patients with an aortic aneurysm, the timing of surgery also depends on the diameter of the ascending aorta (▶ Chap. 15). Treatment usually consists of surgical aortic valve replacement; in patients with an aneurysm of the ascending aorta as the cause of aortic valve regurgitation, a valve-sparing procedure might be possible. TAVI is not suitable for aortic insufficiency due to the usually low or absent calcifications, as embolization of the valve can occur during implantation. Newer TAVI valves specifically designed for the treatment of aortic valve regurgitation by self-anchoring within the aortic leaflets are in development (Jena Valve). TAVI in degenerated aortic valve bioprostheses (*Valve-in-Valve*) is , is increasingly being used, particualrly in large bioprosthesis.

▶ **Practical Management**

Both surgical aortic valve replacement and TAVI can result in peri- or postoperative para- or transvalvular aortic valve regurgitation. Paravalvular leaks occur in TAVI due to inadequate sealing of the aortic valve ring (e.g., in patients with asymmetric calcification of the native valve leaflets or the left ventricular outflow tract) or due to suture insufficiency in surgically replaced valves. Quantifying paravalvular leaks is often difficult because multiple small jets may be present. ◄

9.3 Mitral Valve Stenosis

Definition The normal valve opening area of the mitral valve is 4–6 cm². When the opening area is < 2 cm², a diastolic pressure gradient occurs between the left atrium and the left ventricle. A stenosis is considered significant when the valve opening is ≤ 1.5 cm² (◘ Fig. 9.9).

Epidemiology The prevalence of mitral valve stenosis has decreased with the early diagnosis and antibiotic treatment of streptococcal infections in childhood. In regions with endemic rheumatic heart disease (sub-Saharan Africa, Southeast Asia, Oceania), rheumatic mitral valve stenosis is still quite common.

Etiology The causes of mitral stenosis are:
- **Rheumatic**: the most common form (80% of cases), occurring about 20 years after an episode of rheumatic fever. It leads to an inflammatory fusion of one or both commissures with thickening, fibrosis, and shrinkage of the mitral leaflets. Up to one-third of patients have additional valve involvement (aortic and/or tricusoid regurgitation).
- **Congenital**: usually symptoms already in childhood
- **Degenerative/calcifying**: mainly in older patients and associated with severe renal failure, aortic valve stenosis. Here, calcification of the annulus is primarily observed without commissural fusion of the mitral leaflets.
- **Rare causes**: e.g., in the context of systemic lupus erythematosus, rheumatoid arthritis

Classification The severity of mitral valve stenosis is assessed based on the transvalvular gradient (◘ Table 9.4).

Pathophysiology Due to the reduced opening of the mitral valve, there is a backlog of blood into the atria and lungs, which can lead to an increase in pulmonary venous and arterial pressure and eventually right heart failure. On the other hand, reduced ventricular filling during diastole leads to a reduction in cardiac output. (◘ Fig. 9.12).

Clinical Presentation The symptoms of mitral valve stenosis develop insidiously over the years and are primarily dependent on the severity of the stenosis. Key symptoms are dyspnea (up to pulmonary edema) and arrhythmias (especially atrial fibrillation, particularly with significant dilation of the left atrium). Atrial fibrillation leads to the loss of AV synchrony as well as a further decrease in cardiac output due to the loss of atrial contractility. In severe cases, it can lead to the full clinical picture of severe heart failure. Rheumatic mitral valve stenosis often first manifests in young women during pregnancy. Due to an increase in cardiac output and a reduction in systemic vascular resistance, acute decompensation can occur during pregnancy (◘ Fig. 9.10).

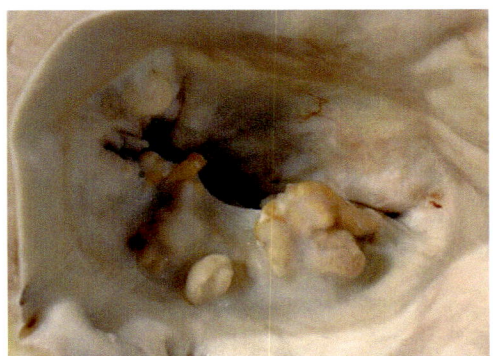

◘ Fig. 9.9 Severely calcified mitral valve. View from the left atrium. (Courtesy of Prof. Dr. Paul Vogt, University Hospital Zurich)

◘ **Table 9.4** Classification of mitral valve stenosis by severity based on the transvalvular pressure gradient, pul-monary arterial pressure increase, and valve opening area

Criterion	Mild	Moderate	Severe
Mean gradient (mmHg)	< 5	5–10	> 10
Systolic pulmonary arterial pressure (mmHg)	< 30	30–50	> 50
Valve opening area (cm²)	> 1.5	1.0–1.5	< 1.0

> Thrombus formation in the left atrium during atrial fibrillation and consequent systemic embolisms (especially to the brain with TIA or stroke) are a feared and not uncommon complication of mitral stenosis. The risk of thromboembolism in patients with rheumatic mitral stenosis is significantly higher than in patients with atrial fibrillation of other etiologies.

Diagnostics Patients with pronounced mitral stenosis often exhibit the typical appearance of "facies mitralis"—bluish-red cheeks and bluish lips. Upon auscultation, a pounding first heart sound, which results from the abrupt closure of the stiff valve, as well as a mitral valve opening sound, which arises from the snapping opening of the valve, can be heard. After the MÖT, a diastolic rumble is audible, caused by the turbulent diastolic blood flow through the valve.

As with all valve defects, transthoracic echocardiography is the method of choice in the diagnosis of mitral valve stenosis. In addition to assessing the morphology of the valve leaflets (◘ Fig. 9.11a), the valve

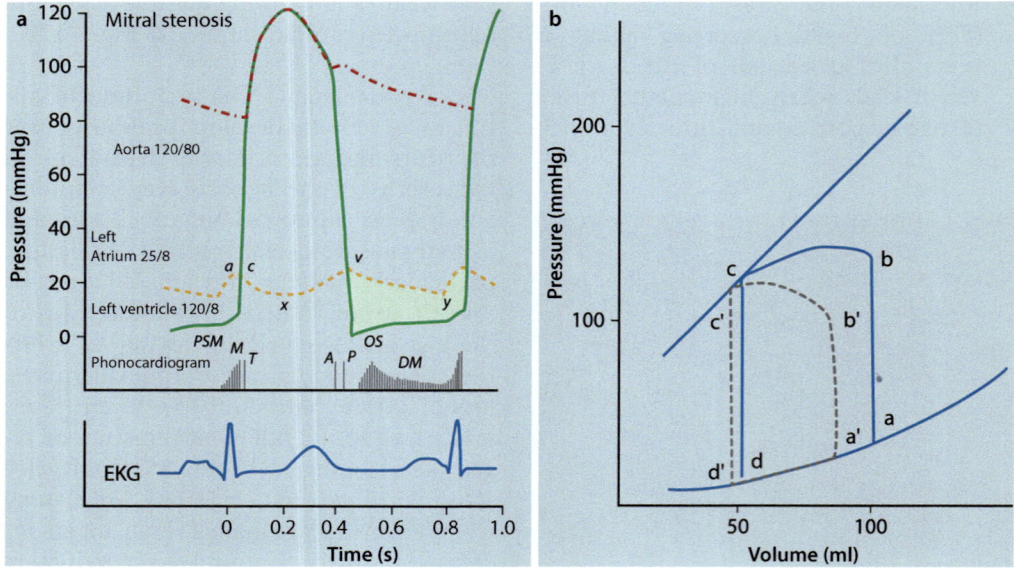

◘ **Fig. 9.10** a, b a **Hemodynamic conditions** of the aorta, left ventricle, and left atrium in relation to the ECG and phonocardiogram in mitral stenosis, b **Pressure-volume curve** in the left ven-tricle in normal condition (solid line) and in mitral valve stenosis (dashed line)

Valvular Heart Diseases

opening area, the gradient across the valve (◉ Fig. 9.11b), and other important parameters (such as regurgitation, atrial size, ejection fraction) are determined. Transesophageal echocardiography is used for further assessement of valve morphology, planning of percutaneous mitral valve valvuloplasty, and exclusion of thrombi in the left atrial appendage. In a detailed invasive examination, the pressure conditions and gradients can be directly determined using combined left and right heart catheterization.

Therapy To alleviate symptoms or control them, diuretic therapy can be initiated. If **atrial fibrillation** is present concomitantly or if a cerebrovascular accident has already occurred, oral anticoagulation with vitamin K antagonists and a target INR of 2–3 is mandatory. NOACs are less effective in mitral valve stenosis than vitamin K antagonists and are therefore not recommended. To maintain atrioventricular synchrony, cardioversion can be performed after appropriate exclusion of intracardiac thrombi (TEE or cardiac CT). Rhythm or rate control optimize the filling time, which often represents the limiting factor of cardiac output in mitral stenosis.

The therapy of choice to reduce valve narrowing, given suitable anatomy, is **percutaneous mitral valve valvuloplasty** (◉ Fig. 9.12). If anatomical and clinical aspects make a successful valvuloplasty unlikely, surgical valve replacement should be considered.

▶ **Practical Aspects**

Mitral Valve Valvuloplasty
In percutaneous mitral valve valvuloplasty, the fused commissurs of the mitral leaflets of the stenotic valve are split using a special balloon (Inoue balloon with differential expansion of the ventricular and atrial balloon halves) (◉ Fig. 9.12), which usually results in a doubling of the valve opening area. For mitral valve valvuloplasty, after transseptal puncture, a balloon is advanced from the femoral vein into the left atrium and antegradely across the mitral valve, where first the distal or ventricular and thereafter the proximal or atrial balloon is inflated. Not every mitral stenosis is suitable for valvuloplasty. The success (which can be estimated using specially developed scores) depends primarily on the degree of calcification, the mobility of the leaflets, and the simultaneous presence of mitral regurgitation. The main risk of mitral valve valvuloplasty is the development of severe mitral regurgitation as a result of valve rupture. ◀

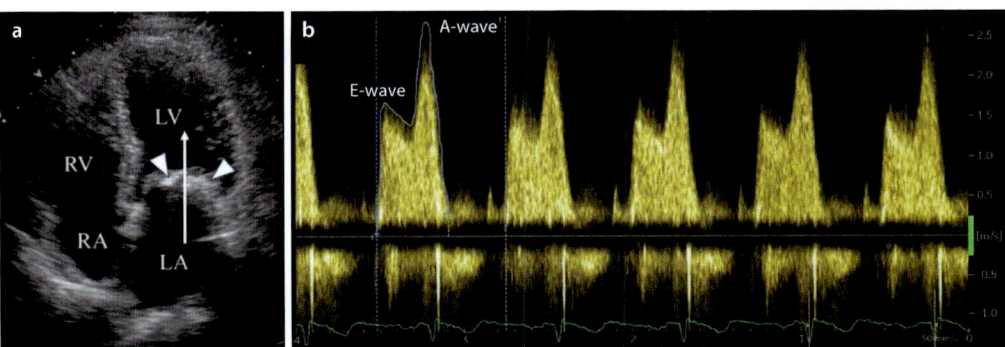

◉ **Fig. 9.11 a, b a** Echocardiographic finding in severely calcified mitral valve in the 4-chamber view. The continuous-wave Doppler measures the mitral inflow with significantly increased flow velocity in early diastole (E-wave) and pronounced atrial kick (A-wave). A maximum flow velocity through the stenotic valve of approximately 2.6 m/sec is observed, with the mean diastolic gradient being approximately 13 mmHg

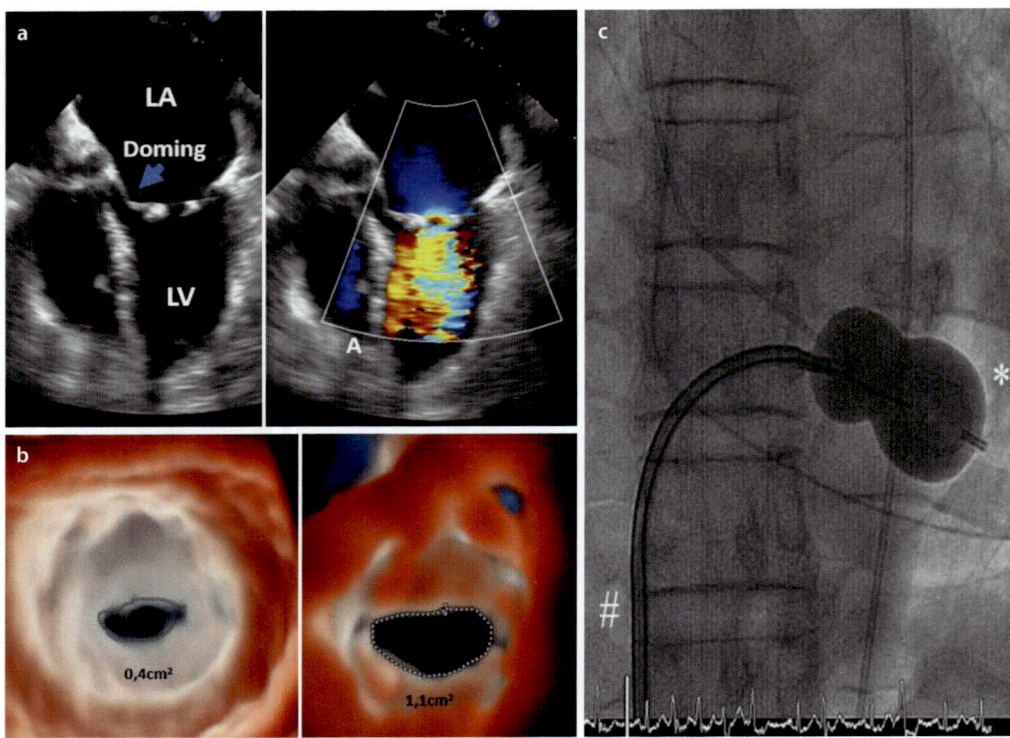

Fig. 9.12 a–c a Transesophageal image of severe mitral valve stenosis with typical doming of the anterior mitral valve leaflet as well as rheumatic thickening of the leaflet edges and flow acceleration in the color Doppler between the left atrium and left ventricle (proximal convergence zone in the LA). **b** Three-dimensional imaging of the anatomical mitral valve opening area before (left; 0.4 cm^2) and after mitral valve balloon valvuloplasty (right; 1.1 cm^2). **c** Fluoroscopic image during a mitral valve valvuloplasty. Transseptal sheath (#), valvuloplasty balloon (*).

9.4 Mitral Valve Insufficiency

Definition In mitral valve regurgitation (short form: mitral regurgtation or MR), there is an inadequate closure of the mitral valve. As a result of the regurgitant volume between the left atrium and left ventricle, there is a volume load of these two cardiac chambers.

Epidemiology For isolated moderate to severe MR, a prevalence of 0.59% in adults without significant gender differences is assumed.

Etiology
- **Primary Mitral Regurgitation** (structural change of the valve apparatus):
  – Mitral valve prolapse
  – Chordal rupture, myxomatous degeneration, Barlow's disease
  – Rheumatic changes
  – Endocarditis (valve perforation, chordal rupture; ▶ Sect. 10.1)
  – Congenital (so-called cleft, anterior/posterior)
  – Papillary muscle rupture (acute MR in infarction)
- **Secondary/functional mitral regurgitation** (initially structurally normal valve apparatus) with coaptation disorder of the mitral leaflets:
  – Ischemic: often papillary muscle dysfunction/tethering of the chordae tendineae

Valvular Heart Diseases

Table 9.5 Classification of mitral regurgitation by severity

Criterion	Light	Moderate	Heavy
Qualitative			
Color-Doppler Jet width	Small, central jet (<4cm² or <20% of the left atrial area)	Between light and heavy	Vena contracta width >0.7 cm with large central jet (>40% of the left atrial area)
Doppler Vena contracta (= narrowest diameter of the flow stream in cm)	<0.3	0.3–0.69	≥0.7
Quantitative (cardiac catheterization or echo)			
Regurgitation volume (ml/beat)	<30	30–59	≥60
Regurgitation fraction (%)	<30	30–49	50
Regurgitation opening (cm²)	<0.20	0.20–0.39	0.40

Color Doppler jet width = width of the mitral regurgitation jet in color Doppler, ◘ Fig. 9.14

- Atrial or ventricular annular dilation and leaflet restriction (tethering), e.g., in dilated cardiomyopathy (▶ Sect. 8.1) or atrial pathologies, e.g., due to heart failure (▶ Chap. 13) or atrial fibrillation (▶ Sect. 12.5)

Classification A distinction is made depending on the time course of development between acute (primarily in papillary muscle rupture in the context of myocardial infarction; Sect. 7.3) and the more common chronic mitral insufficiency. For further classification, see ◘ Table 9.5.

Pathophysiology Mitral regurgitation results from one or more mechanisms involving dysfunction of the annulus, leaflets, chordae, papillary muscles, or the left ventricle and is classified using the Carpentier classification. In MR, the left ventricle pumps a variable portion of the stroke volume back into the atrium due to the leaky mitral valve and the low left atrial resistance. The extent of this regurgitant volume determines the degree of regurgitation and in turn heart rate, left atrial pressure, and left ventricular pressure. Due to the additional filling of the left atrium, the left ventricle is also overfilled during diastole, which means it must consistently eject a larger stroke volume (◘ Fig. 9.13). This leads to long-term dilatation and eccentric hypertrophy of the left ventricle and the development of heart failure and as a consequence an increase in pulmonary pressure.

> Atrial fibrillation often develops secondarily in MR, especially with significant dilatation of the left atrium with atrial fibrillation leading to loss of AV synchrony and associated thromboembolic risk.

Clinical Presentation Chronic MR is usually asymptomatic in mild to moderate cases. Even chronic severe MR often remains oligo- or asymptomatic for a long time (years). Symptoms indicate impairment of left ventricular function and clinically are manifested as exercise intolerance and dyspnea, often with pulmonary congestion. Acute MR can, depending on severity, also lead to the sudden onset of pulmonary edema (so-called *flash pulmonary edema*) up to cardiogenic shock and sudden death.

Diagnostics Upon auscultation, a high-frequency, band-shaped, holosystolic murmur can be heard after the first heart sound

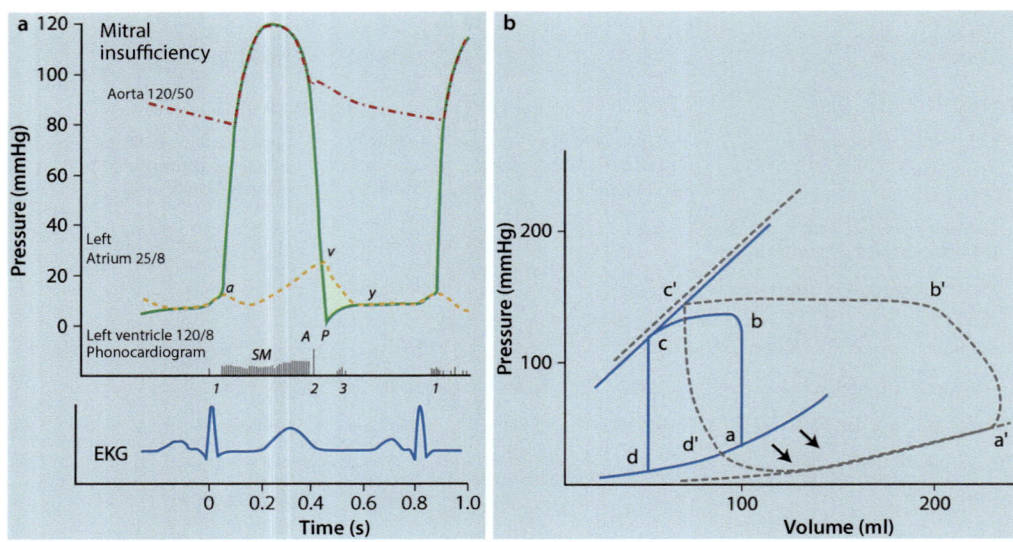

Fig. 9.13 a, b **Hemodynamic conditions** of the aorta, left ventricle, and left atrium in relation to the ECG and phonocardiogram in mitral regurgitation, **b Pressure-volume curve** in the left ventricle in normal condition (solid line) and in mitral regurgitation (dashed line)

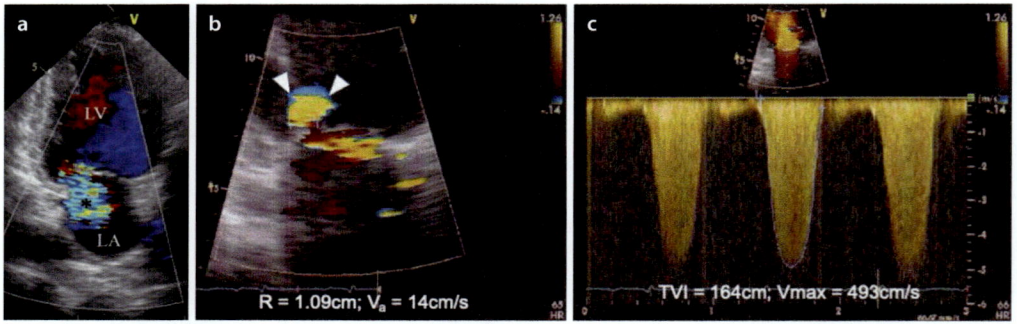

Fig. 9.14 a–c a Color Doppler of mild to moderate mitral regurgitation with a broad signal (*) in the left atrium (*LA*), *LV*: left ventricle). **b** In transesophageal echocardiography, a significant backflow into the left atrium over the mitral valve (arrows) is shown... **c** Continuous-wave Doppler signal over the mitral valve with jet into the left atrium TVI. V_{max}: maximum velocity of the jet over the mitral valve

in MR, corresponding to the backflow of blood into the left atrium and best auscultated in the left lateral position in the axilla.

In severe MR, the loudness of the systolic murmur can be significantly lower than in mild regurgitation due to rapid pressure equalization and a widely open mitral valve (with the absence of turbulence causing the murmur).

> The loudness of the systolic murmur does not indicate the severity of mitral regurgitation.

In addition to the clinical examination, transthoracic echocardiography is also the diagnostic method of choice here (Fig. 9.14). Using echocardiography, valve morphology, the mechanism of insufficiency, the grading of mitral regurgitation can be assessed (◘ Table 9.5), as well as other structural pathologies and left ventricular ejection fraction. Transesophageal echocardiography is used for detailed assessment of the underlying pathology and for planning minimally invasive or surgical therapy. Invasive right heart catheterization can measure left atrial pressure in wedge position and be helpful for typical indications of severe MR (high V-wave).

Therapy The treatment of mitral valve regurgitation is essentially determined by its etiology and severity.

- **Primary Mitral Valve Regurgitation**

In general, the indication for surgery is given in case of symptomatic, severe primary MR. Further surgical indications for primary MR include a drop in ejection fraction ≤ 60%, the occurrence of atrial fibrillation, pronounced left ventricular dilation ≥ 40 mm end-systolic diameter, pulmonary hypertension > 50 mmHg, and pronounced left atrial dilation (in the case of a valve that is highly likely to be reconstructable).

> ▶ **Practical**
>
> Surgical mitral valve reconstruction (MVR) is the treatment of choice for the correction of primary MR, as it is superior to mitral valve replacement in terms of perioperative morbidity and mortality as well as long-term outcomes. In particular, the preservation of the physiological suspension of the mitral leaflets maintains ventricular geometry, which has a favorable effect on ventricular mechanics and corresponding remodeling processes. Another important advantage of MVR is that lifelong anticoagulation is not necessary, while mechanical vlaves require strict anticoagulation due to high thrombogenicity. ◀

Surgical reconstruction of the mitral valve is preferable to valve replacement because it preserves the structure of the left ventricle. Whether a mitral valve is reconstructable depends on both the underlying mechanism of mitral regurgitation and the valve morphology. Acute severe MR (e.g., in the case of leaflet rupture during a myocardial infarction) generally constitutes an emergency indication for surgical repair.

In patients with very high perioperative risk who meet the anatomical requirements for a mitral valve transcatheter edge-to-edge repair (M-TEER), such a procedure should be considered (see below).

- **Secondary Mitral Valve Regurgitation**

Treatment of secondary MR initially consists of optimizing medical heart failure therapy with angiotensin II receptor antagonists and neprilysin inhibitors, beta-blockers, mineralocorticoid receptor antagonists, and SGLT-2 inhibitors (▶ Sect. 13.4). This reduces afterload and increases forward output, which can lead to reverse remodeling of the left ventricle and atrium. Cardiac resynchronization therapy (CRT; ▶ Sect. 13.4) can also reduce the severity of MR and should be performed within the indications (i.e. broad QRS complex with left bundle branch block pattern). Rhythm or rate control can also lead to a significant reduction in MR in the presence of concomitant atrial fibrillation.

Surgical therapy includes mitral valve reconstruction or mitral valve replacement. These are recommended, if another surgical therapy, particularly coronary bypass grafting, is indicated. The mitral valve transcatheter edge-to-edge repair (M-TEER) reduces mortality and hospitalizations due to heart failure in carefully selected patients with severe secondary mitral regurgitation due to left ventricular dysfunction.

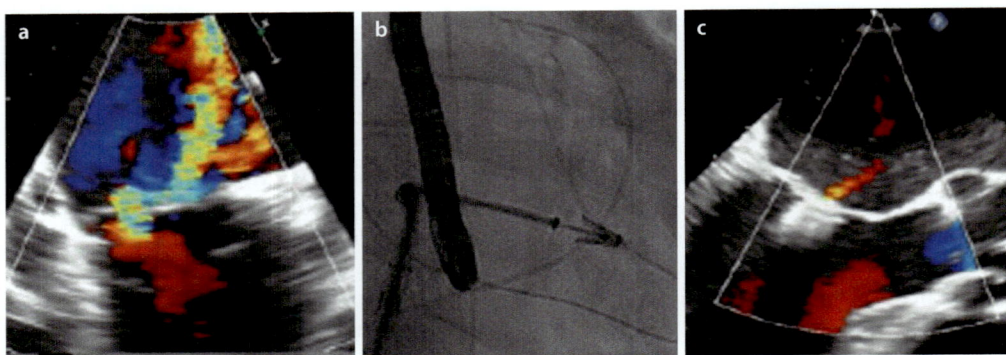

Fig. 9.15 **a–c a** Transesophageal echocardiography with severe eccentric mitral regurgitation due to prolapse of the posterior mitral leaflet, **b** fluoroscopic image during catheter-based mitral valve reconstruction using the edge-to-edge technique, **c** minimal residual mitral valve regurgitation after deployment of the device during catheter-based mitral valve reconstruction

▶ **Practical Aspects**

Interventional Mitral Valve Therapy

In patients with severe mitral regurgitation (◘ Fig. 9.15a) and low procedural risk, catheter-based mitral valve reconstruction (mitral valve edge-to-edge repair; M-TEER) is a very good therapeutic option. Among the catheter-based therapeutic procedures, M-TEER is the best-validated procedure (◘ Fig. 9.15b). In this procedure, a device similar to a clip is placed in the mitral valve via a venous access in the groin and after transseptal puncture (puncture of the interatrial septum), which fuses the anterior and posterior mitral leaflets at specific points, thereby sealing the mitral valve (◘ Fig. 9.15c) (Abbott Mitraclip® and Edwards Pascal™). Percutaneous mitral valve reconstruction is particularly suitable for patients with high surgical risk, as it can be performed without a heart-lung machine and very low per-procedural complications. ◀

9.5 Mitral Valve Prolapse

Definition Mitral valve prolapse (MVP) is based on a pathology of the mitral valve apparatus, the chordae tendineae, the papillary muscles, the mitral annulus, or the valve leaflets themselves.

Epidemiology MVP is common with a prevalence in the population depending on the definition of up to 2.4% and occurs more frequently in women than in men.

Etiology
Causes of mitral valve prolapse:
- familial (most common)
- connective tissue diseases (Marfan syndrome, Ehlers-Danlos syndrome)
- congenital or acquired heart diseases (Ebstein anomaly, atrial septal defect, hypertrophic cardiomyopathy)
- other non-cardiac diseases: hyperthyroidism, von Willebrand-Jürgens syndrome, osteogenesis imperfecta

Clinical Presentation The symptoms are determined by the severity of mitral regurgitation (◘ Table 9.4). The majority of patients with minimal mitral regurgitation are asymptomatic. Occasionally, symptoms such as palpitations, syncope, or chest pain may occur.

Diagnostics On auscultation, a characteristic systolic click and a mid- to late-systolic

9 Valvular Heart Diseases

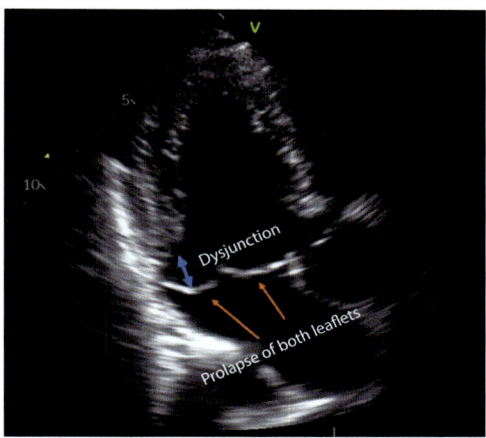

Fig. 9.16 Echocardiographic finding in mitral valve prolapse. It shows a prolapse of both mitral leaflets (red arrows) towards the left atrium beyond the valve plane, as well as an annulo-ventricular disjunction zone (blue arrow)

murmur can be heard. Auscultation, similar to that for mitral regurgitation, is best performed in the left lateral squatting position with the diaphragm of the stethoscope. Accordingly, the characteristic click can be heard earlier (i.e., sooner after S1).

Echocardiographically, the main criterion is the detection of the prolapse of one or both mitral leaflets 2 mm above the mitral annulus (Fig. 9.16). In the case of a systolic leaflet displacement of less than 2 mm, it is referred to as non-diagnostic forms of mitral valve prolapse, which are particularly significant in terms of progression.

Therapy In every patient with clinical fndings consistent with MVP, the diagnosis should be confirmed echocardiographically. With normal cardiac function and in the absence of risk factors or clinical signs of heart failure, the patient can engage in normal activities, but should be monitored echocardiographically every 3 years (earlier if symptoms occur). In the presence of moderate or severe mitral regurgitation, therapeutic steps should be initiated (▶ Sect. 9.4).

Prognosis In the vast majority of patients, the prognosis of isolated MVP is very good. Highly myxomatous valves have an increased risk of chordal rupture and the development of severe mitral regurgitation. Additionally, MVP has been associated with an increased risk of arrhythmias and sudden cardiac arrest or even death. Particularly in the presence of symptoms, long-term ECG monitoring is indicated for further diagnostics. Risk factors for sudden cardiac death in MVP include large numbers of ventricular extrasystoles, late gadolinium enhancement in the inferobasal or papillary muscle region on cardiac MRI, large annulo-ventricular disjunction zones (Fig. 9.16), and high tissue Doppler velocities in the area of the mitral annulus

9.6 Tricuspid Valve Insufficiency

Definition In tricuspid valve regurgitation (short version: tricuspid regurgitation, TR), there is an abnormal closure of the tricuspid valve, usually in connection with a dilation and/or dysfunction of the right ventricle. As a result of the pendulum volume between the right atrium and right ventricle, there is a volume load on these two heart chambers as well as the venous circulation.

Epidemiology A mild TR can be echocardiographically detected as a normal variant in up to 70% of the general population. The frequency of the defect increases exponentially with age and is moderate to severe in more than 4% of the population over 75 years old. TR has been underdiagnosed in the past, although it is associated with a significantly increased risk of mortality and heart failure.

Etiology The following causes of TR are distinguished:
- **Primary**: The primary form of TR is the rarest (about 5%) and usually occurs in

connection with trauma, infective endocarditis (especially intravenous drug use), rheumatic heart disease, carcinoid syndrome, myxomatous valve disease (Barlow's disease), congenital Ebstein anomaly, and iatrogenic valve damage (repeated endocardial biopsies, especially in heart transplant patients).

- **Secondary**: Secondary TR is the most common cause (90%) and arises either due to ventricular dilation or dysfunction or an enlargement of the right atrium as a result of chronic atrial fibrillation (atrial or isolated tricuspid regurgitation). In the majority of patients (about 60%), there is a left-sided problem with secondary pulmonary arterial hypertension or primary or mixed pulmonary arterial hypertension (about 20%).
- **Pacemaker-induced**: Pacemaker-induced TR represents a separate entity due to its specific course and management. About 20–30% of patients who receive a right ventricular pacemaker/ICD/CRT lead can develop significant TR over time, which is mostly due to the interaction of the electrodes with the leaflets.

Classification The classification of the severity of TR is performed using transthoracic echocardiography and follows a multiparametric approach (◘ Table 9.6).

> Particularly noteworthy is the high variability of the regurgitant jet depending on the respiratory cycle, volume status, and intracardiac pressure conditions. This can lead to an underestimation of the severity of the regurgitation, especially in patients with a wide coaptation gap and low jet velocity.

Pathophysiology Most commonly, right ventricular (usually ischemic) damage, right atrial dilation in chronic atrial fibrillation, or pressure overload of the right ventricle in primary or secondary pulmonary arterial hypertension are responsible for the development of TR. The resulting volume overload leads to progressive dilation of the right ventricla and/or atriumand eventually the valvular annulus, which exerts a pull on the leaflets (so-called tethering) and, if untreated, leads to a progression of the severity of TR with a progressive coaptation gap (*"tricuspid regurgitation begets tricuspid regurgitation"*). If there is impaired right ventricular function, this is an additional predictor of a poorer clinical prognosis.

Clinical Presentation As a first manifestation, TR leads to a decrease in cardiac output with dyspnea and reduced exercise performance. In the further course, a gradual diffuse symptomatology with fatigue, appetite disturbance, feeling of fullness, ascites, and leg edema develops. In the late stage, the clinical picture of right ventricular heart failure with diffuse water retention (anasarca) can occur. Laboratory tests show elevated brain natriuretic peptide (BNP), liver enzymes, and renal parameters in the sense of chronic renal failure due to renal congestion. Organ dysfunctions are late consequences of severe TR and are explained by organ congestion due to the increased pressure conditions in the venous circulation. About 70% of patients with significant TR also have chronic atrial fibrillation (Sect. 12.6).

Diagnostics Clinically, patients with severe TI typically show signs of fluid retention, particularly lower leg edema, ascites, and pleural effusions. The neck veins are distended and occasionally pulsatile (Lancisi sign). Upon auscultation, a faint systolic murmur with a maximum in the sternal area can be heard, which increases with inspiration. The second heart sound may be split in the case of pulmonary arterial hypertension. However, a heart murmur is often absent, especially in advanced TI with laminar regurgitation.

Valvular Heart Diseases

Table 9.6 Echocardiographic criteria for the diagnosis of severe tricuspid regurgitation (vena contracta, smallest diameter of the regurgitation jet of an regurgant mitral valve (measured with color Doppler). PISA, proximal isovelocity surface area. EROA, effective regurgitant orifice area)

	Light grade	Medium	Severe
Vena contracta biplan (mm)	< 3	3.1 – 6.9	> 7
PISA radius (mm)	≤ 0.5	0.6 – 0.9	≥ 0.9
EROA (mm²)	< 20	20 – 39	40 – 59
Regurgitation volume (ml)	< 30	30 – 59	≥ 45
Example TTE*			

Transthoracic **echocardiography** is the diagnostic method of choice—not least because TR and the right ventricle are located anteriorly in the thorax and thus are easily accessible for imaging. This allows for the assessment of the morphology of the valve leaflets, the location of the jet (anteroseptal versus posterior), the severity of the regurgitation, the function of the right ventricle, and any interactions of the leaflets with a pacemaker lead. By measuring the pressure difference between the right ventricle and the right atrium (RV/RA gradient), the systolic pulmonary arterial pressure can be estimated (PASP = $4 \times Vmax^2$ plus RA pressure) The detection of systolic regurgitation into the usually dilated hepatic veins is another diagnostic criterion for severe TR. Transesophageal echocardiography is used to further refine the valve morphology, which in about 40% of cases has more than 3 leaflets, and to plan transcatheter interventions.

Right heart catheterization (▶ Sect. 2.7) holds a special place in the diagnosis of TR. In patients with advanced severe TR, ventricularization of the right atrial pressure curve is often observed (◼ Fig. 9.17). The detailed invasive examination of pulmonary pressure conditions with measurement of pulmonary wedge pressure values (wedge pressure) as well as cardiac output and pulmonary and systemic vascular resistances provides clues about the cause of any pulmonary arterial hypertension (primary versus secondary; ▶ Sect. 5.1).

> Since pulmonary arterial pressure values are generally underestimated in the presence of severe tricuspid regurgitation, the calculation of pulmonary vascular resistance is of crucial importance for diagnosing masked primary pulmonary arterial hypertension.

Therapy Due to the strong dependence of the severity of TR on right ventricular dimensions and volume status, therapy with diuretics can be initiated to alleviate or control symptoms. In the case of associated atrial fibrillation, there is also an indication for oral anticoagulation.

> Up until recently, interventions to correct tricuspid regurgitation were rarely performed and generally too late. Early referral of symptomatic patients with significant tricuspid insufficiency to a specialized center is of crucial importance as new treatemnt options became available. Furthermore, evaluation regarding significant left-sided heart valve disease and left ventricular dysfunction is important.

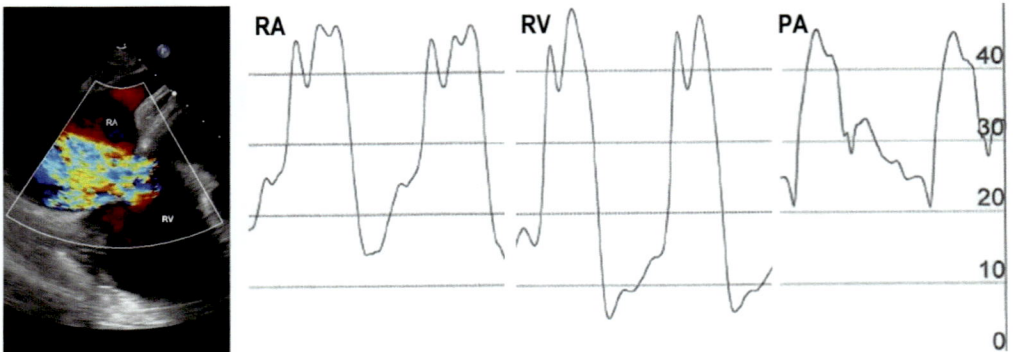

Fig. 9.17 **Hemodynamic conditions in severe tricuspid regurgitation as assessed by echocardiography.** The pressure curves show an equalization of systolic pressure in both right heart chambers and in the pulmonary artery with a massive increase in pressure in the right atrium. The right atrial and right ventricular pressure curves differ only slightly from each other due to the almost absent valve function, which is referred to as "ventricularization" of the right atrial pressure curve. The right ventricular end-diastolic pressure is also elevated as a sign of right ventricular dysfunction. *RA:* right atrium; *RV:* right ventricle; *PA:* pulmonary artery

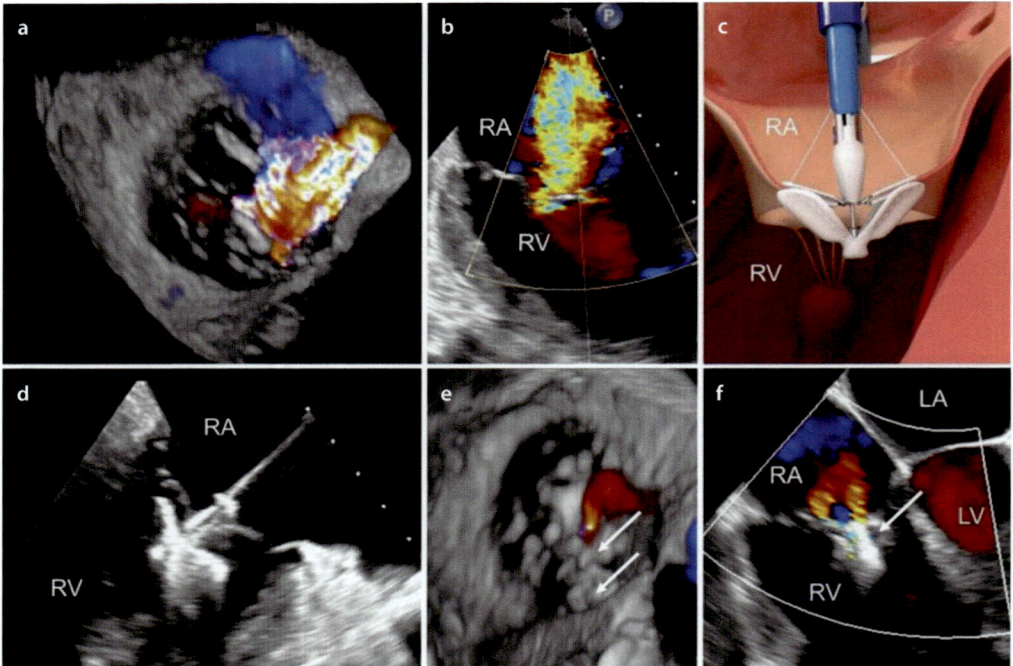

Fig. 9.18 **a–f Example of a transcatheter edge-to-edge reconstruction of the tricuspid valve. a, b** Severe secondary tricuspid regurgitation with predominantly anteroseptal localization; **c** Principle of transcatheter edge-to-edge reconstruction: 2 leaflets of the tricuspid valve are simultaneously grasped and approximated; **d** echocardiographic image during the intervention shortly before grasping the anterior and septal leaflets; **e, f** final result with reduction of tricuspid regurgitation to mild after implantation of 2 TriClip (white arrows = clip)

Although **surgical treatment** is the therapy of choice for patients with primary TR with acceptable surgical risk, its benefit in secondary tricuspid regurgitation is not supported by solid data. Current European guidelines support simultaneous surgical correction of severe symptomatic primary or secondary TR (Class I C) as well as in the presence of annular dilation (> 40 mm, 21 mm/m^2; Class IIa C) in patients undergoing surgery for left-sided cardiac pathology (i.e. mitral valve surgery). If technically feasible, reconstruction with ring annuloplasty is preferred over valve replacement. Although experience has significantly increased over the past two decades, postoperative mortality after isolated tricuspid valve surgery remains relatively high (around 9%), mainly due to the late referral of patients with advanced disease.

As an alternative, new **transcatheter interventions** can be offered for the repair or replacement of the tricuspid valve in selected patients with increased surgical risk (Class IIb C). Among the catheter-based therapeutic procedures, the edge-to-edge technique is most frequently used and leads to an improvement in symptoms and quality of life as well as positive remodeling of the right ventricle by reducing tricuspid regurgitation; however, mortality is not changed using this procedure, at least not in the short-term (Fig. 9.18). Percutaneous tricuspid valve replacement is currently in development with promising early results. A further development is the percutaneous implantation of tricuspid valves that is currently under investigation.

Endocardial Diseases

Alexander Lauten and Thomas F. Lüscher

Contents

10.1 Infectious Endocarditis – 172

10.2 Rheumatic Fever – 180

10.3 Libman-Sacks Endocarditis – 181

References – 182

Earlier versions were also created with the collaboration of David Hürlimann.

© The Author(s), under exclusive license to Springer-Verlag GmbH, DE, part of Springer Nature 2025
T. F. Lüscher and U. Landmesser (eds.), *Cardiovascular System*,
https://doi.org/10.1007/978-3-662-70152-2_10

An inflammation of the heart valves is referred to as endocarditis. This can have numerous causes, with infectious causes being the most common. The latter requires antibiotic therapy for several weeks, is furthermore treated surgically in about 50% of all cases, and still results in death in one out of three patients today (Hill et al. 2007). In contrast to endocarditis, rheumatic fever is a systemic disease in which, after a streptococcal infection, cross-reacting antibodies can lead to an involvement of the heart valves. All these conditions eventually impair valve function and commonly lead to stenosis and/or regurgitation.

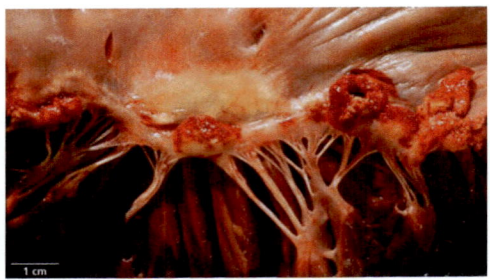

Fig. 10.1 Severe mitral valve endocarditis with hemorrhages and early stage of abscess formation. (Courtesy of Paul Vogt, Institute of Clinical Pathology, University Hospital Zurich)

There are four different **forms of endocardial diseases**:
- Infectious endocarditis (IE): Bacterial infection or fungal infection
- Libman-Sacks-endocarditis and rheumatic fever: Antigen-antibody reaction and immune complex reaction on the endocardium
- endomyocardial fibrosis (rare endocarditis occurring in the tropics with obstruction of ventricular filling) and Löffler endocarditis (▶ Sect. 8.1) – not considered an endocarditis in every classification
- Mixed forms

10.1 Infectious Endocarditis

Definition Infectious endocarditis (IE) is a disease of the endocardium, usually caused by bacteria, only in exceptional cases by fungi. The most important characteristic is infected vegetations deposited on the endocardium, commonly infiltrating the tissue, consisting of pathogens, fibrin, platelets, and infiltrating cells of the immune system. IE may affect one or more heart valves, but can also spread from these to other tissues such as the chordae tendineae or the mural endocardium (◘ Fig. 10.1).

If untreated, the mortality of IE is close to 100%. Despite advances in antimicrobial and surgical therapy, mortality has remained almost unchanged for decades even with optimal treatment. The 30-day mortality for patients with native valve endocarditis, who either are operated early on or treated conservatively, if surgery is not indicated, is still between 10–25%. If a indicated operation is not possible due to comorbidities and high surgical risk, around 1 in 3 patients dies within 30 days. Although IE is one of the rarer cardiovascular conditions, it is estimated to be responsible for ~100,000 deaths annually worldwide (Lozano et al. 2012).

Epidemiology Data on the incidence of IE vary widely. Older data report an incidence of 3.6–7 cases/100,000 life years. However, these figures are not very representative of the current incidence for various reasons.

Due to demographic developments in recent decades with higher age, comorbidities such as valvular heart diseases, cardiovascular implants such as mechanical or biological heart valves, or intravascular foreign body material such as pacemaker electrodes, the prevalence of certain risk factors for endocarditis has increased.

The diagnosis of IE is influenced by a multitude of factors. Ever-improving diagnostic possibilities, such as high-resolution echocardiography or nuclear medicine imaging techniques like ^{18}fluorodeoxyglucose positron emission tomography (^{18}FDG-PET) or leukocyte SPECT, made the diagnosis of IE easier (◘ Fig. 10.2).

Current outcomes data from hospitals in Germany suggest an incidence of 13–15 cases per 100,000 patient-years. These figures are comparable to the incidence observed in other Western industrialized nations.

Around 80% of all infectious endocarditis cases are caused by gram-positive pathogens, mostly staphylococci or streptococci. Although gram-negative pathogens are also frequently found during bacteremia, they rarely lead to endocarditis (◘ Table 10.1)[8].

Pathomechanisms The pathophysiology of IE is only partially understood so far. It is assumed that fibrin and platelets initially adhere to pre-existing endothelial lesions on the valves. This initially results in non-bacterial thrombotic vegetations, which can become secondarily infected in the context of bacteremia. A prerequisite for this is the entry of bacterial pathogens into the bloodstream (i.e. "bacteremia").

In principle, bacteremia occurs daily as a result of minor injuries to the skin or mucous membranes, for example, when brushing teeth or during dental treatments, but usually remains without consequences due to the high resistance of the endothelium against infections and an effective immune defense. A clinical study showed that immediately after brushing teeth, endocarditis-typical pathogens could be detected in the blood in about a quarter of the study

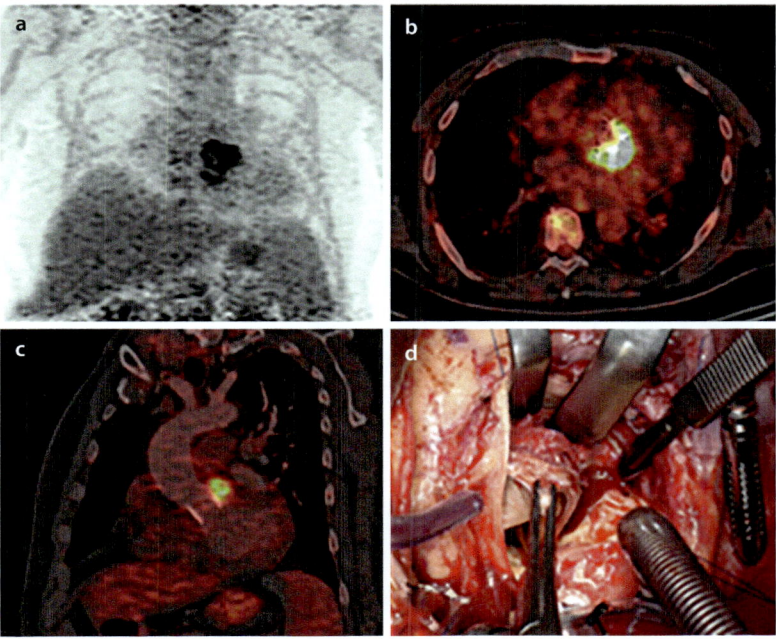

◘ **Fig. 10.2** (a–d) 63-year-old patient who received a biological aortic valve via a minimally invasive approach and recently had a fever of up to 42 °C. Echocardiography suspected a paravalvular abscess. ^{18}FDG-PET/CT showed a pronounced focal metabolic activity within the aortic root in the *Maximum Intensity Projection* (MIP) (a), as shown in the fused PET/CT images (b, c). A large posterior abscess was confirmed during surgery (d). (Courtesy of Ronny Büchel, University Hospital Zurich)

■ Table 10.1 Spectrum of pathogens in bacterial endocarditis

Pathogen	% of patients
Staphylococcus aureus	28
Coagulase-negative staphylococci	13
Viridans streptococci	16
Streptococcus gallolyticus	10
Other streptococcal species	5
Enterococcus species	9
HACEK*	2
Fungi	1
Polymicrobial	1
Culture-negative	10
Others	5

*Bacteria of the HACEK group: Haemophilus, Aggregatibacter, Cardiobacterium, Eikenella, Kingella

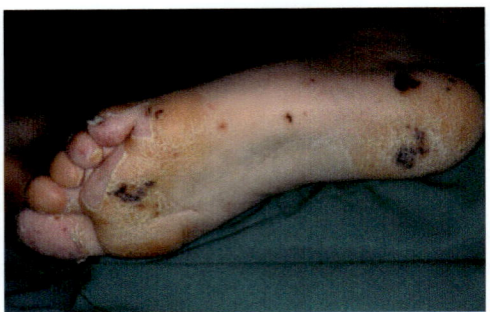

■ Fig. 10.3 Septic emboli as a manifestation of mitral valve endocarditis. (With the kind permission of the Department of Internal Medicine, University Hospital Zurich)

participants, and in almost two-thirds in connection with a tooth extraction.[3,4]

Pathogens of the normal resident flora of the mouth (streptococci of the viridans group) or intestinal mucosa (Streptococcus gallolyticus) are among the most common causes of IE. Since they are generally not pathogenic in these locations, they belong to opportunistic pathogens that only become pathogenic when favorable conditions coincide.

After the initial adhesion of the pathogen to the endothelium in the area of non-bacterial thrombotic vegetations, coagulation activation occurs through the activation of monocytes and endothelial cells, associated with the further attachment of fibrin and platelets. Additionally, bacterial pathogens secrete, among other things, exopolysaccharides and form so-called biofilms. The vegetation consisting of fibrin, platelets, and polysaccharides represents a protective mechanism for the bacteria, acting as a diffusion barrier for antibiotics in the bloodstream as well as for the host's immune system. As a consequence, the pathogens remain protected and metabolically active.[5,6]

Primarily affected are high-pressure areas (mitral or aortic valve) as well as locations distal to narrowings, where blood moves at high speed from a high-pressure to a low-pressure area (e.g., ventricular septal defect). The rule here is: the higher the pressure gradient, the higher the likelihood of infection. In the mitral valve, inflammatory changes are predominantly found on the atrial side, while in the aortic valve, they are predominantly found on the ventricular side.

Clinical Findings The clinical symptoms of infective endocarditis are very non-specific, especially at the onset of the disease process, resembling an infection with an unclear focus. Fever almost always occurs, and systemic emboli in up to 40% of all patients. Splenomegaly occurs more frequently in subacute courses with a longer duration (■ Fig. 10.3). Heart murmurs are usually a sign of an underlying valve disease as a risk factor for IE. Key findings are primarily bacteremia (ideally documented in up to three blood cultures) and endocardial vegetations detected by imaging, com-

Endocardial Diseases

monly by echocardiography. Additionally, a multitude of other symptoms are known to occur in IE (◘ Table 10.2).

The clinical course of IE is variable and is significantly influenced by the type of pathogen. Subacute, rather protracted courses over months up to fulminant courses with severe septsis and lethal outcome within a few days are all possible.

Acute IE is most commonly caused by an infection with Staphylococcus aureus (*S. aureus*) and is characterized by a rapid clinical progression within a few days to weeks with valve destruction, systemic emboli, and infectious metastases up to fulminant septic courses.

Subacute IE ("Endocarditis lenta"), on the other hand, shows protratced clinical courses over weeks to months and is usually caused by less virulent pathogens such as viridans streptococci, enterococci, or coagulase-negative staphylococci (e.g., *S. epidermidis*). Viridans streptococci are the most common causes of subacute and community-acquired endocarditis.

Other clinical signs are vascular findings such as septic emboli, conjunctival hemorrhages, Janeway lesions (non-painful, few millimeters large macular or nodular lesions on the palms or soles; ◘ Fig. 10.3), petechiae, splinter hemorrhages (splinter-shaped hemorrhages under the nail; ◘ Fig. 10.3) as well as immunological phenomena such as Osler's nodes and Roth's spots (oval retinal hemorrhages; ◘ Figs. 10.4 and 10.5).

Community-acquired ("*community-acquired*") and nosocomial ("*hospital-acquired*") endocarditis differ in terms of risk factors, pathogen spectrum, and clinical course.

Diagnosis In addition to the above-mentioned clinical signs of infection, typically elevated laboratory inflammatory markers (CRP, leukocytosis with left shift) are present.

◘ **Table 10.2** Frequency of symptoms and findings of infectious endocarditis. (Modified after[7])

Symptoms	% of patients	Findings	% of patients
Fever	80–85	Fever	80–96
Chills	42–75	Heart murmur	80–85
Sweating	25	Changed or new heart murmur	10–40
Cachexia	25–55	Neurological symptoms	30–40
Weight loss	25–35	Embolisms	20–40
Shortness of breath	20–40	Splenomegaly	15–50
Cough	25	Peripheral manifestations	
Headaches	15–40	Osler nodes	7–10
Nausea or vomiting	15–20	Splinter hemorrhages	5–15
Myalgias or arthralgias	15–30	Janeway lesions	6–10
Chest pain	8–35	Retinal lesions or Roth spots	4–10
Abdominal discomfort	5–15		
Back pain	7–10		
Confusion	10–20		

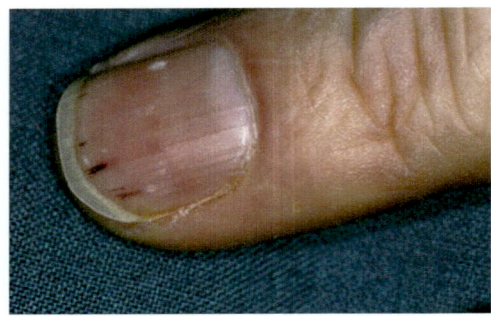

Fig. 10.4 Subungualsplinter hemorrhages. (Courtesy of the Department of Internal Medicine, University Hospital Zurich)

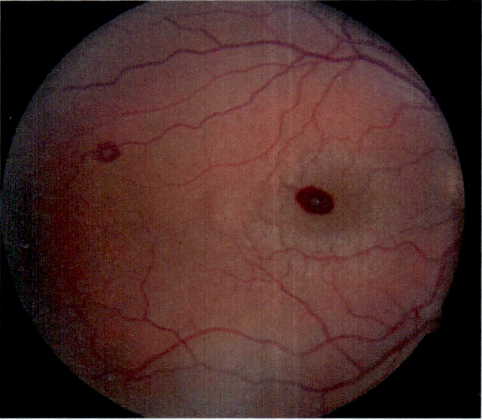

Fig. 10.5 Right eye. Classic Roth's spot temporal to the macula as well as subhyaloid hemorrhage in the area of the fovea. The optic nerve is cut off on the right side of the image. (Courtesy of Dr. R. Eberhard, Department of Ophthamlology of the University Hospital Zurich)

The definitive diagnosis of endocarditis also requires, in addition to pathogen detection, echocardiographic documentation (Fig. 10.6) of a typical vegetation or alternatively confirmation on the pathological specimen after surgical removal of the vegetation or post mortem.

Initially, in case of a clinical suspicion and repeatedly in the further course, the application of the Duke criteria (named after Duke University in North Carolina, USA) allows the diagnosis of IE with high sensitivity and specificity (Table 10.3).

> Endocarditis must always be considered as a possible differential diagnosis in cases of persistent fever, embolisms, or bacteremia.

Special Risk Groups Since certain risk factors increase the likelihood of IE, these should be considered and diagnostically clarified in patients with fever in the presence of one or more of the following findings:

- thromboembolic events,
- bacteremia,
- predisposing risk factors such as cardiac implants,
- history of valvular heart diseases.

In patients with predisposing factors, non-specific symptoms such as weight loss, malaise, and persistent fatigue can also be the only symptoms of IE even without the occurrence of fever. Due to the poor prognosis of IE, especially with delayed initiation of guideline-based treatment, a low threshold for performing echocardiography and, if unclear, further diagnostic procedures (e.g. 18FDG-PET/CT; Fig. 10.2) should be consdered in high risk patients with nonspecific symptoms.

Therapy The therapeutic goal is to eliminate the pathogen within the infected vegetation. If this goal is not achieved, a renewed progression of the infection is to be expected at the latest after the end of antibiotic treatment.

The antibiotic therapy of IE should be targeted to the cause, i.e., pathogen-specific and based on an antibiotic resistance analysis, high-dosed, using a bactericidal antibiotic. Until the antibiogram of the blood cultures is available, a nonspecific empirical antibiotic therapy should be initiated, which must be based on the expected spectrum of pathogens.

Endocardial Diseases

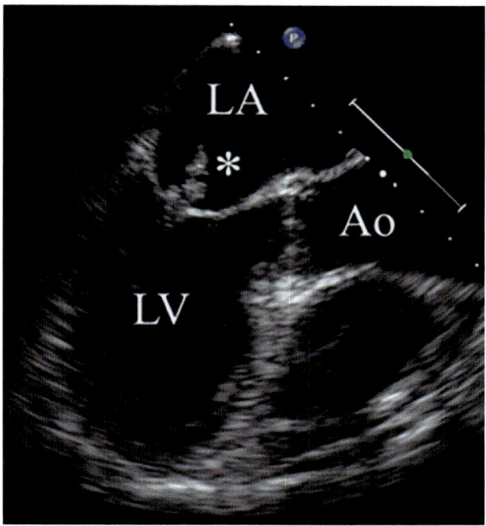

Fig. 10.6 Mitral valve endocarditis in transesophageal echocardiography. A large vegetation (*) is seen on the posterior mitral leaflet

> It is important that blood cultures are always taken initially prior to the start of empirical antibiotic therapy.

For optimal diagnostic yield, collection of 3 pairs of blood cultures at intervals of 30 minutes is recommended. Contrary to early assumptions, these can also be obtained independently of fever spikes to avoid delaying the start of antibiotic therapy. Once the causative pathogen is isolated, the antibiotic therapy must be adjusted according to resistance.

As a rule, antibiotic therapy for native valve endocarditis is carried out for 2–6 weeks, and for prosthetic valve endocarditis for at least 6 weeks in a hospital setting, but depending on the pathogen, clinical presentation, and course, sometimes even longer. Modern therapeutic concepts include the possibility of antibiotic therapy in an outpatient setting after initial hospitalisation in selected patients with confirmed effective antibiotic treatment and a controlled infection *(i.e. no fever, regression of inflammatory marks in bold; OPAT = Outpatient Parenteral Antibiotic Therapy)*.

Antibiotic Regimen for Initial Therapy of Infectious Endocarditis

Empirical Therapy for Culture-Negative Endocarditis
- For native valves or late prosthetic valve endocarditis (≥ 12 months after implantation):
  - Ampicillin 12 g/d IV in 4–6 divided doses **plus**
  - Flucloxacillin 12 g/d IV in divided dosages **plus**
  - Gentamicin 3 mg/kg BW/d IV or IM single dose
- For patients with penicillin allergy:
  - Vancomycin 30–60 mg/kg/d IV in 2–3 dasages
  - Gentamicin IV: 3 mg/kg/d IV or IM as a single dose
- For culture-negative early prosthetic valve endocarditis (i.e., within 12 months after implantation):
  - as for patients with penicillin allergy **plus** additionally Rifampicin IV, 900–1200 mg/d in 2–3 doseges for 4–6 weeks

Therapy for Penicillin-Sensitive Streptococci (minimum inhibitory concentration MIC ≤ 0.125 mg/l)*
- Penicillin G IV: 12–18 million U/d, in 4–6 dosages for 4 weeks **or**
- Amoxicillin 3–4 × 2–4 g IV **or**
- Ceftriaxone 2–4 g/d IV in 1–2 dosages

* For strains with relative penicillin resistance (MIC 0.25–2 mg/l), different dosages or combination treatments apply.

Therapy for Staphylococcal Endocarditis
- *Methicillin-sensitive:*
  - Oxacillin IV: 12 g, in 4–6 divided dosages over 4 weeks
- *Methicillin-resistant (MRSA):*
  - Vancomycin IV: 30–60 mg/kg/d, in 4–6 divided dosages for 6 weeks
- Alternatively:

Table 10.3 Duke criteria for infective endocarditis

Definitive infectious endocarditis	Pathological criteria	Detection of microorganisms by culture or histology of a local or embolized vegetation or in an intracardiac abscess **or** pathological lesion: vegetation or intracardiac abscess with histologically confirmed active endocarditis
	Clinical criteria according to the classification below	2 major criteria or 1 major criterion and 3 minor criteria or 5 minor criteria
Possible infectious endocarditis		1 major criterion plus 1 minor criterion or 3 minor criteria
Diagnosis rejected if		confirmed alternative diagnosis or explanation for the manifestations of suspected endocarditis or persistent resolution of the manifestations of suspected endocarditis after antibiotic therapy for less than 5 days or lack of pathological evidence of endocarditis during surgery or autopsy after antibiotic therapy for less than 5 days
Diagnostic criteria of infectious endocarditis		
Major criteria	Positive blood cultures	Typical microorganisms of infectious endocarditis in 2 separately taken blood cultures	Streptococcus viridans, Streptococcus bovis, HACEK group (see text) or Staphylococcus aureus or community-acquired enterococci in the absence of a primary focus
		or	
		Persistently positive blood cultures (microorganisms consistent with infectious endocarditis) in	≥ 2 blood cultures taken at intervals of > 12 h or 3/3 or more than half of 4 or more separately taken positive blood cultures (time interval between first and last blood culture at least 1 h)
		1 positive blood culture for Coxiella burnetii or anti-phase 1 IgG antibody titer > 1:800	

(continued)

Endocardial Diseases

Table 10.3 (continued)

Major criteria	Evidence of endocardial involvement	Positive echocardiography (ideally TEE, especially in valve prostheses or complicated infectious endocarditis)
		New valve regurgitation (increase or change of a pre-existing heart murmur is not sufficient)
		Oscillating intracardiac mass on the valves or valve apparatus or in a regurgitation jet or on implanted material (in the absence of an alternative anatomical explanation) or Abscess or new dehiscence of a valve prosthesis
Minor criteria	Predisposition: predisposing heart condition or intravenous drug abuse	
	Fever ≥ 38.0 °C	
	Vascular phenomena: major septic emboli, septic pulmonary infarcts, mycotic aneurysms, intracranial hemorrhages, Janeway lesions	
	Immunological phenomena: glomerulonephritis, Osler's nodes, Roth's spots, rheumatoid factor	
	Microbiological evidence	Positive blood culture, which however do not meet the major criteria or serological evidence of an active infection consistent with infectious endocarditis

TEE = transesophageal echocardiography

- Daptomycin 10 mg/kg/d IV once daily

Therapy for Prosthetic Valve Endocarditis with Staphylococci
- *Methicillin-sensitive:*
  - Oxacillin IV: 12 g/d, in 4–6 dosages for 6 weeks **plus**
  - Gentamicin IV: 3 mg/kg BW/d, in 1–2 dosages for 2 weeks **plus**
  - Rifampicin IV: 900–1200 mg/d, in 2–3 dosages for 6 weeks
- *Methicillin-resistant (MRSA):*
  - Vancomycin IV: 30–60 mg/kg BW/d, in 2–3 dosages for 6 weeks **plus**
  - Gentamicin IV: 3 mg/kg BW/d, in 1–2 dosages for 2 weeks **plus**
  - Rifampicin IV: 900–1200 mg/d, in 2–3 dosages for 6 weeks

(mod. according to European Society of Cardiology Guidelines on Endocarditis)

Endocarditis Prophylaxis According to current recommendations, endocarditis prophylaxis is only required for patients at the highest risk, provided they are undergoing a high-risk procedure. The following are considered high-risk patients.

Endocarditis High-Risk Patients
- Patients with prosthetic valves including transcatheter valves or with reconstructed valves using prosthetic material
- Patients with a history of endocarditis
- Patients with congenital heart defects:
  - any cyanotic defects
  - up to 6 months after surgical or interventional correction of defects using prosthetic material or lifelong in the case of residual shunt or valve insufficiency

For other valve diseases or congenital heart defects, prophylaxis with antibiotics is not recommended.

Currently, **dental procedures** that involve manipulation of the gingiva or the periapical region of the teeth or perforation of the oral mucosa are considered high-risk procedures. For these procedures in the aforementioned patient group, endocarditis prophylaxis should be administered as a single dose, 60 minutes before the procedure (orally) or 30–60 minutes before the procedure (intravenously).

Additionally, **perioperative prophylaxis** is recommended during the implantation of a pacemaker, an ICD, a heart valve prosthesis, or other cardiac foreign material.

These overall restrictive recommendations are based on the recognition that transient bacteremia regularly occurs during daily activities. Therefore, targeted endocarditis prophylaxis, e.g., during dental procedures, would only prevent a negligible number of infections. Furthermore, the effectiveness of endocarditis prophylaxis has only been demonstrated in animal studies; prospective randomized studies in humans are lacking.

10.2 Rheumatic Fever

Definition Rheumatic fever is an inflammatory systemic disease that occurs after an infection with hemolytic group A streptococci, usually streptococcal pharyngitis.

Epidemiology Acute rheumatic fever has become rare in the Western world. However, in older patients and immigrants from Mediterranean and Third World countries, valve defects as sequelae of a prior rheumatic fever are still commonly found.

Etiology, Pathophysiology Rheumatic fever is an immune response to bacterial structures or surface proteins (M, T, and R proteins), which cross-react with human glycoproteins due to structural homologies, ultimately leading to autoimmune reactions (antigen mimicry). In the heart, this typically results in endocardial involvement such as verrucous vegetations on the valves and/or inflammatory infiltration of the left ventricular endocardium, and subsequently granulomatous infiltration of the myocardium and pericardium (Aschoff bodies).

Clinical Findings, Diagnostics The diagnosis of rheumatic fever is based on the Jones criteria.

> **Jones Criteria**
> - **Major criteria:** carditis, migratory polyarthritis, chorea minor, subcutaneous nodules, erythema marginatum
> - **Minor criteria:** fever, arthralgia, elevated C-reactive protein (CRP) or erythrocyte sedimentation rate

Rheumatic fever is likely, if a streptococcal infection preceded it (positive throat culture, positive detection of streptococcal antigen, or rising streptococcal antibody titer) and 2 major criteria or 1 major criterion and 2 minor criteria are present.

Therapy Therapy is causal in nature using antibiotics for pathogen eradication.

> For all streptococcal infections, penicillin is the drug of choice, administered acutely for 10 days and as long-term prophylaxis, depending on the situation, for up to 10 years or lifelong.

Additionally, depending on the clinical scenario, symptomatic therapy for arthritis (aspirin) and chorea minor (noise isolation, possibly carbamazepine or valproate) is recommended. In patients with impaired left ventricular function, medical therapy for heart failure should be initiated, possibly supplemented by corticosteroids.

10.3 Libman-Sacks Endocarditis

Libman-Sacks endocarditis is a non-infectious inflammation that primarily occurs as an involvement of the endocardium in the context of systemic diseases such as systemic lupus erythematosus (SLE), antiphospholipid syndrome, or cancer.

Libman-Sacks endocarditis is characterized by fibrinoid necrotic warty endocardial thickenings, so-called verrucae, which are preferably found on the underside of the valve leaflets (Fig. 10.7).

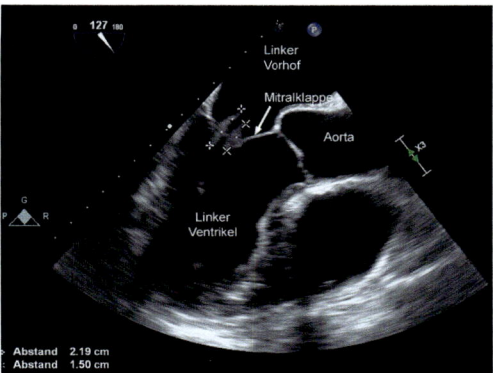
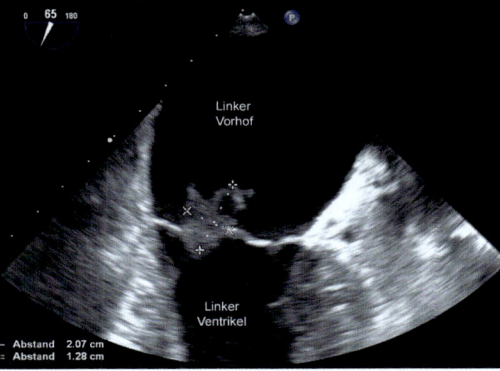

Fig. 10.7 Mitral valve endocarditis of the Libman-Sacks type with a large deposit on the posterior leaflet

Patients with Libman-Sacks endocarditis are often asymptomatic, and the endocardial involvement is discovered accidentely during the diagnostic work-up of systemic lupus erythematosus (SLE) using echocardiography. Date on the frequency of the condition are inconsistent; however, endocardial involvement up to Libman-Sacks endocarditis is found in 10–50% of all SLE patients. The vegetations can be the source of systemic emboli and, in individual cases, can lead to acute heart failure through valve destruction.

There is no specific therapy for Libman-Sacks endocarditis, except for the treatment of the underlying disease and symptomatic therapy of relevant valve defects. Prophylaxis of bacterial colonization of the verrucae in the sense of "infective endocarditis prophylaxis" is also advisable.

References

Bonow RO MD, Zipes DP, Lippy P, founding editor and online editor Eugene Braunwald. Braunwald's Heart Disease : a Textbook of Cardiovascular Medicine. Philadelphia, PA :Elsevier/Saunders, 2012. 2012;9th Edition:Page 1547.

Hill EE, Herijgers P, Claus P, Vanderschueren S, Herregods MC and Peetermans WE. (2007) Infective endocarditis: changing epidemiology and predictors of 6-month mortality: a prospective cohort study. Eur Heart J. 2007;28:196–203.

Lockhart PB, Brennan MT, Sasser HC, Fox PC, Paster BJ and Bahrani-Mougeot FK. Bacteremia associated with toothbrushing and dental extraction. Circulation. 2008;117:3118–25.

Lozano R, Naghavi M, Foreman K, Lim S, Shibuya K, Aboyans V, Abraham J, Adair T, Aggarwal R, Ahn SY, Alvarado M, Anderson HR, Anderson LM, Andrews KG, Atkinson C, Baddour LM, Barker-Collo S, Bartels DH, Bell ML, Benjamin EJ, Bennett D, Bhalla K, Bikbov B, Bin Abdulhak A, Birbeck G, Blyth F, Bolliger I, Boufous S, Bucello C, Burch M, Burney P, Carapetis J, Chen H, Chou D, Chugh SS, Coffeng LE, Colan SD, Colquhoun S, Colson KE, Condon J, Connor MD, Cooper LT, Corriere M, Cortinovis M, de Vaccaro KC, Couser W, Cowie BC, Criqui MH, Cross M, Dabhadkar KC, Dahodwala N, De Leo D, Degenhardt L, Delossantos A, Denenberg J, Des Jarlais DC, Dharmaratne SD, Dorsey ER, Driscoll T, Duber H, Ebel B, Erwin PJ, Espindola P, Ezzati M, Feigin V, Flaxman AD, Forouzanfar MH, Fowkes FG, Franklin R, Fransen M, Freeman MK, Gabriel SE, Gakidou E, Gaspari F, Gillum RF, Gonzalez-Medina D, Halasa YA, Haring D, Harrison JE, Havmoeller R, Hay RJ, Hoen B, Hotez PJ, Hoy D, Jacobsen KH, James SL, Jasrasaria R, Jayaraman S, Johns N, Karthikeyan G, Kassebaum N, Keren A, Khoo JP, Knowlton LM, Kobusingye O, Koranteng A, Krishnamurthi R, Lipnick M, Lipshultz SE, Ohno SL, Mabweijano J, MacIntyre MF, Mallinger L, March L, Marks GB, Marks R, Matsumori A, Matzopoulos R, Mayosi BM, McAnulty JH, McDermott MM, McGrath J, Mensah GA, Merriman TR, Michaud C, Miller M, Miller TR, Mock C, Mocumbi AO, Mokdad AA, Moran A, Mulholland K, Nair MN, Naldi L, Narayan KM, Nasseri K, Norman P, O'Donnell M, Omer SB, Ortblad K, Osborne R, Ozgediz D, Pahari B, Pandian JD, Rivero AP, Padilla RP, Perez-Ruiz F, Perico N, Phillips D, Pierce K, Pope CA, 3rd, Porrini E, Pourmalek F, Raju M, Ranganathan D, Rehm JT, Rein DB, Remuzzi G, Rivara FP, Roberts T, De Leon FR, Rosenfeld LC, Rushton L, Sacco RL, Salomon JA, Sampson U, Sanman E, Schwebel DC, Segui-Gomez M, Shepard DS, Singh D, Singleton J, Sliwa K, Smith E, Steer A, Taylor JA, Thomas B, Tleyjeh IM, Towbin JA, Truelsen T, Undurraga EA, Venketasubramanian N, Vijayakumar L, Vos T, Wagner GR, Wang M, Wang W, Watt K, Weinstock MA, Weintraub R, Wilkinson JD, Woolf AD, Wulf S, Yeh PH, Yip P, Zabetian A, Zheng ZJ, Lopez AD, Murray CJ, AlMazroa MA and Memish ZA. (2012) Global and regional mortality from 235 causes of death for 20 age groups in 1990 and 2010: a systematic analysis for the Global Burden of Disease Study 2010. Lancet. 2012;380:2095–128.

Murdoch DR, Corey GR, Hoen B, Miro JM, Fowler VG, Jr., Bayer AS, Karchmer AW, Olaison L, Pappas PA, Moreillon P, Chambers ST, Chu VH, Falco V, Holland DJ, Jones P, Klein JL, Raymond NJ, Read KM, Tripodi MF, Utili R, Wang A, Woods CW, Cabell CH and International Collaboration on Endocarditis-Prospective Cohort Study I. Clinical presentation, etiology, and outcome of infective endocarditis in the 21st century: the International Collaboration on Endocarditis-Prospective Cohort Study. Arch Intern Med. 2009;169:463–73.

Roberts GJ. Dentists are innocent! „Everyday" bacteremia is the real culprit: a review and assessment of the evidence that dental surgical procedures are a principal cause of bacterial endocarditis in children. Pediatr Cardiol. 1999;20:317–25.

Veltrop MH and Beekhuizen H. Monocytes maintain tissue factor activity after cytolysis of bacteria-infected endothelial cells in an in vitro model of bacterial endocarditis. J Infect Dis. 2002;186:1145–54.

Veltrop MH, Beekhuizen H and Thompson J. Bacterial species- and strain-dependent induction of tissue factor in human vascular endothelial cells. Infect Immun. 1999;67:6130–8.

Pericardial Diseases

Thomas F. Lüscher, Matthias Greutmann and Jan Steffel

Contents

11.1 Pericarditis – 186

11.2 Pericardial Effusion and Tamponade – 188

© The Author(s), under exclusive license to Springer-Verlag GmbH, DE, part of Springer Nature 2025
T. F. Lüscher and U. Landmesser (eds.), *Cardiovascular System*,
https://doi.org/10.1007/978-3-662-70152-2_11

Pericarditis is an inflammation of the pericardium (▶ Chap. 1) due to infectious or non-infectious causes. The accumulation of fluid in the pericardial sac is referred to as pericardial effusion. The presentation and course of a pericardial effusion are variable and range from a harmless, asymptomatic incidental finding to life-threatening pericardial tamponade.

11.1 Pericarditis

Definition Pericarditis is an inflammation of the pericardium due to infectious or non-infectious causes. When the inflammation spreads to the myocardium, it is referred to as perimyocarditis.

Etiology There are multpile forms of pericarditi:

- **Idiopathic** (around 50% of cases): The majority of so-called idiopathic pericarditis is triggered by viruses or autoimmune diseases that can not or no longer be identified.
- **Infectious:** Most commonly caused by viruses (Coxsackievirus A and B, adenoviruses, echoviruses, HIV). Bacteria (Mycobacterium tuberculosis, Staphylococcus aureus, streptococci) are less commonly involved.
- **Covid-19:** Adaptive immune reactions with peri- and more frequently perimyocarditis occurred frequently during the Covid-19 pandemic and very rarely after vaccination (significantly < 1%).
- **Collagenoses:** Autoimmune diseases such as systemic lupus erythematosus, periarteritis nodosa, Kawasaki syndrome, and other forms from this disease entity can lead to pericarditis.
- **Post-myocardial infarction syndrome:** Pericarditis epistenocardiaca is now rare due to timely revascularization with primary percutaneous intervention in myocardial infarction (▶ Sect. 7.5).
- **Dressler syndrome:** is an autoimmune reaction after cardiac surgery (formerly also after myocardial infarction, see above) and occurs mainly after cardiac surgical procedures involving opening of the pericardium.
- **Uremia:** Pericarditis with effusion, important dialysis indication
- **Malignant diseases** (▶ Sect. 15.2): Primary tumors are extremely rare, but more common as a result of metastases (most commonly in breast, lung, and esophageal carcinoma as well as lymphoma and leukemia).
- **Trauma** to the pericardium
- **Radiation therapy:** Occurring most comminly n tumors of the breast, mediastinum, and lung. Today, very rare due to site targeted radiation therapy.

Clinical Findings Commonly, pericarditis presents with non-specific symptoms such as fever and reduced eercise performance as well as pleuritic pain, which is more pronounced when lying down, therefore patients with pericarditis prefer to sit and leaning forward. Clinically, a distinction is made between dry and wet pericarditis.

A *dry (fibrinous) pericarditis* is most commonly encountered in the initial stage of acute pericarditis and frequently in the context of pericarditis associated with myocardial infarction. Clinically, it presents as a sharp retrosternal pain that is exacerbated when lying down, during deep inspiration, and when coughing. Therefore, these patients usually sit leaning forward in the emergency room.

❗ The most important differential diagnosis of pericarditis is myocardial infarction, where the symptoms are generally not exacerbated when lying down, during deep inspiration, and when coughing.

On auscultation, a scraping friction sound (locomotive sound) can be heard, which typically has 3 components: ventricular systole, ventricular diastole, atrial systole.

Often, dry pericarditis progresses into a *wet*(**exudative**) **form**. Inflammation leads to the formation of a pericardial effusion, which can vary in size. Clinically, the typical pain decreases and can even disappear completely under these conditions, as the resulting pericardial effusion reduces or even prevents the (painful) friction of the pericardial layers. During examination, the heart sounds become softer, the typical friction sound decreases, and may completely disappear. If complete healing does not occur, pericarditis can progress to a chronic form (chronic pericarditis, see below).

Diagnostics In *acute* **pericarditis**, ST-segment elevations are typically found (▶ Fig. 11.1), which must be distinguished from ST-segment elevations in acute myocardial infarction. In pericarditis, the changes are usually detectable in all ECG leads (unlike in acute myocardial infarction, where a regional distribution of ST elevations with "mirror-image" ST depressions is typically observed; ▶ Sect. 7.3). Additionally, an increase in C-reactive protein (as an expression of inflammation) and cardiac enzymes (e.g., troponins, creatine kinase; ▶ Sect. 7.3) can be present, especially with myocardial involvement (i.e., perimyocarditis), which can further complicate the differential diagnosis.

Therapy The treatment depends on the cause or any existing comorbidities (e.g., antibiotics in tuberculosis, dialysis in uremic pericarditis, steroids in autoimmune diseases, etc.). Otherwise, the therapy is primarily symptomatic with nonsteroidal anti-inflammatory drugs (e.g., diclofenac or ibuprofen) for pain management. In cases of severe inflammation and recurrences, glucocorticoids or, less commonly (though very effective), colchicine may be used. In t-resistant pericarditis and pericarditis constrictiva, surgical intervention via pericardiectomy must be considered.

- **Pericarditis constrictiva**

> In constrictive pericarditis, infectious or inflammatory processes lead to scar-like thickening of the pericardium with calci-

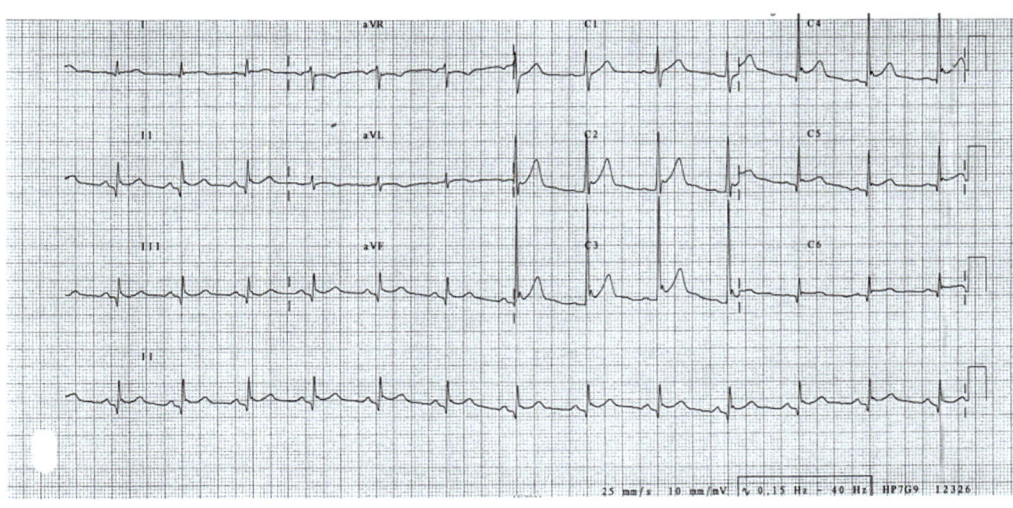

Fig. 11.1 ECG in pericarditis

fications, resulting in a so-called armored heart. As a consequence, the filling of the ventricles is increasingly impaired and heart failure-like symptoms develop..

Despite preserved systolic function, heart failure develops due to impaired diastolic filling (diastolic dysfunction, **diastolic heart failure;** ▶ Sect. 13.2). Due to the impaired expansion of the ventricle, rapidly and persistently high filling pressures occur during diastole ("*dip-and-plateau" ventricular filling pressure curves*). Typically, the right heart is compromised (due to lower filling pressures), leading to the development of peripheral edema, ascites, and even congestive cirrhosis (▶ Sect. 13.2).

At the **clinical examination**, an increase in central venous pressure during inspiration with jugular vein distention is typical (so-called Kussmaul's sign) is notable. About one-third of patients exhibit pulsus paradoxus (a drop in blood pressure during inspiration), especially with additional pericardial effusion.

The gold standard in the **diagnosis** of constrictive pericarditis is hemodynamic assessment with evidence of constriction, either via invasive pressure measurement (right heart catheterization; ▶ Sect. 2.7) or echocardiography. Additionally, pericardial thickening can be best assessed using cardiac CT or MRI (◘ Fig. 11.2). In the chest X-ray overview, a calcified pericardium can occasionally be seen, especially in constrictive pericarditis.

The only causal therapy for constrictive pericarditis is the surgical removal of the pericardium (**pericardiectomy**). However, this procedure is associated with a significant complication rate and a perioperative mortality of 6–12%. Nevertheless, symptomatic improvement can be achieved in 80% of patients postoperstively. Additionally, early removal of the pericardium is also expected to provide a prognostic advantage.

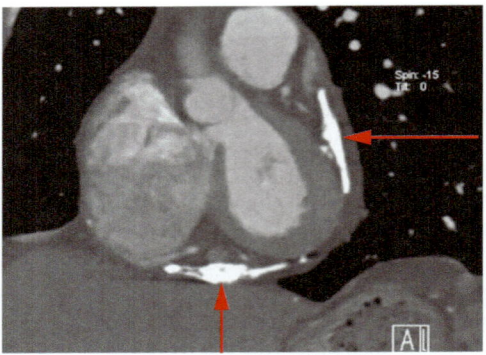

◘ **Fig. 11.2 Computed tomography in chronically calcified pericarditis.** The calcified pericardial parts (white structures; arrows) are clearly visible. (Courtesy of Thomas Frauenfelder, Institute of Radiology, University Hospital Zurich)

11.2 Pericardial Effusion and Tamponade

Definition Pericardial effusion refers to the accumulation of fluid in the serous space between the pericardium and the epicardium. If a pericardial effusion significantly impedes the filling of the heart, it is referred to as a pericardial tamponade.

Etiology One of the most important complications of pericarditis is pericardial effusion. However, other conditions can also be involved, such as tumor infiltration, vasculitis, traumatic lesions, or a prior cardiac surgical procedure.

Pathophysiology Pericardial effusion, once it reaches a certain size, leads to an impairment of cardiac function, particularly of the right heart chambers as filling pressures are much lower here. The hemodynamic spectrum of a pericardial effusions reaches from irrelevant to tamponade, but may be dynamic over time.

> Whether and when a pericardial effusion becomes hemodynamically relevant and tamponades primarily depends not on

Pericardial Diseases

the amount of effusion but rather on the speed of its development.

For instance, an acute effusion of 200 ml (e.g., in the context of an iatrogenic ventricular perforation) can lead to the full picture of tamponade within a very short time. In contrast, a pericardial effusion that develops over a longer period of up to 1000 ml or more (e.g., in the context of tuberculosis) can be hemodynamically well tolerated.

Clinical Findings A hemodynamically irrelevant pericardial effusion is generally not symptomatic. Nevertheless, signs of an underlying disease that may be causing it (tuberculosis, tumor conditions, etc.) can be present and should be searched for.

If there is compression of the cardiac chambers (pre-tamponade and tamponade), this leads to low blood pressure (**hypotension**), which leads to a compensatory increase in heart rate (i.e. tachycardia). Due to the backlog of blood in front of the right ventricle, there is jugular vein distention, and in the case of a backlog in front of the left ventricle, dyspnea and pulmonary edema ensue. Additionally, a drop in systemic blood pressure during inspiration by more than 10 mmHg is often observed (i.e. *pulsus paradoxus*). Pathophysiologically, this is due to an increase in venous return to the right ventricle during inspiration with a consequent shift of the septum to the left, which may occur in the context of tamponade during diastolic pressure equalization (unlike the physiological situation where increased left ventricular filling pressure prevents such a phenomenon). However, such an inspiratory blood pressure drop can also be observed after nitrate administration and in hypovolemia. The negative predictive value of pulsus paradoxus is very high, i.e. in its absence, a pericardial tamponade is very unlikely (exception: localized pericardial effusion, such as after cardiac surgical procedures).

> Beck's Triad of severe tamponade: muffled heart sounds, hypotension, jugular vein distention

Diagnostics Upon auscultation, heart sounds are dampened and muffled by the effusion. The ECG shows low voltage.

The diagnostic method of choice is echocardiography (◘ Fig. 11.3; ▶ Sect. 2.3).

Even with an amount of only 50 ml, an effusion is clearly visible with echocardiography, whereas in chest X-ray it is only visible with 400 ml or more (◘ Fig. 11.4). Furthermore, echocardiography can assess the filling patterns of the right and left ventricles, compression of the right atrium and ventricle (◘ Fig. 11.5), the respiratory variability of the inferior vena cava, as well as other structural heart diseases (e.g., direct evidence of tumor infiltration, etc.).

> Although echocardiography provides valuable clues for the diagnosis, a diagnosis of pericardial tamponade should

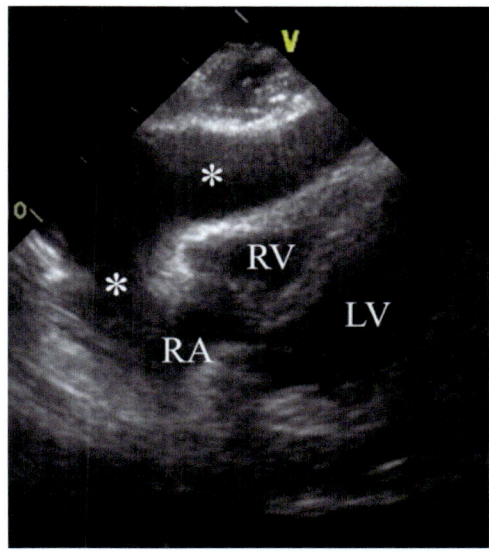

◘ **Fig. 11.3** Echocardiographic finding in large pericardial effusion (*). Compare with normal anatomy in ◘ Fig. 2.4 (▶ Sect. 2.3)

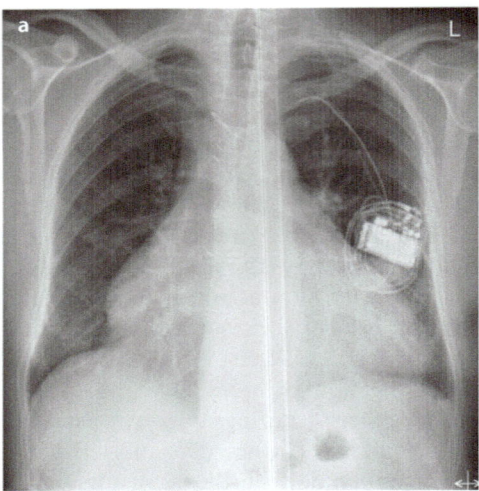 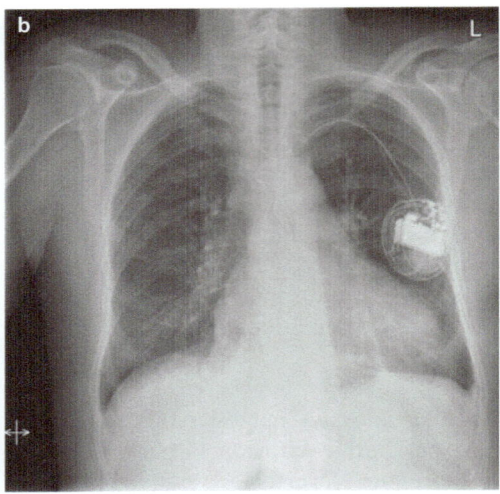

◘ **Fig. 11.4** (**a, b**) **Chest X-ray**. (**a**) Before pericardiocentesis, a significantly widened cardiac silhouette is visible, which (**b**) normalizes again after puncture

only be made in combination with the clinical context.

Therapy In the case of *hemodynamically insignificant* pericardial effusion, the therapy should focus on the underlying disease (e.g. dialysis in uremia, etc.). If necessary, a puncture can be performed for diagnostic purposes.

> A hemodynamically significant pericardial effusion, on the other hand, must be drained, and in the context of pericardial tamponade, this is a vital emergency procedure.

▶ Practical

Pericardiocentesis
Normally, a pericardiocentesis can be performed subxiphoidally, e.g., under echocardiographic control or fluoroscopy. The patient is draped sterilely and access is visualised echocardiographically using a subxiphoid window under sterile conditions. At the ideal site (locally large pericardial effusion, short distance from the skin to the effusion, no parts of the liver interposed), the skin is punctured with a long needle after infiltration with local anesthesia and advanced towards the left shoulder under aspiration. If the effusion is successfully punctured with the needle, a guidewire is advanced into the pericardial sac using the Seldinger technique, and the actual drainage catheter is inserted over the lead wire (after dilation). If the position of the puncture needle is uncertain, the correct position can be checked before (!) dilation and insertion of the drainige catheter, e.g., by injecting foamed NaCl solution (so-called *bubbles*) or contrast medium to visualize the punctured cavity. Depending on the question and clinical indication, the drainage remains in place for a few hours to a few days before it is removed. Complications such as liver injury or accidental puncture of a heart chamber are rare with correct technique, especially in the presence of a large pericardial effusion.

With longer-standing pericardial effusion, septations and partial organization of the ef-

Pericardial Diseases

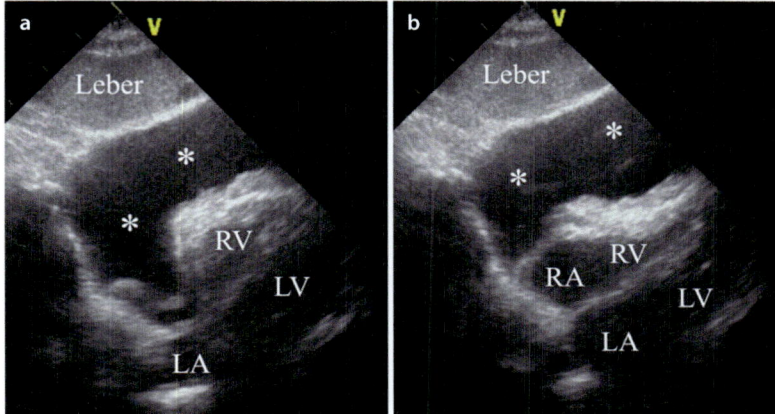

Fig. 11.5 Large pericardial effusion (*) with signs of tamponade in the echo. During systole, there is a clear compression of the right atrium (left) and in diastole, a compression of the right ventricle (right). Additionally, fibrin deposits are found on the free wall of the RV. *RA:* right atrium, *RV:* right ventricle, *LA:* left atrium, *LV:* left ventricle

fusion can occur, making percutaneous puncture no difficult or longer possible. In these cases, a surgical procedure may be required. In chronically recurrent pericardial effusions, a so-called pericardial window with drainage into the pleura or peritoneum may be necessary. ◄

Conduction System Diseases—Cardiac Arrhythmias

Jan Steffel and Thomas F. Lüscher

Contents

12.1 Physiology – 195

12.2 ECG – 195
12.2.1 Rhythm – 196
12.2.2 P-wave and PQ duration – 196
12.2.3 QRS Complex – 197
12.2.4 Repolarization – 198
12.2.5 Extrasystoles – 199
12.2.6 Bundle Branch Blocks – 200

12.3 Antiarrhythmics – 202

12.4 Cardiac Arrhythmias – 203
12.4.1 Sinoatrial Block (SA Block) – 204
12.4.2 Atrioventricular Block (AV Block) – 205

12.5 arrhythmias – 208
12.5.1 Sinus tachycardia – 208
12.5.2 Atrial fibrillation – 209
12.5.3 Atrial Flutter – 213
12.5.4 Pre-excitation and Wolff-Parkinson-White Syndrome (WPW) – 214

Earlier versions with the collaboration of C. Brunckhorst

© The Author(s), under exclusive license to Springer-Verlag GmbH, DE, part of Springer Nature 2025
T. F. Lüscher and U. Landmesser (eds.), *Cardiovascular System*,
https://doi.org/10.1007/978-3-662-70152-2_12

12.5.5 AV Node Reentrant Tachycardias – 217
12.5.6 Ventricular Tachycardia – 219
12.5.7 QT Interval Prolongation and Torsade de Pointes Arrhythmia – 221
12.5.8 Ventricular Fibrillation – 221

Conduction System Diseases—Cardiac Arrhythmias

Herzrhythmusstörungen Cardiac Arrhythmias are disturbances in heart rhythm in frequency, regularity, origin, and/or conduction. A distinction is made between bradyarrhythmias (e.g., sick sinus syndrome, AV blocks; usually < 60/min) and tachyarrhythmias (e.g., atrial fibrillation, ventricular tachycardias; usually > 100/min). Furthermore, arrhythmias are classified according to their anatomical origin into supraventricular and ventricular arrhythmias. Various antiarrhythmic drugs, catheter ablation, pacemakers, and implantable cardioverter defibrillators (ICD) as well as, if necessary, anticoagulation to prevent peripheral embolisms and stroke are used to treat arrhythmias.

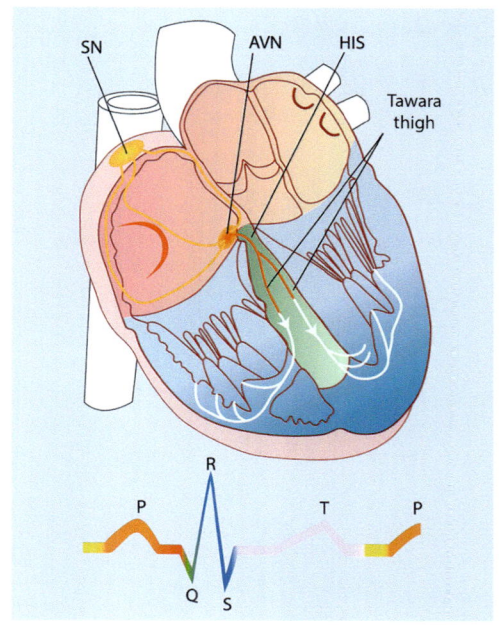

Fig. 12.1 Course of conduction in the heart and temporal correlation with the ECG. *SN:* sinus node, *AVN:* AV node, *HIS:* His bundle

12.1 Physiology

The sinus node is the primary pacemaker of the heart with a physiological depolarization frequency of 60–100/min. If it fails, the AV node or the AV junction zone ("AV Junction") with an intrinsic frequency of about 40–50/min acts as a secondary pacemaker. If it also fails, the ventricular myocardium takes over as a tertiary pacemaker with a frequency of about 20–40/min, which, however, is usually insufficient for an adequate cardiac output.

The **sinus node** consists of specialized cells located in the crista terminalis of the right atrium. The spontaneous depolarization of its pacemaker cells (that are calcium-dependent, express I_F channels, but no sodium channels) leads through the transition cells to a coordinated electrical impulse that initiates the depolarization and thus the contraction of the atria.

After the atria, the **AV node** is excited, which, thanks to its decremental conduction characteristic with its ability to block conduction above a certain heart rate (so-called Wenckebach point), assumes an important filtering function at high atrial rates and allows to coordinate electrical acitivity with hemodynamic events in the atria and the ventricle.

From the AV node, the excitation is transmitted to the **His bundle**, which passes through the annulus fibrosus and further divides into the anterior and posterior left and right bundle branches, and finally transmits the excitation via Purkinje fibers to the working myocardium (Fig. 12.1).

12.2 ECG

To begin with, the principles of ECG interpretation are briefly reviewed (▶ Chap. 2.2; Table 12.1 and Fig. 12.2); for more in-depth study, we refer to the textbooks of physiology.

Table 12.1 ECG-normal values

Parameter	Normal value
P wave	< 120 ms
PQ	120–200 ms
QRS	< 120 ms
QTc	Women: < 460 ms*, Men: < 440 ms*

* inconsistent

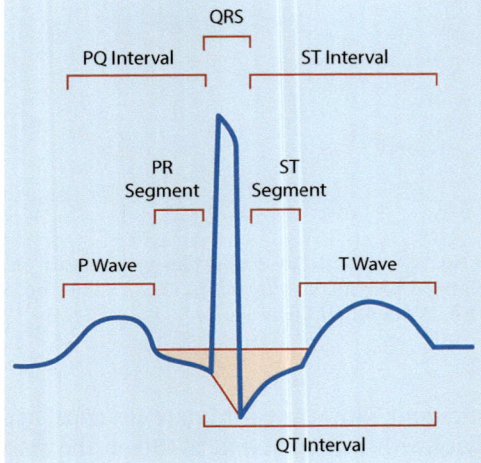

Fig. 12.2 ECG segments and normal values

Systematic EKG-Basic Evaluation
1. Rhythm: Regular? Irregular? "Regularly irregular"?
2. P-waves? Axis of the P-waves?
3. Is each P-wave followed by a QRS complex?
4. PQ time (< 120 ms = shortened, > 200 ms AV block I°), pre-excitation?
5. QRS axis type
6. QRS duration (normal < 120 ms)
7. Pathological Q-waves? Normal R/S transition over the anterior wall?
8. Repolarization
   - QT time or QTc time?
   - ST segment depression/elevation?
   - T-wave inversion?

12.2.1 Rhythm

The analysis of the EKG begins with the **analysis of the heart rhythm**. If it is irregular, the next question is whether there is regularity in the irregularity ("regularly irregular") or if there is absolute arrhythmia ("**un**regularly irregular"). In the latter case, the suspicion of atrial fibrillation/flutter is high, so attention should be particularly focused on the search for fibrillation or flutter waves. However, caution is required Frequent supraventricular or ventricular extrasystoles can also make an otherwise regular sinus rhythm appear irregular.

If the rhythm is regular, the next focus is on the **P-waves**. The regular sequence of P-waves, each followed by a QRS complex, in most cases indicates a sinus rhythm. This is "proven" by the axis of the P-wave, which is determined similarly as the axis of the QRS complex (see below). If the axis of the P-wave corresponds to an indetermint or steep type (positive in I, II, avF), a sinus rhythm is very likely present.

Following the rhythm analysis, it is advisable to systematically analyze the EKG "from left to right," i.e., from the **P-wave to the T-wave**. This approach avoids overlooking important features of the ECG tracingthe.

12.2.2 P-wave and PQ duration

The **P-wave** corresponds to the excitation of the atria, normally lasting up to 120 ms. Any prolonged or morphologically altered P-wave can be a sign of a disturbance in atrial excitation or conduction. In right atrial hypertrophy, the P-wave is elevated in leads II and III (> 0.25 mV, so called P dextroatriale), in left atrial hypertrophy, the P-wave is prolonged (> 120 ms in II, usually with a prominent "notch," and markedly biphasic in V1, so-called P sinistroatriale, ◘ Fig. 12.3).

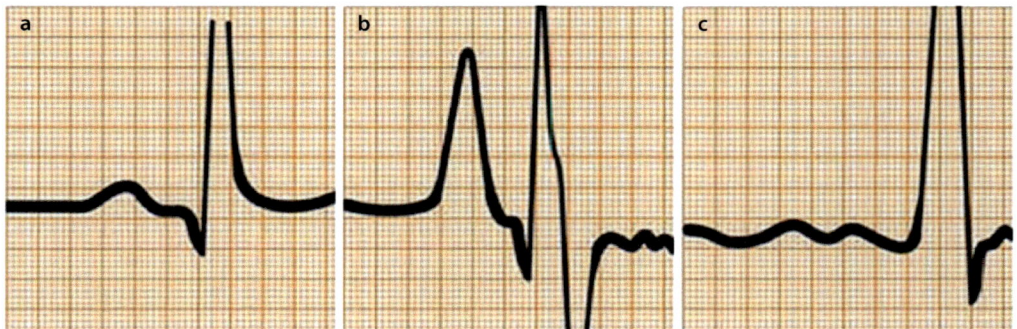

Fig. 12.3 (a-c) Changes in the P-wave. (a) Normal configuration, (b) P-dextroatriale and (c) P-sinistroatriale

The **PQ time** corresponds to the sum of atrial excitation and physiological conduction delay in the AV node and normally lasts 120–200 ms. In ectopic atrial rhythm, supranormal AV conduction, or the presence of an accessory pathway, it can be shortened ("Short PQ-Syndrome"); in first-degree AV block, it is prolonged (> 200 ms).

12.2.3 QRS Complex

The QRS complex corresponds to ventricular depolarization; several aspects of the QRS complex must be systematically evaluated. The QRS complex normally has a duration of 60–120 ms. If it lasts 120 ms or longer, it is referred to as a complete bundle branch block.

Furthermore, the **axis type of the QRS complex** has to be determined, which corresponds to the electrical heart axis. The axis type of the QRS complex is determined by the projection of the QRS complex (or its main deflection) towards the limb leads according to Einthoven and Goldberger (Fig. 12.4a). As an example, the left axis type and the extreme left axis type are depicted in Fig. 12.4b. An QRS axis of −30° or more, is referred to as the extreme left axis type. The lead that is orthogonal to the line rotated by −30° is referred to as Einthoven ("Roman") II. The green vector corresponds to a left axis type; it projects in the lead direction towards II, hence a positive deflection is seen in II for the left axis type.

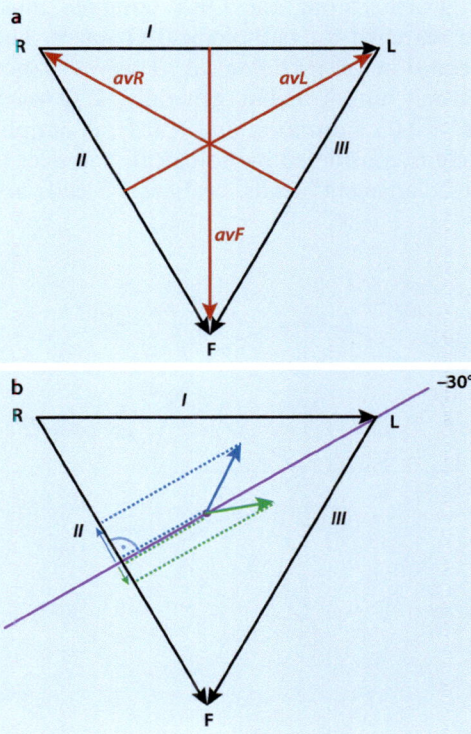

Fig. 12.4 (a, b) Cabrera triangle (a) and projection in left axis/extreme left axis (b). See text for details. Black: Einthoven lead, red: Goldberger leads, green: left axis type, blue: extreme left axis type, violet: line at −30° (transition point LT/ELT), which is orthogonal to II

In contrast, for the extreme left axis type, the QRS vector projects into the opposite direction towards the lead direction II; accordingly, a negative deflection is seen in II in case of an extreme left axis type. ◘ Fig. 12.4 shows the different axis types with their respective defining leads, whose polarity turns from positive to negative (or vice versa) towards the next axis type. For instance, again based on the left axis type: In the transition to the extreme left axis type, II turns from positive to negative (green); in the transition from the left axis type to the horizontal type, aVF turns from negative to positive (blue). Based on the Cabrera triangle (◘ Fig. 12.4a), each axis type and its characteristic leads can be reconstructed as are summarized in ◘ Fig. 12.5.

Furthermore, the QRS complex must be searched for pathological Q waves. The definition of pathological Q waves is not entirely uniform, but generally, a Q wave of > 0.03 s duration and > 0.1 mV amplitude is considered pathological, if it occurs in 2 "adjacent" leads. "Adjacent" leads are II–III–aVF ("inferior leads"), V4–V6 ("anterolateral leads"), and I–aVL–V6 ("lateral leads"). Q waves are physiologically observed in aVR and V1. The description of Q waves can be indicative of a prior myocardial infarction; however, it should be noted that this finding is neither very sensitive nor specific: infarctions can occur without Q waves; on the other hand, Q waves can also occur in other pathologies (e.g., left bundle branch block).

Finally, the so-called **R/S transition** is described, i.e., the lead in which the amplitude of the R wave becomes greater than that of the S wave. Normally, this occurs in V3 or V4. A delayed R/S transition can again be a sign of a prior myocardial infarction (but can also occur in LBB, Wolf-Parkinson-White (WPW) syndrome, among others); an early R/S transition is observed, for example, in right bundle branch block and right heart strain.

12.2.4 Repolarization

The **QT interval** corresponds to the time from the beginning of ventricular excitation to the end of repolarization. The physiological QT duration is frequency-dependent, which is why the frequency-corrected QT interval (QTc) is used as a better measure. To calculate the QTc, the QT interval (in sec) is divided by the square root of the RR interval (in sec).

$$Bazett\ Formel: QTc(\sec) = \frac{QT(\sec)}{\sqrt{RR(\sec)}}$$

❯ A prolongation of the QTc increases the risk of torsade de pointes tachycardia, as the likelihood of triggered activity during repolarization is increased.

During the **ST segment**, the ventricle is depolarized. A significant elevation or depression of the ST segment above or below the level of the isoelectric line is pathological

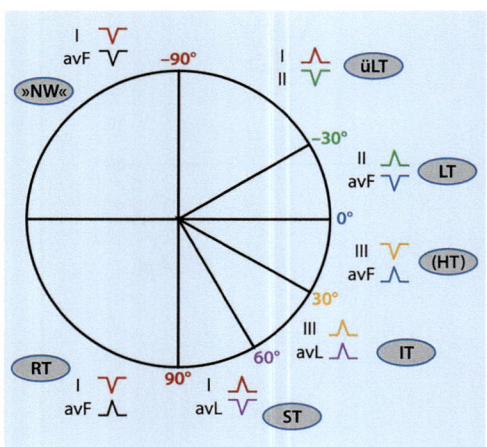

◘ **Fig. 12.5** Axis types and their "characterizing" leads. See text for details. *ELT*: extreme left axis type, *LT*: left axis type, *HT*: horizontal type, *IT*: indeterminate type, *ST*: steep type, *RT*: right axis type, *NW*: "Northwest" territory (extremely extreme left/right axis type). In clinical practice, HT and LT are often generally summarized as "left axis type"

Conduction System Diseases—Cardiac Arrhythmias

in most cases. In the case of ST elevation, a distinction must be made as to whether it originates from the descending R (typical for an infarction, ▶ Chap. 7.5) or from the ascending S (typical for pericarditis, Section. 11). ST depression is typically observed in myocardial ischemia, but can also have a number of other (partly nonspecific) causes.

The **T wave** essentially corresponds to ventricular repolarization. Compared to depolarization, repolarization is based on an opposite polarity **and** direction of the excitation process, which is why the vector of the T wave is physiologically aligned concordantly to the main vector of the QRS complex. Numerous changes, both specific and nonspecific, can be observed: For example, a high, peaked T wave can occur in an acute myocardial infarction or in hyperkalemia. An isolated T wave inversion in adjacent leads may indicate a prior (non-transmural) infarction.

An **U wave** may appear after the T wave and can be misleading especially if it arises from the T wave, as in this case, it is considered part of the T wave and thus may give rise to an falsly prolonged QT interval.

12.2.5 Extrasystoles

Extrasystoles are heart beats outside the physiological basic rhythm. They are classified according to their anatomical site of origin into supraventricular and ventricular extrasystoles.

In the case of **supraventricular**extrasystoles (◘ Fig. 12.6), the excitation focus is in the atrium. In this case, ventricular excitation occurs via the physiological pathway through the AV node and His bundle, resulting in a narrow QRS complex (in the absence of a pre-existing ventricular conduction delay). It may happen that the next excitation originating from the sinus node falls into the absolute refractory period of the preceding atrial excitation, resulting in a compensatory pause. Only with the next normal sinus action is the P wave followed by a regular QRS complex.

> Supraventricular extrasystoles are common, in most cases harmless, and therefore do not require any therapy in a healthy heart. In cases of severe symptoms, beta-blockers or verapamil-type calcium antagonists, as well as possibly ablation treatment, are used.

In the case of a **ventricular**extrasystole (VES; ◘ Fig. 12.7), the QRS complex is wide due to pathological ventricular excitation. A VES from the left ventricle usu-

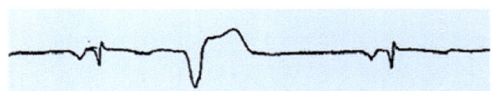

◘ **Fig. 12.7** Ventricular extrasystole

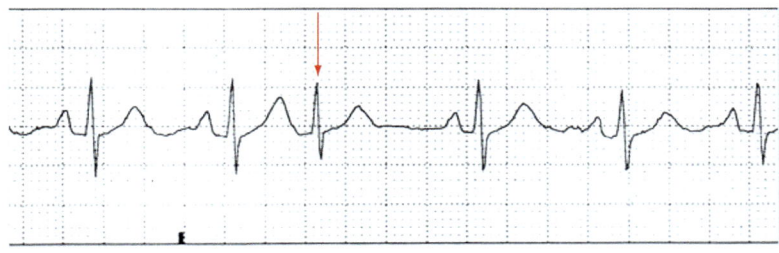

◘ **Fig. 12.6** Supraventricular extrasystole (arrow)

ally has the morphology of a right bundle branch block, while a VES from the right ventricle has the morphology of a left bundle branch block. The excitation can also spread retrogradely from the ventricle through the AV node to the atrium, so a negative P wave may appear on the ECG. In this case, too, a compensatory pause commonly occurs after an extrasystole. If a VES occurs after every normal beat, it is called **bigeminy**. With a **couplet**, 2 extrasystoles occur in succession, and in a **triplet**, 3 extrasystoles occur in succession. Apart from occasional palpitations, isolated ventricular extrasystoles generally do not cause symptoms per se. In the case of early-onset VES, a peripheral pulse deficit and thus symptoms of relative bradycardia can occur as the ventricle is not yet refilled with blood.

12.2.6 Bundle Branch Blocks

Definition A bundle branch block is a conduction block distal to the bundle of His.

Depending on the location of the block, a distinction is made between a **complete** right or left bundle branch block, as well as a left anterior and a left posterior hemiblock. A complete bundle branch block has a QRS duration > 120 ms. A right bundle branch block pattern with a QRS duration < 120 ms is referred to as **incomplete** right bundle branch block.

ECG Changes
- **Right bundle branch block**: The QRS complex is M-shaped deformed in V1 and V2 and has a blunt S in I, aVL, and V6 (◘ Fig. 12.8).
- **Complete left bundle branch block**: There is a broad and deep S wave in V1 and V2 as well as a characteristic RsR' in V5 and V6 (◘ Fig. 12.9).
- **Left anterior hemiblock**: The QRS duration is < 120 ms, there is an extreme left axis deviation, qR in aVL (◘ Fig. 12.10).
- **Left posterior hemiblock (LPHB)**: The QRS duration is < 110 ms; there is a

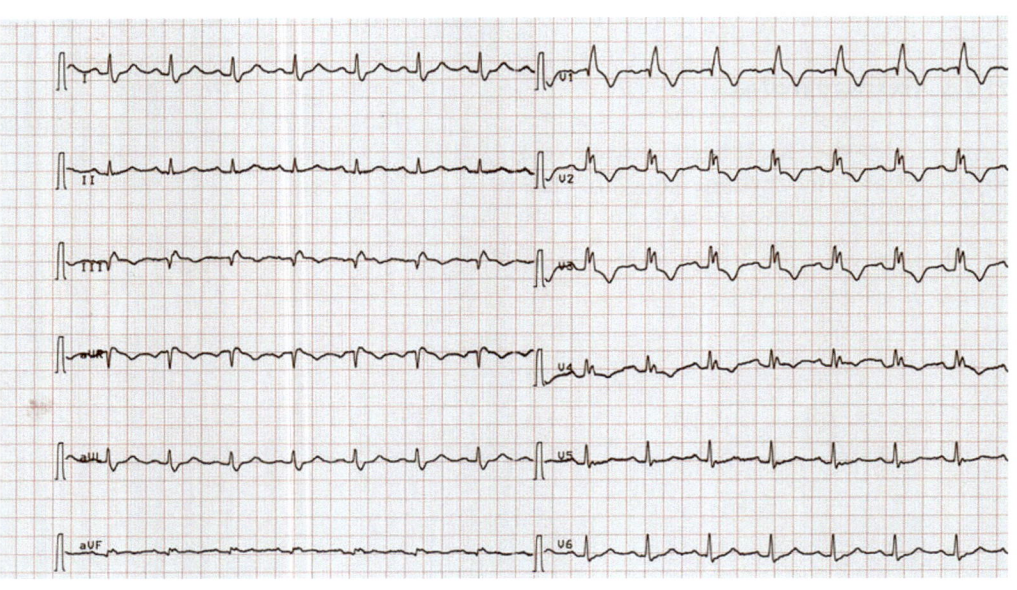

◘ **Fig. 12.8** Complete right bundle branch block

Conduction System Diseases—Cardiac Arrhythmias

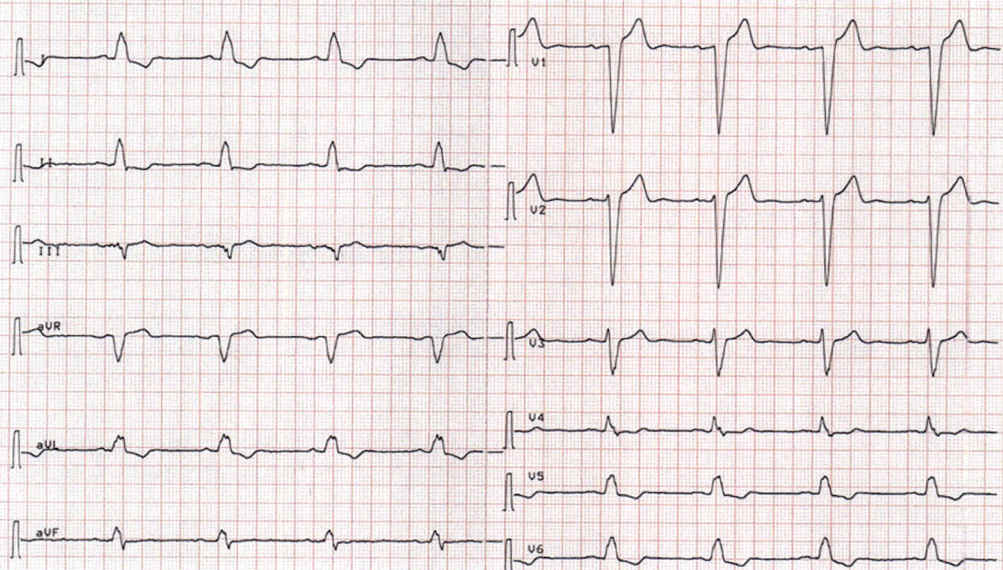

Fig. 12.9 Complete left bundle branch block

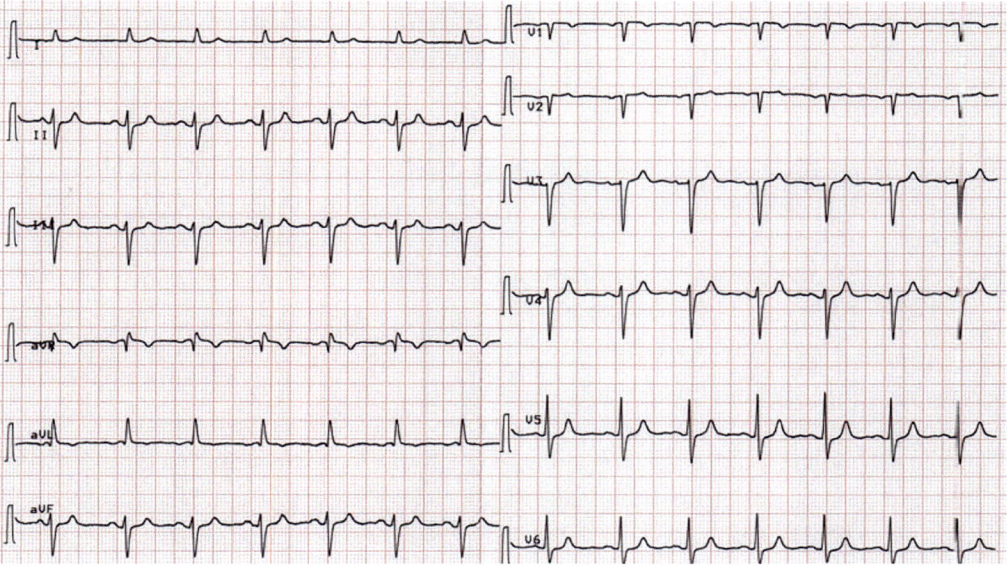

Fig. 12.10 Left anterior hemiblock

> right axis deviation or extreme right axis deviation with an rS pattern in I and aVL as well as qR in II, III, avF.

▸ The diagnosis of an left posterior hemiblock (LPHB) can only be made if right heart strain, which can be associated with similar ECG changes, is excluded.

Etiology Typical underlying causes of a bundle branch block are:

— Ischemia: CAD (▶ Chap. 7.2) and myocardial infarction (▶ Chap. 7.5), especially with typical symptoms and newly onset LBB,
— Hypertrophy of the left ventricle (▶ Sect. 4 and ▶ Chap. 8.1),
— Right heart overload: Pulmonary embolism (▶ Chap. 17.3), pulmonary hypertension (especially with RBB; ▶ Chap. 5.3),
— Myocarditis (▶ Chap. 8.2),
— idiopathic.

Clinical Findings In general, isolated bundle branch block does not lead to any detectable symptoms.

Therapy If possible, the underlying condition should be treated.

12.3 Antiarrhythmics

Numerous drugs can be used for rhythm control. Their specific area of application is discussed within the context of the respective medical conditions. Traditionally, antiarrhythmics are divided into 4 classes according to Vaughan-Williams (◻ Table 12.2 and ◻ Fig. 12.11).

▸ All antiarrhythmics can exhibit proarrhythmic side effects in addition to their intended antiarrhythmic effect.

Regarding the exact, detailed mechanisms of action of antiarrhythmics, we refer to pharmacology textbooks.

◻ **Table 12.2** Antiarrhythmics

Class	Mechanism	Examples
I	Sodium channel blockers; reduction of depolarization speed	
Ia	Slowing of depolarization speed (Phase 0) by blocking sodium channels Prolongation of repolarization duration by blocking potassium channels	Quinidine, Procainamide
Ib	Shortening of AP duration	Lidocaine, Mexiletine
Ic	Marked slowing of AP depolarization speed	Flecainide, Propafenone
II	Beta blockers	Metoprolol, Bisoprolol, etc.
III	Potassium channel blockers, prolongation of repolarization duration	Amiodarone, Dronedarone, Sotalol, Ibutilide
IV	Calcium channel blockers (Verapamil type); mainly affect the sinus and AV nodes	Verapamil, Diltiazem

AP: Action potential

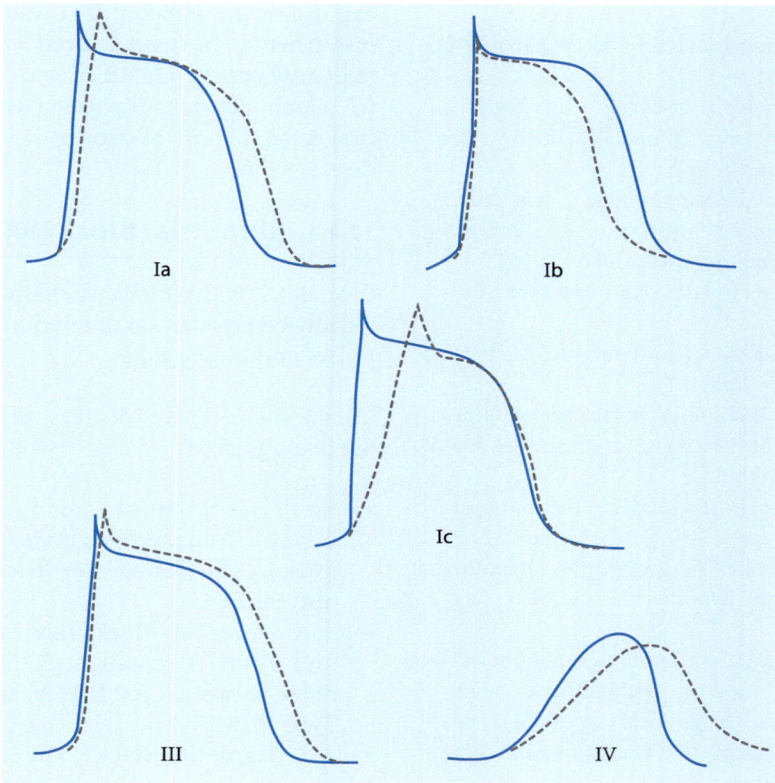

Fig. 12.11 Action potentials (solid line) and their changes under the influence of various classes of antiarrhythmics (dashed lines; according to Vaugham-Williams). Ventricular (Ia, Ib, Ic, III) and AV node action potentials (IV) are shown

12.4 Cardiac Arrhythmias

Definition A reduction in heart rate < 60 beats/min is referred to as bradycardia.

Pathophysiology, Etiology In bradycardia, there is initially a compensatory increase in stroke volume to maintain cardiac output. With a significantly reduced heart rate (usually < 40/min), a reduction in cardiac output commonly occurs. However, especially in highly trained athletes, resting heart rates < 30/min can also be associated with a normal cardiac output.

Bradycardia most commonly occurs in the context of sinus or AV node pathology. The causes may vary, but they often occur physiologically (e.g., in athletes or with high vagal tone). In the latter case, action is only required if the patient is symptomatic.

Causes of Sinus Bradycardia
- Idiopathic/degenerative (with increasing age; most common cause)
- Increased vagal tone: vasovagal syncope, hypersensitive carotid sinus
- Physical training (sports)
- Hereditary disease

- Ischemic heart disease (▶ Chap. 7.2 and 7.3)
- Infiltrative diseases: amyloidosis, sarcoidosis, hemochromatosis, etc. (▶ Chap. 8.1)
- Rheumatic/autoimmune spectrum: rheumatoid arthritis, systemic lupus erythematosus, scleroderma
- Muscle diseases, e.g., myotonic dystrophy
- Trauma/status post-surgical intervention (▶ Sect. 9.1)
- Infectious causes: borreliosis, diphtheria, Chagas disease, endocarditis, sepsis, typhoid
- Electrolyte disturbances (hypo-/hyperkalemia)
- Metabolic derangements: hypothyroidism, hypothermia, anorexia nervosa
- Medication-induced: negative chronotropic and/or bathmotropic medications (beta-blockers, calcium antagonists of the Varapamil- or Diltiazem-type, Digoxin, etc.; ▶ Sect. 13.3)
- Neurological diseases: increased intracranial pressure, CNS tumors
- Obstructive sleep apnea

Therapy The treatment of bradycardia disturbances depends on the overall clinical picture.

In an **emergency situation**, in case of hemodynamic instability or complete sinus arrest, the administration of sympathomimetics and, if necessary, implantation of a provisional pacemaker, possibly bridged by external pacing, is the therapy of choice.

The **long-term therapy** depends on the presence or absence of an underlying cause of bradycardia. If this can be successfully treated (e.g., by discontinuing bradycardic medications), a pacemaker implantation can usually be avoided. If it cannot or only insufficiently be treated, or if no underlying cause can be identified even after careful search, permanent pacemaker implantation is the therapy of choice.

12.4.1 Sinoatrial Block (SA Block)

Definition A SA-Block is characterized by a disturbed formation or conduction of impulses in the sinus node.

Classification Three degrees of SA-block are distinguished:

- 1st degree SA-Block: Conduction of the impulse from the sinus node to the atrial myocytes is slowed, not detectable in a normal ECG
- 2nd degree SA-Block: intermittent failures of atrial excitation. A distinction is made between Type I (Wenckebach) and Type II (Mobitz).
- 3rd degree SA-Block: The conduction of impulses from the sinus node is completely blocked (like sinus arrest). Either a replacement rhythm (AV node or further distal) or asystole is present.

In **2nd degree Type I SA-Block (Wenckebach)**, the conduction delay increases from impulse to impulse until finally an impulse is not conducted at all. Since the impulse generation in the sinus node is regular, but the delay increase becomes less from beat to beat, a shortening of the PP interval can be seen in the ECG, followed by a PP pause interval that is shorter than the sum of the two preceding PP intervals.

In **Type II Mobitz**, there are intermittent failures of the P wave in a constant ratio (◘ Fig. 12.12).

Etiology, Therapy For etiology and therapy see ▶ Chap. 12.3.

12.4.2 Atrioventricular Block (AV Block)

Definition An AV block, is characterized by a delay in impulse conduction at the level of the AV node.

Classification Three degrees of severity are distinguished:

- 1st degree AV-Block (PR interval > 200 msec.)
- 2nd degree AV-Block
  - Type I (Wenckebach, Mobitz I)
  - Type II (Mobitz or Mobitz II)
- 3rd degree AV-Block (complete interruption of AV conduction, AV dissociation)

In **AV Block 1st degree** (◘ Fig. 12.13), the conduction time is prolonged (> 200 ms),

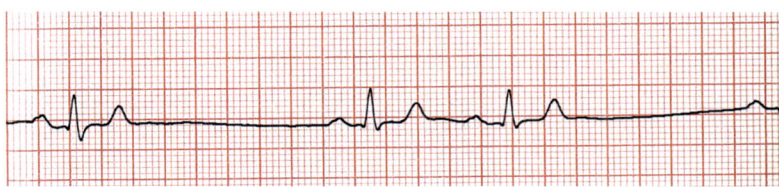

◘ **Fig. 12.12** Intermittent sinoatrial block Type II (Mobitz). With pronounced sinus arrhythmia, the PP interval of the sinus pause is slightly longer than the sum of the "normal" PP intervals

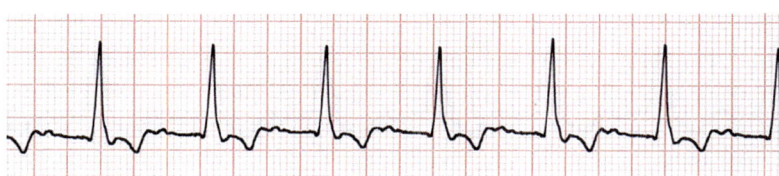

◘ **Fig. 12.13** AV Block 1st degree with significantly prolonged PQ time (280 ms)

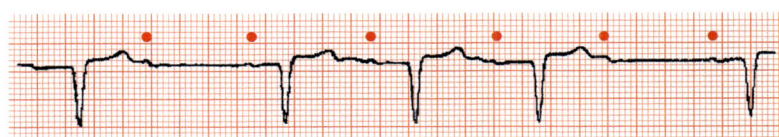

◘ **Fig. 12.14** Second-degree AV block Wenckebach type. There is a successive prolongation of the AV conduction time, every 4th P wave is not conducted to the ventricle

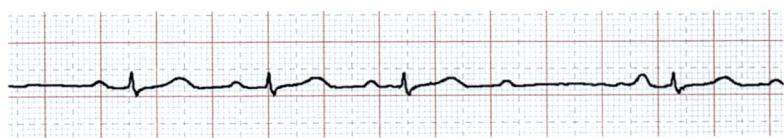

◘ **Fig. 12.15** Mobitz block. Unlike the Wenckebach block (◘ Fig. 12.14), there is no PQ time prolongation from beat to beat. Also, no AV reciprocity is observed

but all atrial excitations are conducted to the ventricle. In the ECG, a QRS complex follows each P wave.

The **second-degree AV block** is characterized by the occurrence of individual conduction blockages.
- In **Wenckebach type** (◐ Fig. 12.14), the conduction time typically increases successively until an atrial excitation is no longer conducted, after which this periodicity starts again. This shows the characteristic picture of "AV reciprocity": The PQ time **before** the blocked P is longer than the PQ time **after** the blocked P.
- In the (rarer) **Mobitz type** (◐ Fig. 12.15), the atrioventricular conduction is blocked in a constant ratio, e.g., in a 3:1 ratio. In this case, every 3rd P wave is not conducted to the ventricle in the ECG. The PQ time before and after the blocked excitation, however, is the same, so unlike the Wenckebach block, there is **no** prolongation of the PQ time (no AV reciprocity). The Mobitz type AV block is often associated with a structural disease, and the risk of progressing to a complete AV block is significantly increased.

▶ In a 2:1 block of AV conduction (◐ Fig. 12.16), i.e., conduction of only every 2nd P wave to the ventricle takes place. In this case, the distinction between second-degree AV block Wenckebach type and Mobitz type is not easily made and usually requires the addition of further diagnostic tools (carotid sinus pressure, administration of atropine, exercise, etc.).

A so-called "high-degree" AV block is present when more than one P wave in a row is not conducted. However, unlike third-degree AV block, intermittent conduction occurs. This block is often confused with second-degree AV block Mobitz type, in which only one P wave conduction fails, but not two (or more) in a row. Clinically, the "high-degree" AV block almost always has the same consequences as a third-degree AV block.

In **third-degree AV block** (◐ Fig. 12.17), there is a complete interruption of conduction from the atrium to the ventricle. As a substitute, a pacemaker located further distally takes over the function of impulse formation with a frequency of 30–40/min (rarely up to 60/min in high Hisian escape rhythm). In the ECG, usually widened but regular QRS complexes appear, which are completely independent of the P waves (complete AV dissociation).

A complete block of both the left and right bundle branches corresponds in its

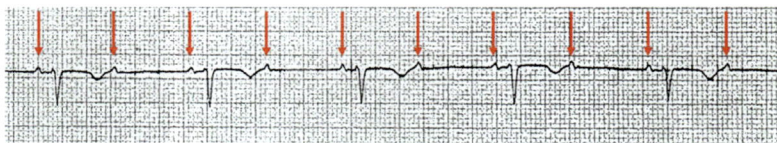

◐ **Fig. 12.16** Second-degree AV block with 2:1 conduction

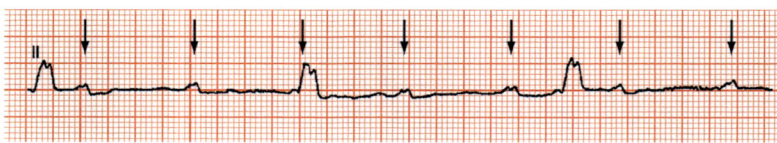

◐ **Fig. 12.17 Third-degree AV block.** Complete AV dissociation of atrial excitations (marked in black) and ventricular complexes

manifestation and clinical consequence to third-degree AV block and is referred to as a **trifascicular block**. Occasionally, the term "trifascicular block" is also used when a bifascicular block and a first-degree AV block are present simultaneously, which, however, should be avoided due to the propaedeutic inaccuracy and the potential for misinterpretation.

Etiology The causes of AV conduction disorders largely correspond to those listed in the overview (▶ Chap. 12.4) of the causes of bradycardia. Common causes include:

- increased vagal tone (Valsalva maneuver, carotid pressure)—especially in AVB I° and Wenckebach Block II°, significantly less in Mobitz type AVB II° and AVB III°,
- medications: Digitalis, beta-blockers, calcium antagonists of the Verapamil or Diltiazem type,
- electrolyte disturbances, especially hyperkalemia,
- ischemia, acute myocardial infarction,
- myocarditis,
- cardiomyopathies,
- history of cardiac surgery, e.g., aortic valve replacement, TAVI (▶ Chap. 9.1)
- congenital heart disease (e.g. atrial septal defect, Ebstein's anomaly),
- hypothyroidism,
- idiopathic fibrosis of the conduction system,
- sarcoidosis, scleroderma, amyloidosis, lupus erythematosus.

Clinical Findings First-degree AV block is mostly asymptomatic. In third-degree AV block, as well as occasionally in higher-grade second-degree AV block and/or pronounced bradycardia, there may be exercise intolerance, dizziness, or even syncope.

Therapy In AV block, as in SA block and bradycardic rhythm disturbances in general, a treatable cause must be excluded or, if present, treated.

In first-degree AV block and Wenckebach type second-degree AV block, further therapy is determined by the patient's clinical presentation. If symptoms that impair quality of life are present, the indication for pacemaker implantation may be given. Additionally, caution is advised when using bradycardic medications (e.g. beta-blockers, amiodarone, etc.).

In patients with Mobitz type second-degree AV block, high-degree AV block, and (acquired) third-degree AV block, there is an indication for pacemaker implantation from a prognostic perspective.

▶ Practical Recommendations

Principle of Pacemaker Therapy

A modern pacemaker detects the heart's own actions (sensing) and, if no intrinsic actions are detectable within a set time interval, delivers impulses (pacing), which then leads to the contraction of the atrium or ventricle, respectively (◘ Table 12.3). The primary goal is to prevent the heart rate from falling below the programmed base rate. By parallel sensing in the atrium and stimulation in the ventricle, AV synchrony is maintained in the case of total AV block. Ventricular sensing prevents a pacemaker-delivered impulse from falling into the relative refractory period of the preceding beat in the event of an intrinsic action or the occurrence of ventricular extrasystoles, thus avoiding the triggering of a ventricular rhythm disturbance. Modern pacemakers also have the capability to increase the stimulated heart rate, for example, when the patient exercises (i.e. rate adaptive pacing). Through a special mechanisms, the patient's ventilation rate and/or the relative acceleration of the pacemaker unit (accelerometer) are usually measured; based in that information, the patient's activity level is extrapolated, resulting in an adjustment of the pacemaker rate. ◀

■ **Table 12.3** Standardized Pacemaker Coding

1	2	3	4
Stimulation	Sensing	Mode of Operation	Rate Adaptation
0 (none)	0 (none)	0 (none)	0 (none)
A (atrium)	A (atrium)	T (triggered)	R (adaptive)
V (ventricle)	V (ventricle)	I (inhibited)	
D (dual A + V)	D (dual A + V)	D (dual T + I)	

12.5 arrhythmias

Definition Tachycardia is defined as an increase in heart rate > 100 beats/min.

Classification Depending on their anatomical site of origin, supraventricular and ventricular tachycardias are distinguidshed. Based on the mechanism, a distinction is made between automaticity (abnormal acceleration of phase IV activity), reentry (circulating excitation), and triggered activity (triggered by "afterdepolarization" falling on a preceding action).

12.5.1 Sinus tachycardia

Definition Sinus tachycardia is originating from the sinus node (or structures near the sinus node).

Etiology Sinus tachycardia can appear physiologically during physical exertion or psychological stress. On the other hand, it can also occur as a result of a systemic disease (e.g., hyperthyroidism, pulmonary embolism, etc.) or as demand tachycardia (e.g., in hypovolemia, anemia, fever, pregnancy, etc.).

Rarely, sinus tachycardia is based on a **sinus node dysfunction**, i.e., a functional disorder of the sinus node itself (so-called **inappropriate sinus tachycardia**, IST). In this heterogeneous and overall insufficiently characterized disease pattern, there is a permanently elevated heart rate at rest and an excessive increase under stress. There is evidence of a genetic origin in some cases (e.g. Familial Inapropriate Sinus Tachycardia). A special case is Postural Orthostatic Tachycardia Syndrome (POTS; typically in the context of Long Covid) where an inappropriate increase in heart rate acurrs upon standing with blood pressure decrease, dizzines up to (pre-)syncope.

Therapy If sinus tachycardia is based on a pathological cause (e.g. hyperthyroidism among others), this must primarily be treated and **not** primarily using bradycardic medications (beta-blockers, Ivabradine etc.).

▶ Bradycardic medications may even worsen symptoms, as tachycardia in these situations (e.g. anemia among others) represents a physiological reaction of the organism to maintain cardiac output or the increased basal metabolic rate.

In inappropriate sinus tachycardia (IST), symptomatic administration of bradycardic medications (e.g. beta-blockers, Verapamil- or Diltiazem-type calcium antagonist, If-channel blocker) may be indicated, but this must be done cautiously in the presence of pronounced intermittent bradycardia and occasionally requires simultaneous pacemaker implantation to protect against sinus arrest or higher-grade AV block.

12.5.2 Atrial fibrillation

Definition In atrial fibrillation, focal activity and micro-reentries within the atria develop, which in most cases originate in the pulmonary veins, lead to extremely high atrial frequencies (> 350/min); this results basically in a standstill of the atrial musculature. Since the AV node only irregularly transmits these high atrial frequencies to the ventricle, an absolute arrhythmia with ventricular frequencies usually around 70–110/min, but sometimes up to 180/min., occurs.

> If an accessory conduction bundle is present at the same time (→ WPW), it can, in extreme cases, lead to very rapid transmission of atrial potentials to the ventricle, resulting in ventricular tachycardia with possible degeneration into ventricular fibrillation (so-called "FBI tachycardia": Fast—Broad—Irregular).

Epidemiology Atrial fibrillation is by far the most common tachycardia. The prevalence of atrial fibrillation increases with age: in adults over 60 years, it averages about 0.5%, and in those over 75 years, it rises to about 9%. The incidence also increases with age: one-quarter of all adults over 40 years will experience at least one episode of atrial fibrillation in their lifetime.

Etiology Atrial fibrillation can occur in heart-healthy patients as a degenerative conditione of the atrium or pulmonary veins, respectively. However, it is often accompanied by any form of structural heart disease, e.g., arterial hypertension (▶ Sect. 4), CAD (▶ Chap. 7.2), mitral valve disease (▶ Chap. 9.4) or heart failure (▶ Chap. 13.2). Additionally, exogenous causes such as systemic diseases (e.g. hyperthyroidism, pulmonary embolism; ▶ Chap. 17.3; history of-cardiac surgery) as well as alcohol consumption in predisposed individuals can trigger atrial fibrillation (so-called *Holiday Heart Syndrome*). Hereditary causes have also been described, e.g., the 10q22-q24 mutation on chromosome 10, which usually leads to atrial fibrillation at a younger age and occurs frequently in families.

Pathophysiology The development and maintenance of atrial fibrillation require both a trigger (i.e., an initiator) and a substrate for maintenance (◘ Fig. 12.18).

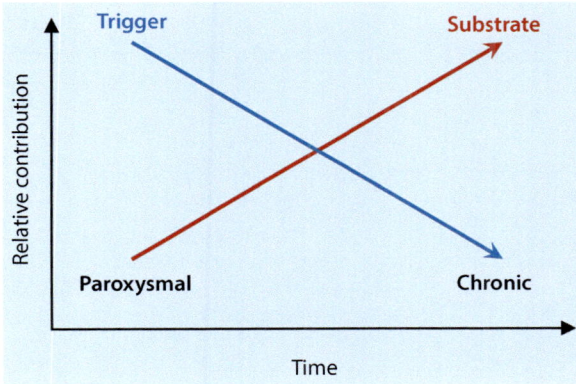

◘ Fig. 12.18 Relative contribution of trigger and substrate in the development and maintenance of atrial fibrillation

Automatically discharging ectopic excitation foci in the pulmonary veins are the most common triggers of atrial fibrillation. The substrate for maintaining atrial fibrillation sometimes consists of structurally altered atrial areas in the context of structural heart disease, e.g., in the form of atrial fibrosis in long-standing hypertension, but it can also be absent, especially in early forms of atrial fibrillation. On the other hand, atrial fibrillation itself leads to structural remodeling processes of the atria with fibrosis formation (so-called Remodeling), so that especially in long-standing atrial fibrillation, these remodeling processes significantly contribute to the maintenance of atrial fibrillation (*"Atrial fibrillation begets atrial fibrillation,"*). The remodeling processes occur in parallel and synergistically in the form of electrical, anatomical, and functional remodeling.

Atrial fibrillation can, simply put,
— occur paroxysmally (as sudden attacks),
— persistently (< 7 days), or
— permanently (no cardioversion possible).

With increasing duration and development from paroxysmal to permanent atrial fibrillation, the relative contribution of the latter continuously increases in the interplay of trigger and substrate (◘ Fig. 12.18).

Clinical Findings Occasionally, patients are only mildly symptomatic with effective rate control. Symptoms are mainly noticed at high heart rates. The patient experiences palpitations, occasionally radiating to the neck, and at higher frequencies chest pain, dyspnea, or dizziness and even syncope may occur. Due to the decreasing cardiac output exercise intolerance is often observed. Due to atrial overload, there is an increased release of atrial natriuretic peptide (ANP), which can lead to polyuria.

> In principle, any increase in heart rate shortens the time for myocardial perfusion, as coronary blood flow occurs almost exclusively during diastole. Thus, with pronounced or prolonged tachycardia, angina pectoris can occur due to the resulting ischemia, especially in the context of pre-existing coronary artery disease.

Diagnostics During clinical examination, a pulse deficit is noticeable, i.e., there is a difference between the heart rate as obtained during auscultation and the radial pulse. The ECG shows absolute arrhythmia with fibrillation waves and absent P-waves (often most clearly seen in II and V1; ◘ Fig. 12.19).

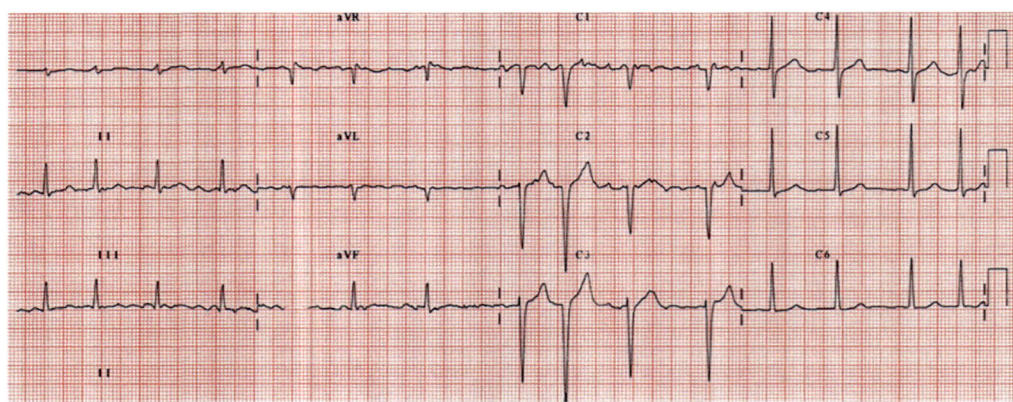

◘ **Fig. 12.19 ECG in atrial fibrillation** shows absolute arrhythmia, a regular P-wave is not detectable, but coarse fibrillation waves are noticable in V1

Conduction System Diseases—Cardiac Arrhythmias

Therapy If possible, an underlying systemic disease (e.g., hyperthyroidism, pulmonary embolism; ▶ Sect. 17.3) or heart failure (▶ Sect. 13.3) should be treated. Indeed, ablation of atrial fibrillation in HFrEF improves outcomes.

Otherwise, the management of atrial fibrillation consists of 3 components:
- Anticoagulation,
- Control of symptoms (rate control or rhythm control)
- Treatment of risk factors and comorbidities.

The exact pathophysiology of the increased risk of stroke in atrial fibrillation is not always clear. In addition to the altered flow properties of the blood during atrial standstill during atrial fibrillation, systemic factors also seem to play a decisive role.

▶ A decisive proportion of mortality and particularly morbidity in atrial fibrillation is due to thromboembolic events, especially stroke.

Therefore, in atrial fibrillation, there is an indication for blood thinning through oral **anticoagulation**—depending on the patient's risk profile, which is determined using the so-called CHA_2DS_2-VASc score:
- Chronic Heart Failure (heart failure; ▶ Chap. 13.3)
- Hypertension (▶ Sect. 4)
- Age ≥ 75 years (2 points), age ≥ 65 years (1 point)
- Diabetes,
- Status post-stroke (CVI/TIA; ▶ Chap. 7.5) (2 points)
- Vascular disease (▶ Sect. 7.5),
- Female sex is no longer considered important

Depending on the score, the recommended treatment for blood thinning is determined: At 0 points, no oral anticoagulation (OAC) is recommended; at 1 point, it should be considered (risk-benefit assessment; bleeding vs. embolism); and from 2 points, it is clearly recommended. The factor "female sex" is a special case: This only constitutes an indication for OAC in combination with at least one other risk factor; according to CHA_2DS_2-VASc, no OAC is recommended for women with no other risk factors.

Today, oral anticoagulation is primarily carried out with one of the Novel Oral AntiCoagulants (**NOAC**s; Apixaban®, Dabigatran®, Edoxaban® or Rivaroxaban®). Large studies have shown that NOACs, which selectively inhibit factor Xa (Apixaban, Rivaroxaban, Edoxaban) or thrombin (Dabigatran), have a better benefit-risk profile compared to vitamin K antagonists and are also more patient-friendly (no INR controls as with the vitamin K antagonists). Therefore, they are recommended as the preferred therapy for anticoagulation in atrial fibrillation.

However, certain limitations and caveats exist, particularly in patients with severe renal failure as well as in patients with mechanical heart valves or mitral stenosis (where they are contraindicated and Vitamin K antagonists should be used; ▶ Sect. 9.3) and others. In contrast, aspirin is no longer recommended for stroke prevention in atrial fibrillation in practically any patient due to its low efficacy.

For patients with a strong indication for anticoagulation, but simultaneous contraindications (especially after a severe bleeding event), an interventional method for stroke prevention is available with **percutaneous left atrial appendage closure**. Here, a catheter introduced transseptally via the femoral vein is used to close the left atrial appendage with a umbrella-shaped device,. Indeed, the main source of thromboembolism in atrial fibrillation is the left atrial appendix which can be effectively closed with a special device (◘ Fig. 12.20). Alterna-

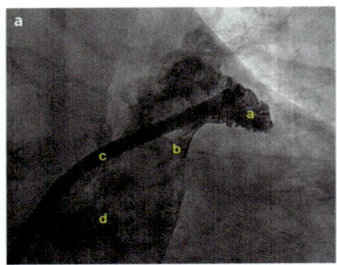 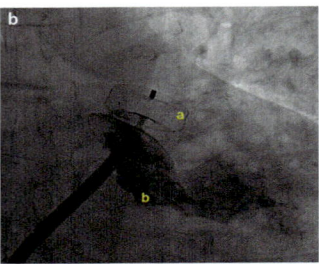 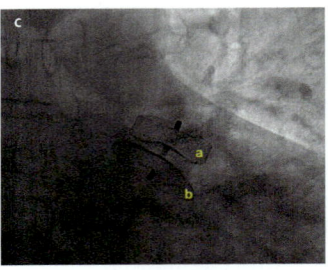

Fig. 12.20 (a–c) **LAA closure.** (a) Angiographic representation of the LAA (a = left atrial appendage, b = left atrial appendage neck; c = sheath; d = LA); (b) Implantation of the occluder (a), b = LA. (c) LAA occluder in situ (a = disc, b = lobe). (Courtesy of Fabian Nietlispach)

tively, the left atrial appendage can be surgically closed during a heart operation. This therapy is currently mainly used in patients with absolute contraindications for anticoagulation (high bleeding risk, history of cerebral or subdural hemorrhage, etc.).

For **frequency control**, beta-blockers, calcium antagonists of the Verapamil- or Diltiazem-type, or Digitalis (in case of heart failure, but less effective in rate control) can be used. This therapeutic concept is practiced today only in patients who are demonstrably "asymptomatic" with regard to their atrial fibrillation even after an electrical cardioversion, and in whom no consequences are expected even with the likely progression of the disease in later years.

In **rhythm control**, acute and chronic management are distinguished:
- If there is hemodynamic instability in the **acute phase**, there is an indication for immediate cardioversion to sinus rhythm using electrical energy and/or intravenous antiarrhythmics.
- The **chronic** rhythm control can be managed pharmacologically with the use of antiarrhythmics. Here, primarily class Ic antiarrhythmics (▶ Chap. 12.3, in the absence of structural heart disease) as well as class III antiarrhythmics (e.g. Amiodarone) are used.
- Alternatively, nowadays and generally preferred in larger centers, there is the option of **catheter-based ablation** using radiofrequency energy, cryoablation, or electroporation (▶ Sect. 12.5.5) for symptomatic atrial fibrillation. Due to numerous technical improvements in recent years, this procedure is increasingly being used and, according to several guidelines, can also be considered as first-line therapy in suitable patients. In patients with heart failure (HFrEF), ablation can be prognostically favorable in addition to its pronounced symptomatic benefit. It is important that the procedure is performed in any case by experienced operators and in centers specifically designed for this purpose.

Prior to a cardioversion, whether pharmacological or electrical, except in an emergency situation (see above), anticoagulation in the therapeutic range must be carried out for at least 3 weeks or an atrial thrombus must be excluded by transesophageal echocardiography (▶ Sect. 2.5). Also, after a successful cardioversion, anticoagulation must be continued for another 4 weeks, among other things because the standstill of the atrial walls (*atrial stunning*) can persist for some time despite restored sinus rhythm, thus the risk of thromboembolism remains.

If there is a risk (according to the CHA_2DS_2-VASc score), anticoagulation must also be continued in patients with rhythm

Conduction System Diseases—Cardiac Arrhythmias

control, among other things because in these situations, many patients have intermittent, partly asymptomatic atrial fibrillation with a corresponding risk of thrombus formation and peripherla or cerbera embolisation and stroke.

Prognosis The prognosis of atrial fibrillation primarily depends on the presence or absence of structural heart diseases. The prognosis of "idiopathic" atrial fibrillation was long considered to be generally good, but data now show that atrial fibrillation per se is associated with a worse prognosis, which is why it cannot be dismissed as "harmless" and should be treated accordingly.

12.5.3 Atrial Flutter

Definition Atrial flutter is characterized by an atrial frequency of 240–350/min, with no isoelectric line between the individual P-waves on the ECG.

Pathophysiology Typical atrial flutter is sustained by a macro-reentry in the right atrium, which includes the isthmus between the entry of the inferior vena cava and the tricuspid valve (so-called cavo-tricuspid isthmus). In atypical atrial flutter, this macro-reentry circuit can practically be located anywhere in the right or left atrium.

Clinical Findings Patients with atrial flutter are usually more symptomatic than those with atrial fibrillation; otherwise, the clinical presentation is similar.

Diagnostics The ECG features typical counter-clockwise isthmus-dependent atrial flutter with a sawtooth pattern between normally shaped QRS complexes in leads II, III, aVF (◘ Fig. 12.21).

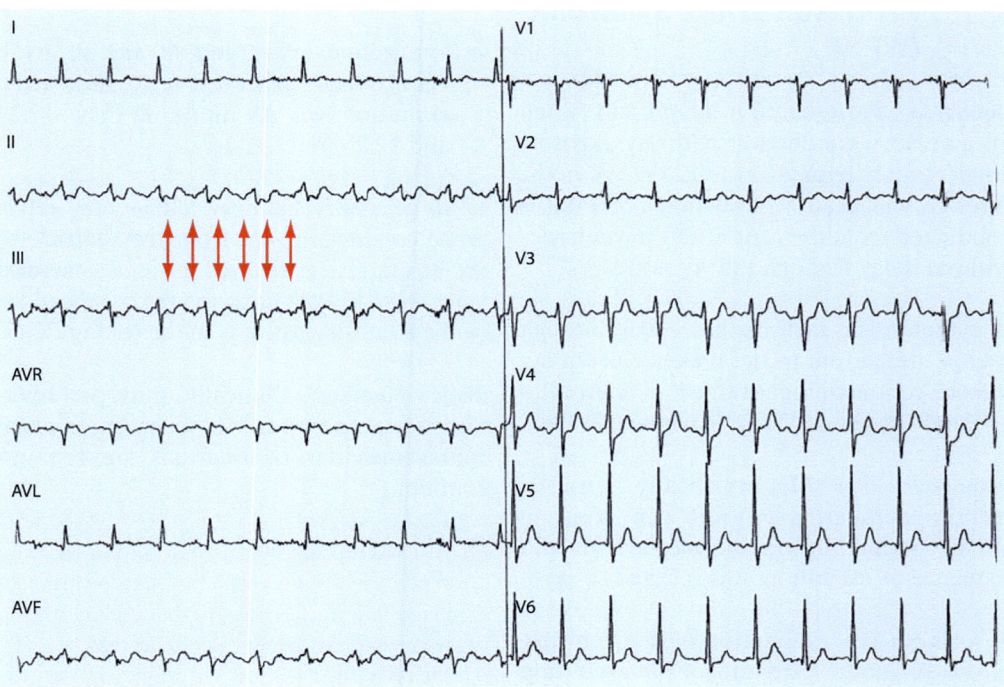

◘ **Fig. 12.21** ECG in typical atrial flutter. The flutter waves are best seen in leads II, III (red arrows), and aVF

› Therapy

The management of atrial flutter is similar to that for fibrillation in terms of stroke prevention.

In the **acute situation**, emergency cardioversion is indicated in case of hemodynamic instability. Otherwise, the same guidelines for cardioversion and anticoagulation apply as for atrial fibrillation.

For the **long-term therapy of atrial flutter**, catheter ablation of the underlying reentry circuit at the cavo-tricuspid isthmus has a high success rate and is the first-line therapy for typical atrial flutter. To do so, tissue is heated and replaced by scar tissue using a **radiofrequency catheter** (▶ Sect. 12.5.5), thereby interrupting the electrical circuit underlying the flutter. Frequency control is generally not promising in atrial flutter, nor is medical rhythm therapy.

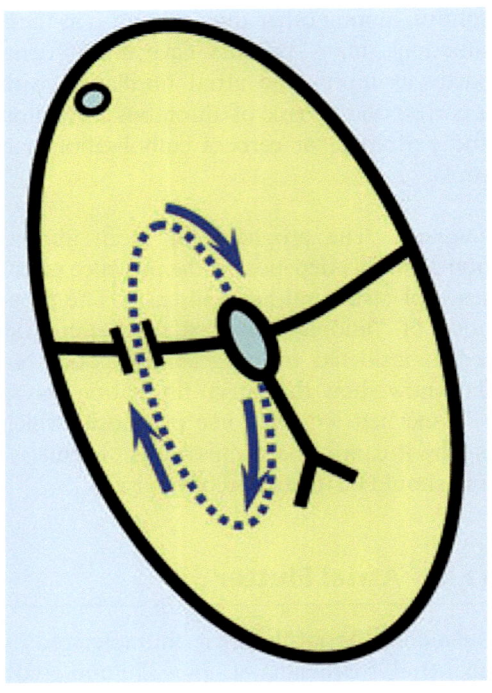

Fig. 12.22 Mechanism of orthodromic AVRT

12.5.4 Pre-excitation and Wolff-Parkinson-White Syndrome (WPW)

Definition Pre-excitation is present when an accessory conduction pathway exists as an electrical "bypass" around the AV node, through which an atrial action potential is conducted from the atrium to the ventricles without delay through the AV node.

If symptomatic tachycardias occur through such a mechanism in the presence of an accessory conduction pathway, it is referred to as **Wolff-Parkinson-White Syndrome (WPW)**.

Pathophysiology Mechanistically, an AV reentry tachycardia (AVRT) can occur in WPW. Depending on the mechanism and sequence of excitation, it is referred to as

— orthodromic (excitation of the ventricle via AV node, retrograde atrial excitation via accessory bundle, ◘ Figs. 12.22 and 12.23) or

— antidromic (excitation of the ventricle via accessory pathway, retrograde atrial excitation via AV node, ◘ Figs. 12.24 and 12.25) referred to.

If an accessory pathway allows only retrograde conduction (i.e., from the ventricle to the atrium), it is referred to as a **concealed** (*concealed*) **WPW**, as there are no indications of the accessory pathway in the resting ECG.

Clinical Findings Clinically, pure preexcitation is asymptomatic; however, paroxysmal supraventricular tachycardias are not uncommon.

› If atrial fibrillation is present at the same time, ventricular fibrillation can be triggered via the accessory bundle in extreme cases, as the physiological delay in the AV node is bypassed and there is very rapid conduction to the ventricle ("FBI tachycardia").

Conduction System Diseases—Cardiac Arrhythmias

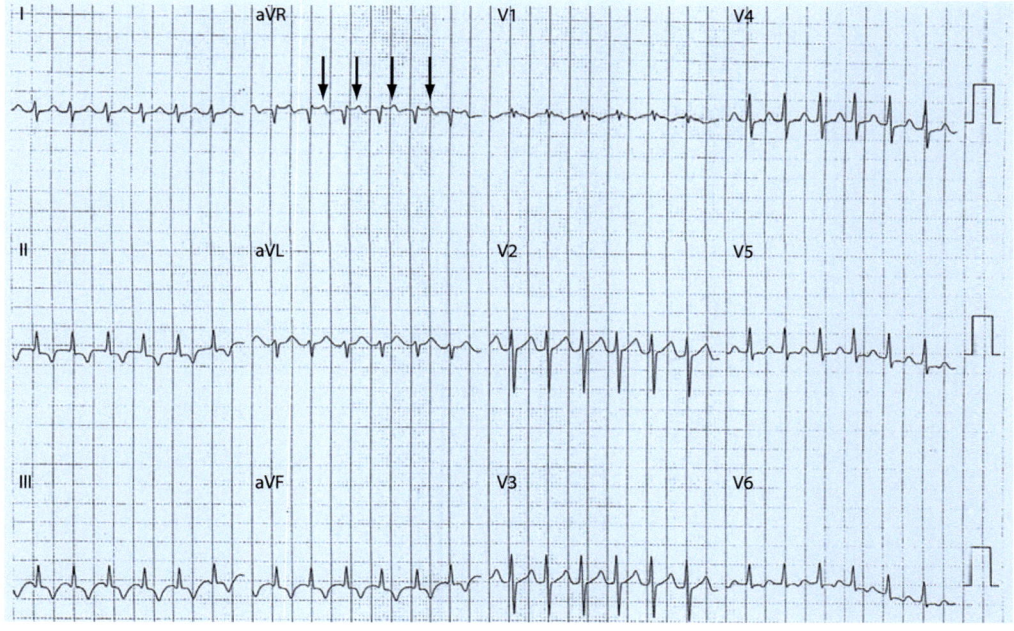

Fig. 12.23 Orthodromic AV reentrant tachycardia (AVRT). The arrows mark the retrograde atrial excitation following the QRS complex

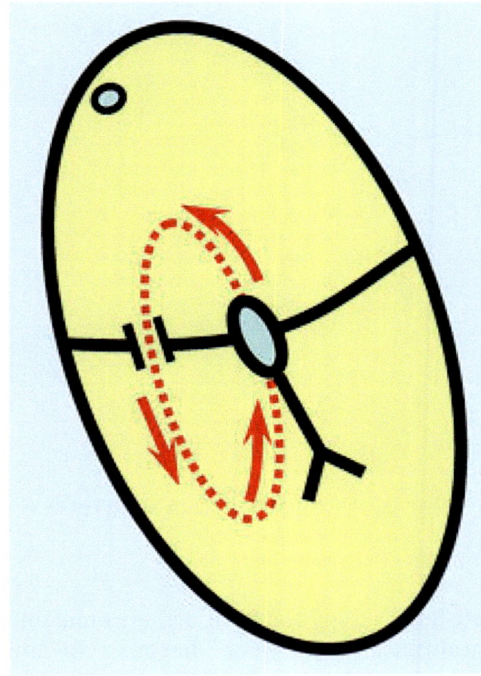

Fig. 12.24 Mechanism of antidromic AVRT

Diagnostics In **preexcitation**, the ECG shows a shortening of the PQ time to less than 120 ms and a delta wave (broadening of the QRS complex "forward" as an expression of early ventricular excitation via the accessory pathway, ● Fig. 12.26). The morphology of the QRS complex can already provide clues to the location of the accessory pathway in the resting ECG.

In **orthodromic AVRT of WPW**, retrograde atrial excitation following ventricular excitation can be detected in the ECG (● Fig. 12.23), which follows at a certain distance from the QRS complex ("long-R-P" tachycardia). In **antidromic AVRT**, ventricular excitation is maximally preexcited, resulting in the appearance of a wide complex tachycardia (● Fig. 12.25), whose QRS vector corresponds to that of the delta wave. P waves are either not visible or can be identified within the QRS complex.

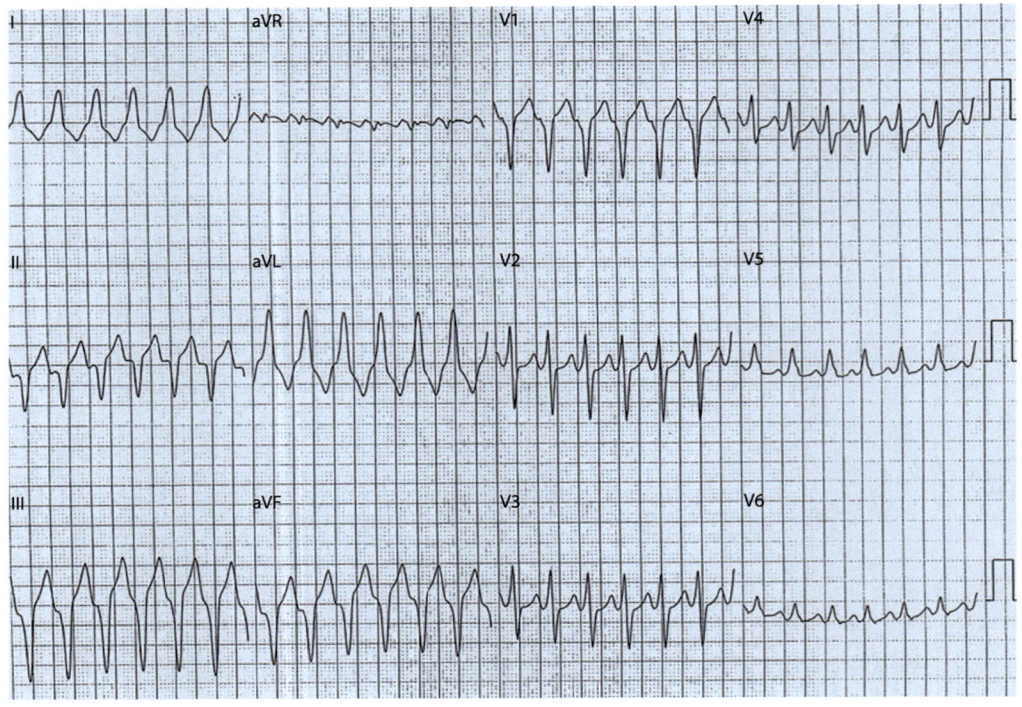

Fig. 12.25 Antidromic AV reentrant tachycardia (AVRT) in WPW syndrome

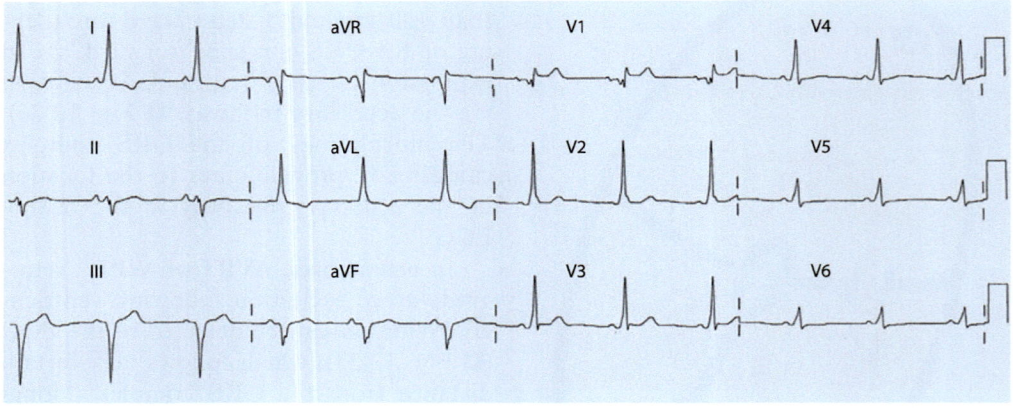

Fig. 12.26 Ventricular preexcitation in the presence of an accessory conduction pathway, which is visible as a delta wave in the resting ECG

Therapy In the acute phase, the administration of adenosine (6 mg, 12 mg up to 18 mg as a rapid bolus) is recommended as first-line therapy for both orthodromic and antidromic AVRT. The diagnosis of antidromic AVRT can be difficult, as it is a wide complex tachycardia. Alternatively, class Ic antiarrhythmics have proven effective (except in the presence of concurrent structural heart disease such as CAD). In cases of concurrent atrial fibrillation with rapid conduction (where adenosine administration is ineffective and may be counterproductive) and hemodynamic instability, cardioversion is the first-line therapy.

❗ Digitalis and Verapamil are relatively contraindicated in WPW, as they block the AV node and thus may promote rapid conduction via the accessory pathway.

In principle, catheter ablation is indicated in the presence of an accessory pathway, as the potential for rapid ventricular conduction can lead to life-threatening arrhythmias. Catheter ablation can now be performed with a high success rate and low complication rate.

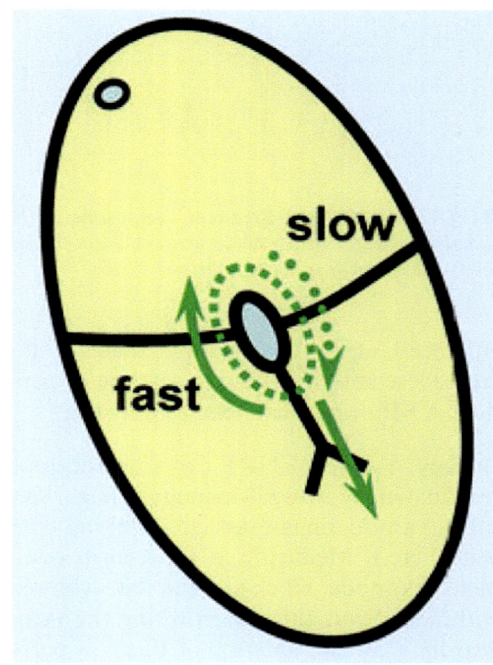

Fig. 12.27 Mechanism of AVNRT with typical slow-fast pattern

12.5.5 AV Node Reentrant Tachycardias

Definition The AV Node Reentrant Tachycardia (AVNRT) is a supraventricular arrhythmia characterized by a reentrant circuit within the AV node.

Epidemiology Women are more frequently affected than men, accounting for 70% of cases, and tend to have AVNRTs at a younger age.

Pathophysiology In 20% of the population, there is a dual conduction physiology in the AV node with pathways that conduct at different speeds. Typically, there is a slow pathway with a short refractory period and a fast pathway with a longer refractory period. An inopportune atrial extrasystole can lead to a reentrant circuit within the AV node, triggering an AVNRT. In 90% of cases, the slow pathway conducts anterogradely and the fast pathway retrogradely (so-called slow-fast type, **Fig. 12.27**). In about 10% of cases, it is the reverse (fast-slow type) or there are two slow pathways (slow-slow type).

Clinical Findings Patients with AVNRT report palpitations as a correlate of the intermittently occurring supraventricular tachycardias. Simultaneous excitation of the ventricle and atrium can lead to atrial contraction against the closed AV valve, resulting in a pulsation in the neck.

Diagnostics The typical frequency of AVNRT is between 140–220/min. In the ECG, narrow QRS complexes are seen, and P waves may be hidden within the QRS complex or detectable shortly after the QRS complex (**Fig. 12.28**; "short R-P" tachycardia). Due to the tachycardia with

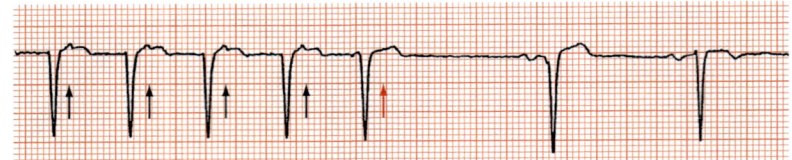

Fig. 12.28 **AV Node Reentrant Tachycardia (AVNRT).** The retrograde atrial excitation following the QRS complex is clearly visible (black arrows). After the last complex, there is no retrograde atrial excitation (red arrow), and the tachycardia terminates

enhanced atrial contraction, there is increased secretion of atrial natriuretic peptide (ANP), which can lead to polyuria.

Therapy Acute AVNRT can sometimes be terminated by a vagal maneuver (e.g., Valsalva, carotid sinus massage, drinking cold water, etc.). Medically, a short-term complete AV node blockade can be achieved with adenosine, thus interrupting the tachycardia. Catheter ablation of the slow pathway ("*slow pathway*" ablation) is the treatment of choice, which can be performed with a high success rate and low complication rate.

> ▶ **Practical Recommendation**
>
> **Electrophysiological Study (EPS) and Radiofrequency Ablation (RFA)**
> While in the past, drug therapy was practically the only treatment option for most arrhythmias, nowadays many rhythm disorders can be effectively and safely treated using invasive catheter techniques, and thus in many cases, can be definitively cured.
> For this purpose, several electrophysiological catheters are first placed via the femoral vein in the right atrium, in the right ventricle, at the His bundle, and if necessary, in the coronary sinus, with which the rhythm disorder is characterized using special stimulation protocols.
> During ablation, tissue is specifically heated (radiofrequency ablation), cooled (e.g., cryo-balloon catheter), or the cell membrane is destroyed (electroporation) using a special catheter, resulting in scar formation. Various therapeutic strategies are used in the treatment of specific rhythm disorders:
>
> – In **atrial fibrillation**, the pulmonary veins, which as mentioned, in most cases represent the focus of the fibrillation, are primarily electrically isolated. For this purpose, circular scars are drawn around the mouth of the pulmonary veins using radiofrequency energy (heat), cryoenergy, or electroporation (Pulse Field or cold ablation), thus electrically isolating the veins from the atrium. The rhythm disorder is therefore not resolved at its origin, but its spread to the atria is prevented.
> – In **atrial flutter**, the substrate is a macro-reentry circuit, which (in typical atrial flutter) includes the isthmus between the tricuspid valve ring and the inferior vena cava. By drawing an ablation line (usually using radiofrequency energy) across this isthmus, the reentry circuit can be interrupted and the atrial flutter resolved.
> – In the presence of an accessory pathway, it is first carefully localized using an electrophysiological study. By targeted radiofrequency energy delivery (rarely focal cryoenergy) the pathway can then be ablated, thus resolving the rhythm disorder.
> – In **AVNRT**, ablation of the slow pathway of the AV node is performed. This eliminates a critical component of the reentry circuit necessary for maintaining the tachycardia, thus usually curing the tachycardia. ◀

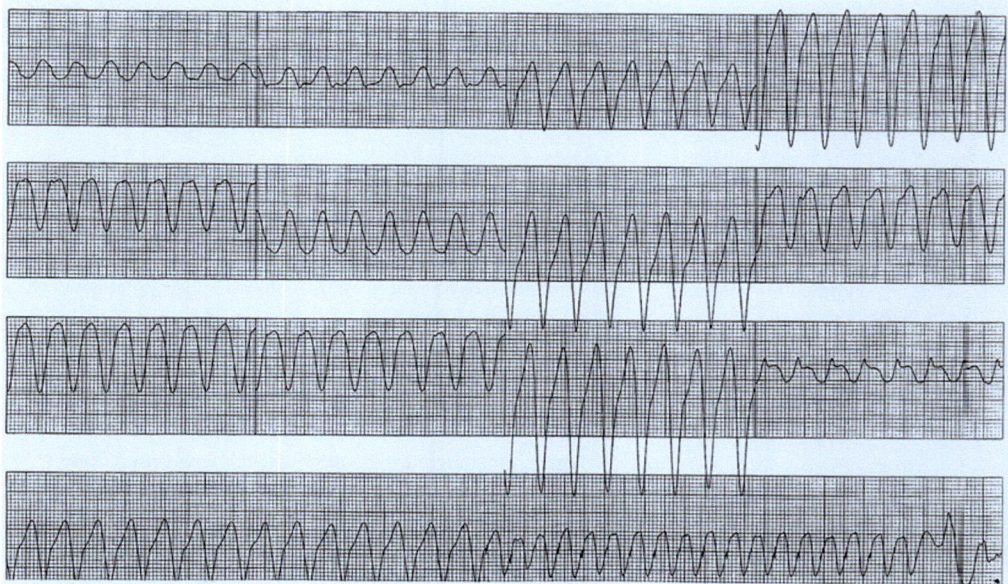

◘ Fig. 12.29 Ventricular Tachycardia

12.5.6 Ventricular Tachycardia

Definition The occurrence of 4 or more ventricular extrasystoles (VES) in succession is formally referred to as ventricular tachycardia (VT) (◘ Fig. 12.29). At higher rates of ventricular tachycardia, it is referred to as ventricular flutter (250–350/min) or fibrillation (> 350/min; ◘ Fig. 12.31). The transition from ventricular flutter to ventricular fibrillation is fluid. The term ventricular flutter has largely been replaced by the term "fast VT" in the ICD era.

Classification, Differential Diagnosis Sustained ventricular tachycardia lasts longer than 30 s, while non-sustained VT lasts < 30 s. In monomorphic VT, each QRS complex is identically configured, whereas in polymorphic VT, it is not.

Occasionally, it can be difficult to distinguish a ventricular tachycardia from a supraventricular tachycardia conducted in the presence of a bundle branch block, as both present as wide complex tachycardia. However, there are some indications that suggest one or the other genesis (◘ Table 12.4).

Etiology and Pathophysiology While ventricular extrasystoles can also frequently occur in healthy individuals, VTs are often an expression of structural heart disease. As the most common electrophysiological mechanism, monomorphic VTs consist of reentry mechanisms that revolve around a ventricular substrate and maintain the tachycardia. The most common cause is a previous myocardial infarction, where regional abnormal propagation and excitability of the myocytes occur in the (border) zone of the infarction. Other substrates for the development (and maintenance) of a VT can be other local scars, ventricular dilation in heart failure, fibrosis, inflammation, and structural changes in the context of cardiomyopathies (▶ Sect. 8.1) as well as cardiac manifestations in sarcoidosis, amyloidosis, Chagas disease, Fabry disease, etc.

◻ **Table 12.4** Differential diagnosis of wide complex tachycardia. (Supraventricular with bundle branch block vs. ventricular tachycardia)

More likely supraventricular tachycardia with bundle branch block	More likely ventricular tachycardia
Onset with premature atrial excitation (P wave)	Onset with premature QRS complex
QRS complexes similar to those in sinus rhythm (axis, morphology)	QRS complexes similar to ventricular extrasystoles during sinus rhythm (axis, morphology)
QRS morphology consistent with aberrant conduction (V1, V6)	QRS morphology rather not consistent with aberrant conduction (V1, V6)
Gradual onset or gradual slowing	**AV dissociation**
Slowing/termination with vagal maneuvers	**Fusion beats** (intrinsic ventricular excitation via AV node coincides with VT complex)
	Atrial excitation intermittently coincides with excitable ventricular myocardium and is conducted normally (***Capture beats***)
	Atypical left axis (especially position between −90 and 180°)
	Concordant R-wave pattern in the precordial leads (especially negative concordance)
	No RS complex in the precordial leads
	QRS duration > 140 ms

Bold—indicative of VT (AV dissociation, fusion beats, capture beats)

In addition, there are the relatively benign idiopathic ventricular tachycardias (often from the area of the right or left ventricular outflow tract) with focal automaticity as a mechanism, which also occur in healthy hearts and generally have a good prognosis. Causes of polymorphic VTs include acute myocardial infarction (▶ Sect. 7.3), ischemias (▶ Sect. 7.2), electrolyte imbalances, acidosis, hypoxia, etc.

❗ In patients with hypertrophic cardiomyopathy (HCM), there is an increased risk of sudden cardiac death due to ventricular fibrillation, especially during physical exertion (HCM = most common cause of death in young athletes).

Therapy In the case of hemodynamic instability, there is an indication for electrical cardioversion (see below). Furthermore, a triggering cause, particularly ischemia or another structural heart disease, must be sought or excluded and, if present, treated accordingly. For the pharmacological therapy of structural VTs, amiodarone or class Ib antiarrhythmics are generally used, which are relatively effective on the one hand, but associated with numerous side effects on the other. Alternatively, ablation treatment is increasingly being performed for ventricular tachycardias, although this generally involves a slightly higher risk and lower success rates than the ablation of supraventricular arrhythmias.

12.5.7 QT Interval Prolongation and Torsade de Pointes Arrhythmia

Definition The Torsade de Pointes Arrhythmia is a distinct form of ventricular tachycardia, triggered by a prolonged repolarization time of the ventricles (i.e. a prolonged QT interval), which results in triggered activity in phase III of the action potential (◘ Fig. 12.30).

Etiology A prolongation of the QT interval can be congenital (long QT syndrome) or acquired. Typical causes for the latter are electrolyte disturbances (e.g., hypokalemia) as well as various medications (e.g., quinidine, antihistamines, antibiotics, many psychotropic drugs) and certain antiarrhythmics (see ► http://www.qtdrugs.org for details).

Diagnostics In the ECG, a rapid VT with continuous rotation of the electrical heart axis in the tachycardia is shown, resulting in the typical spindle-shaped ECG curve (*torsade de pointes* = twisting of the points).

12.5.8 Ventricular Fibrillation

Etiology and Pathogenesis Ventricular fibrillation, like polymorphic VT, is in most cases caused by ischemia, whether due to CAD or a myocardial infarction (the latter being the most common cause!) or another macro- (e.g coronary spasm) or microcirculatory disorder. Since no effective filling and emptying of the ventricles occurs under these conditions, ventricular fibrillation corresponds to a (hyperdynamic) cardiac arrest.

❗ Without immediate resuscitation measures (chest compressions and defibrillation), ventricular fibrillation consistently leads to cardiac death.

Diagnostics In the ECG, ventricular fibrillation manifests as irregular excitation formation and regression without a recognizable ECG-typical pattern (◘ Fig. 12.31).

Therapy In the acute situation, the restoration of a sinus rhythm by means of cardioversion or defibrillation has the highest priority in cases of rapid ventricular tachycardia, ventricular flutter, or ventricular fibrillation.

► Practical Recommendations

Cardioversion, Defibrillation
In cardioversion (for ventricular tachycardia) or defibrillation (for ventricular fibrillation), an electric shock is usually delivered externally to the thorax. The difference between the two methods is that in cardioversion, this shock is triggered on the R-wave

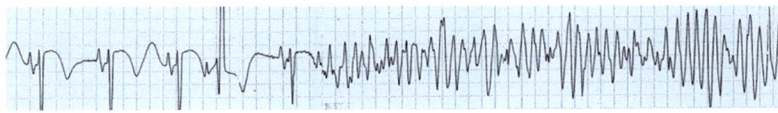

◘ **Fig. 12.30** Torsade de Pointes

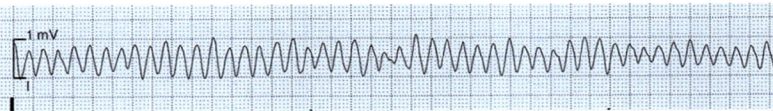

◘ **Fig. 12.31** Ventricular Fibrillation

in the simultaneously derived ECG (synchronized). This prevents the risk of delivering a shock during the vulnerable phase of ventricular repolarization (and thus triggering ventricular fibrillation). In ventricular fibrillation, there is no orderly depolarization and repolarization, so the shock must be delivered unsynchronized. Both cardioversion and defibrillation cause an instantaneous depolarization of all muscle cells that are not currently in the absolute refractory period. This interrupts the arrhythmia and allows the normal conduction system to resume orderly ventricular depolarization. ◄

Prevention In the case of survived sudden cardiac death (in the absence of a triggering secondary event such as myocardial infarction; ► Sect. 7.5), the implantation of a cardioverter-defibrillator (*Implantable Cardioverter-Defibrillator*, ICD) is indicated for secondary prophylaxis to immediately trigger overpacing or an internal defibrillation in the event of a recurrent ventricular arrhythmia (► Sect. 13.3). Additionally, concomitant medication therapy (e.g., with amiodarone and/or beta-blockers) is often initiated.

Heart Failure

Bettina Heidecker and Otmar Pfister

Contents

13.1   Definition and Epidemiology – 224

13.2   Etiology and Pathophysiology – 224

13.3   Diagnostics – 229

13.4   Therapy – 231

Earlier versions were created with the collaboration of G. Noll, A. Flammer, J. Steffel, T. F Lüscher.

© The Author(s), under exclusive license to Springer-Verlag GmbH, DE, part of Springer Nature 2025
T. F. Lüscher and U. Landmesser (eds.), *Cardiovascular System*,
https://doi.org/10.1007/978-3-662-70152-2_13

Heart failure is characterized by the inability of the heart to adjust its output to meet the demands of the organism. Heart failure can be due to reduced contractility with reduced ejection fraction, so-called heart failure with reduced ejection fraction (HFrEF). On the other hand, the filling of the heart can be impeded by a compliance disorder of the ventricle (diastolic dysfunction), so-called heart failure with preserved ejection fraction (HFpEF). The increase in cardiac filling pressures is considered a central hemodynamic sign of heart failure. Treatment is primarily involves medications (e.g. diuretics, ACE inhibitors, angiotensin receptor-neprilysin inhibitors [ARNI], sartans, beta-blockers, mineralocorticoid receptor antagonists [MRA], SGLT-2 inhibitors, among others) as well as in advanced stages using rhythm management devices (i.e. CRT and/or ICD). As a last resort, implanting a ventricular assist system ("artificial heart") or heart transplantation (HTX) may be considered.

13.1 Definition and Epidemiology

Definition Heart failure occurs when the heart is no longer able to adjust its output to meet the demands of the organism without increasing cardiac filling pressures. Generally, based on the left ventricular ejection fraction (LVEF), a distinction is made between heart failure with reduced ejection fraction (LVEF ≤ 40 % HFrEF), heart failure with mildly reduced left ventricular ejection fraction (LVEF 41–49 %; HFmrEF), and heart failure with preserved ejection fraction (LVEF ≥ 50 %; HFpEF).

For the **diagnosis of heart failure** according to the definition of the European Society of Cardiology from 2021 and 2023, the presence of the following findings is required for all subgroups:

- typical symptoms (e.g., dyspnea, orthopnea, bendopnea, nocturia) **AND**
- typical findings on clinical examination (e.g., distended neck veins, peripheral edema, tachypnea, pulmonary crackles)
- increased levels of natriuretic peptides (e.g. NT-proBNP ≥ 125 pg/mL or BNP ≥ 35 pg/mL).

For **HFrEF** and **HFmrEF**, objective evidence of a reduced ejection fraction (e.g., by echocardiography) is further necessary.

For **HFpEF**, the following evidence is further required:
- evidence of an LVEF ≥ 50 % with normally sized, i.e., non-dilated ventricles **AND**
- a structural abnormality (hypertrophy and/or enlargement of the left atrium and/or diastolic dysfunction) **AND**
- a moderate increase in natriuretic peptides.

Epidemiology The prevalence of heart failure is age-dependent; on average, 2% of adults in the Western world are affected. Among those over 65 years of age, 6–10% suffer from heart failure. In Europe and North America, 1 in 5 adults will develop heart failure over the course of their lifetime. Men are more frequently affected by HFrEF than women of the same age (ratio 60;40%), while women are more often affected by HFpEF than men (60:40).

13.2 Etiology and Pathophysiology

Etiology In principle, any structural heart disease can be the cause of heart failure. In fact, strictly speaking, heart failure per se is not a disease but merely a clinical syndrome due to an underlying heart disease.

Heart Failure

> The most common cause of HFrEF, accounting for about 60% of cases, is myocardial infarction (or multiple infarctions) as a result of coronary artery disease (CAD).

Not infrequently, the chain of events hypertension → coronary heart disease → heart attack → heart failure are the underlying causes (Fig. 13.1).

Common causes of heart failure
- Coronary heart disease (CCS or ACS); (▶ Chap. 7.3 and 7.5)
- Hypertensive heart disease (▶ Chap. 4)
- Dilated cardiomyopathy (mostly due to genetic causes) (▶ Chap. 8.1)
- Hypertrophic cardiomyopathy (genetically determined; ▶ Chap. 8.1)
- Restrictive cardiomyopathy (▶ Chap. 8.1)

- Valvular cardiopathies (▶ Chap. 9)
- Constrictive pericarditis (▶ Chap. 11)
- Myocarditis (▶ Sect. 8.2)
- Storage diseases, e.g., amyloidosis, hemochromatosis, Fabry disease
- Stress-induced Takotsubo syndrome (previously *Broken Heart Syndrome*)
- Congenital heart disease (▶ Chap. 14)

Pathophysiology The pathophysiological development of heart failure is primarily determined by the underlying heart disease and the body's reactions to the reduced cardiac output.

> The development of heart failure successively leads to a remodeling of the heart chambers with hypertrophy of the myofibrils and fibrosis, especially of the left ventricle, which is referred to as remodeling.

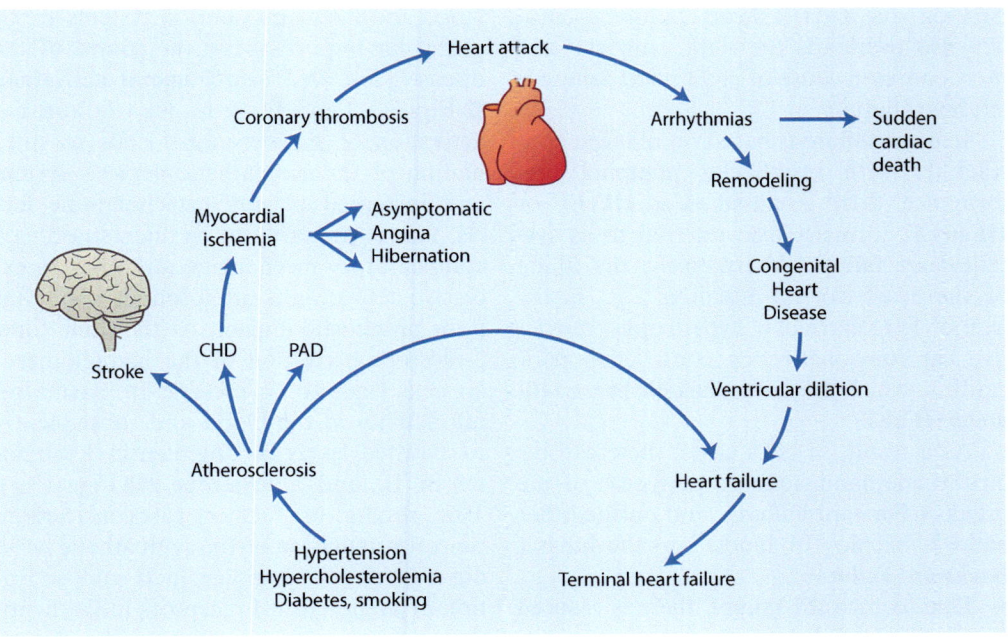

Fig. 13.1 Heart failure as the final stage of CHD. *CHD:* Coronary heart disease, *PAD:* Peripheral arterial disease

This **remodeling** process is usually progressive and, depending on the predominant physical load (pressure versus volume load), leads to myocardial hypertrophy and/or an increasing dilation of the left ventricle. According to Laplace's law, an increase in ventricular dilation is associated with an increase in wall tension. This leads to an increased myocardial oxygen demand. An increasing end-diastolic left ventricular volume leads, according to the Frank-Starling mechanism, to an increase in myocardial contractility up to a certain point. However, with further increasing dilation, the ejection fraction (normal $\geq 55\%$) successively decreases. With increasing severity of the disease, a decrease in cardiac output follows after an initially compensated stage, with corresponding clinical consequences.

Topographically, **left** and **right heart failure** can be distinguished. Isolated left heart failure occurs much more frequently than isolated right heart failure. However, in advanced heart failure, a combination is usually found clinically, as the chronic backlog due to left heart failure eventually also overloads the right ventricle—the most common cause of right heart failure is left heart failure.

If heart failure is based on reduced contractility with insufficient pumping performance, there is classified as **HFrEF** or **HFmrEF**, formerly also referred to as **systolic heart failure**. Alternatively, the filling of the heart can be impaired, e.g., in the case of left ventricular hypertrophy, restrictive cardiomyopathy, or constrictive pericarditis, which leads to **diastolic heart failure or HFpEF**.

As a result, in both cases, there can be, on the one hand, reduced perfusion of the organs (**Forward Failure**), and on the other hand, a backlog of blood into the lungs (**Backward Failure**):

- Due to forward failure, there is **reduced perfusion of the organs** and corresponding consequences and symptoms, e.g., acute or chronic renal failure and/or reduced muscle and cerebral perfusion. This leads to general fatigue, weakness, and reduced exercise performance.
- Backward failure, on the other hand, in the case of left heart failure causes **pulmonary venous congestion** up to pulmonary edema, which over time eventually leads to right heart strain and in extreme cases to cor pulmonale with right heart failure (◘ Fig. 13.2).
- Right ventricular backward failure leads to a venous backlog of blood in the venous systemic circulation (superior and inferior vena cava) and thus to jugular vein distention as well as liver congestion (in extreme cases to portal hypertension with all its consequences such as ascites, congestive liver damage up to cirrhosis; i.e. *cirrhose cardiaque*), peripheral edema, and pleural effusions.

Although the primary cause of heart failure is a functional disorder of the heart itself, the adaptations of the peripheral circulation and the neurohumoral systems are of particular importance in the course of the disease (so-called **neurohumoral activation**, ◘ Figs. 13.3 and 13.4). In heart failure, the activation of baroreceptors leads to stimulation of the sympathetic nervous system and increased plasma catecholamine levels. This is primarily to be understood as a compensatory mechanism, although an excessive activation is often found, which has poor prognostic impact. At the same time, β-receptor activation in the juxtaglomerular cells leads to an increase in plasma renin activity in the blood and subsequently to elevated levels of angiotensin I, angiotensin II, and aldosterone (◘ Fig. 13.3). This results in further vasoconstriction, central stimulation of the sympathetic nervous system (via angiotensin II and activation of angiotensin I receptors in the hypothalamus), as well as sodium and water retention with edema formation in the lungs

Heart Failure

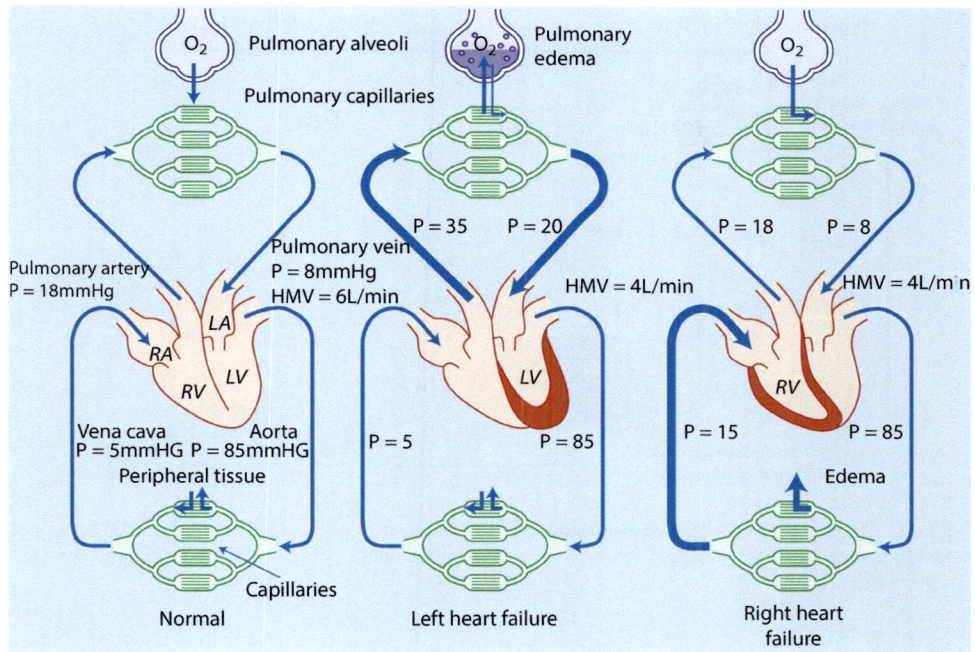

◘ **Fig. 13.2 Hemodynamics in heart failure.** *LA:* left atrium, *RA:* right atrium, *LV:* left ventricle, *RV:* right ventricle, *CO:* cardiac output, *P:* pressure

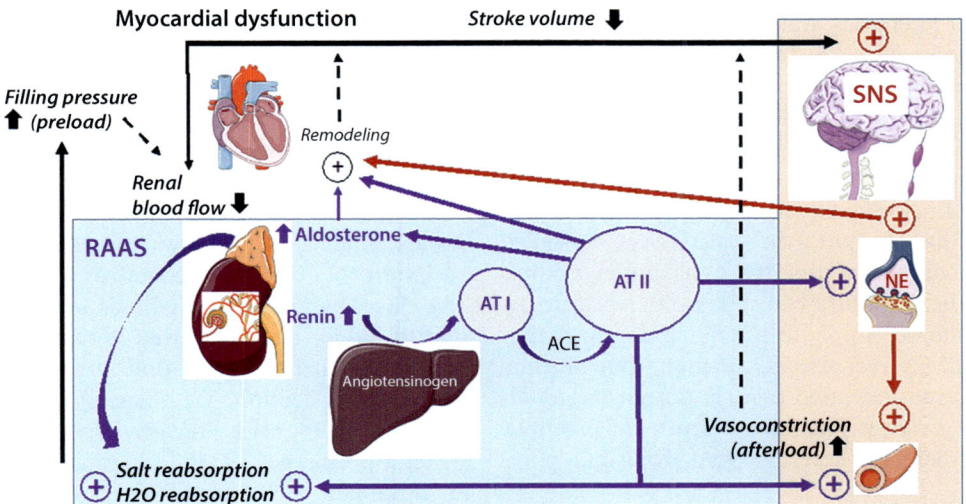

◘ **Fig. 13.3 Neuroendocrine machansism activated in heart failure.** *ACE*: Angiotensin-converting enzyme, *ACEI*: Angiotensin-converting enzyme inhibitor, *ANP*: Atrial natriuretic peptide, *AT I*: Angiotensin I, *AT II*: Angiotensin II, *ARB*: Angiotensin receptor blocker, *ARNI*: Angiotensin receptor neprilysin inhibitor, = Beta-blocker, *BNP*: Brain natriuretic peptide, *MRA*: Mineralocorticoid receptor antagonist, *NE*: Norepinephrine, *SGLT2I*: Sodium glucose co-transporter 2 inhibitor, *SNS*: Sympathetic nervous system

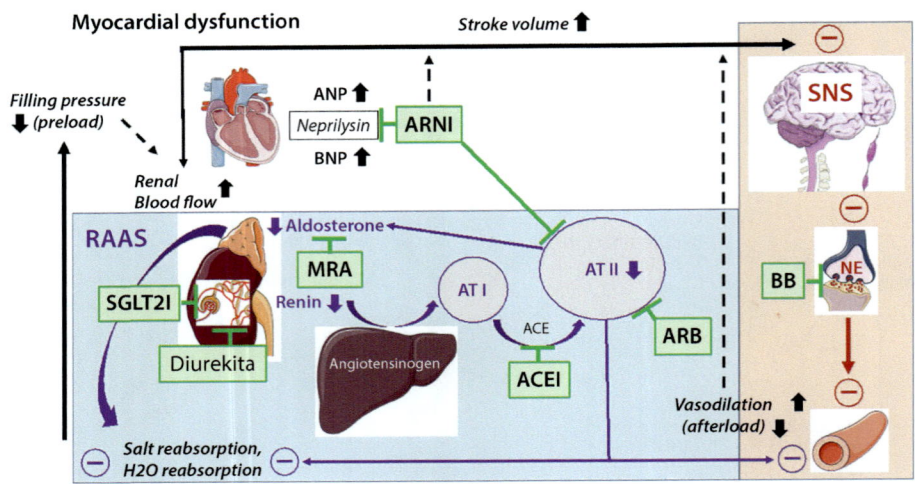

Fig. 13.4 Mechanisms of action of medications in the treatment of chronic heart failure. *ACE* = Angiotensin-converting enzyme, *ACEI* = Angiotensin-converting enzyme inhibitor, ANP = Atrial natriuretic peptide, *AT I* = Angiotensin I, *AT II* = Angiotensin II, *ARB* = Angiotensin

and periphery. These effects are further enhanced by aldosterone, which among other things leads to hypokalemia and fosters fibrosis of tissues. Additionally, there is an increased release of vasopressin, which further increases water retention in the kidney's collecting ducts as well as vasoconstriction. As a result, hyponatremia often occurs in end stage of heart failure, which is extremely unfavorable prognostically.

In contrast to heart failure with reduced cardiac output (the usual case, so-called *low-output failure*), the signs and symptoms of heart failure can also occur with inadequate O_2 supply to the tissue due to pathologically increased O_2 demand and normal or even increased cardiac output (*high-output failure*). The latter occurs, for example, in anemia or severe hyperthyroidism.

Clinical FIndings Typical clinical symptoms of heart failure are:

- Exercise intolerance,
- Exertional dyspnea (NYHA I–IV),
- Paroxysmal nocturnal dyspnea attacks,
- Nocturia (pronounced nighttime urination),
- Peripheral edema (in extreme cases: anasarca),
- Orthopnea (dyspnea while lying down, which disappears or significantly improves upon sitting up),
- Bendopnea (dyspnea when bending over, "tying shoes"),
- Fatigue.

To describe the **severity** of heart failure, the 4-stage schema of the New York Heart Association (NYHA) has become established. The classification is mainly based on the extent of subjectively perceived dyspnea. The American Heart Association proposed a further classification, i.e. Stage A (at risk of heart failure; HF), Stage B (Pre-HF with structural changes of the heart), Stage C (symptomatic HF), Stage D (advanced HF)

> **NYHA Classification of Heart Failure**
> - **NYHA I:** no physical limitation due to the disease. No occurrence of dysp-

nea, inadequate exhaustion, arrhythmias, or angina pectoris even under exertion, but left ventricualr dysfunction.
- **NYHA II:** slight limitation of physical performance due to the disease. Everyday, moderate physical activities such as long walks, prolonged uphill walking, or forced stair climbing cause symptoms, especially dyspnea.
- **NYHA III:** significant limitation of physical performance. Symptoms during activities with low activity levels (brushing teeth, dressing, walking on flat ground, etc.), but no complaints at rest
- **NYHA IV:** symptoms at rest, bedridden

13.3 Diagnostics

At clinical examination, the following findings are typically found in the context of decompensated heart failure:
- 3rd (or 4th) heart sound,
- possibly widened apical impulse,
- pulmonary congestion with coarse crackles,
- jugular venous distension (Fig. 13.5) or positive hepatojugular reflux,
- enlarged, tender liver (congested liver),
- peripheral edema (Fig. 13.6).

> The individual differences of the clinicial presentation of heart failure are significant, e.g. depending on the pathogenesis or severity or medication, some symptoms are more pronounced, while others may be completely absent.

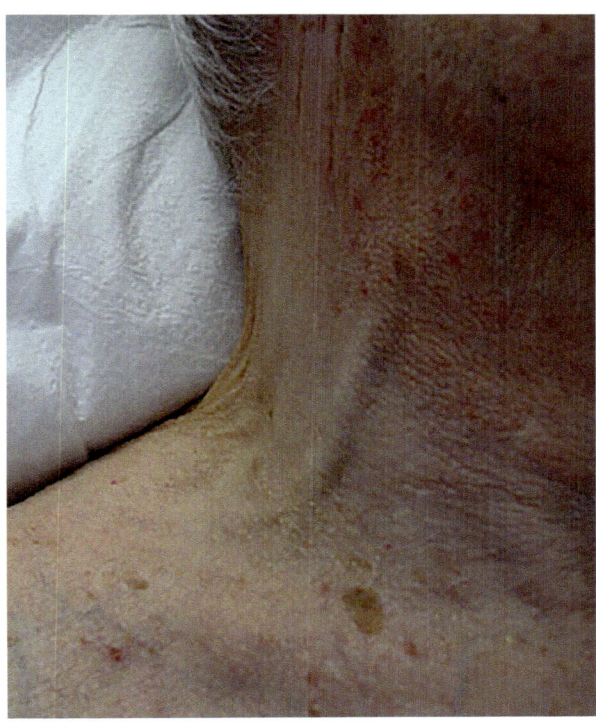

Fig. 13.5 Jugular venous distension

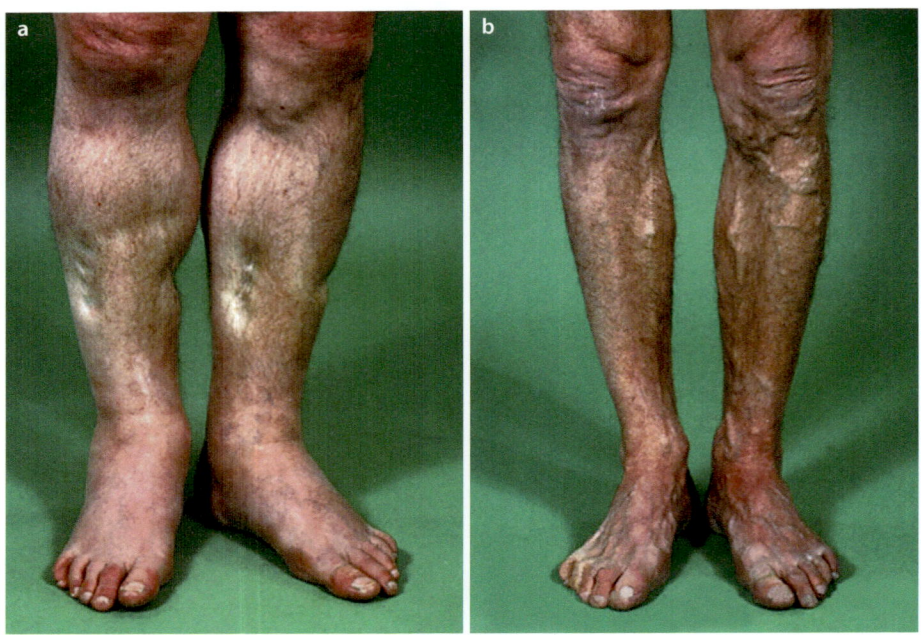

Fig. 13.6 (**a**, **b**) **Peripheral edema**. (**a**) Before and (**b**) after diuretic therapy in right-sided decompensation. (Courtesy of the Image Archive, Department of Internal Medicine, University Hospital Zurich)

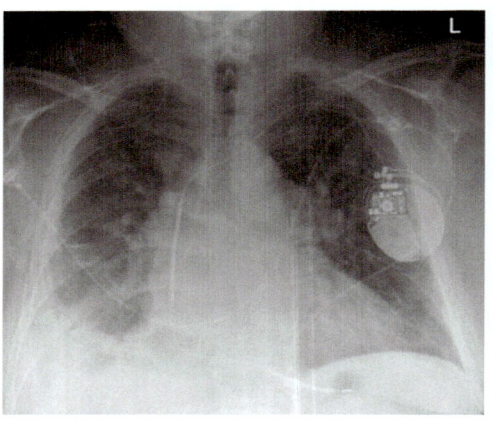

Fig. 13.7 Chest X-ray in decompensated heart failure with heart enlargement, basoapical redistribution, and right pleural effusion. Incidental finding of status post ICD implantation in the left pectoral region with correct positioning of the electrode tip at the bottom of the right ventricle

In the **chest X-ray** (Fig. 13.7), significant cardiac enlargement (cardio-thoracic ratio > 0.5) can be seen in HFrEF. However, a normal heart size does not exclude heart failure, especially not in HFpEF.

❗ Cardiomegaly on X-ray always requires further investigation.

The **laboratory examination**, reveals an increase in Brain Natriuretic Peptide (BNP). This is a cardiac hormone that is secreted as a result of increasing ventricular stretching. Due to its high sensitivity and specificity, BNP has become diagnostic in heart failure; thus, with a normal BNP, heart failure is very unlikely. However, it is known that in certain patient groups, particularly patients with obesity, BNP values are often lower, in some cases even normal or near normal despite the presence of heart failure. **Clinical examination** is paramount. Furthermore, it is suitable for monitoring the course and estimating the prognosis, as it in the presence of normal kidney function clinical signs correlate well with the severity of heart failure. Recently,

NT-proBNP (N-terminal proBNP) is increasingly being determined instead of BNP, as it has a more consistent serum concentration and its serum levels are not influenced by angiotensin receptor-neprilysin inhibitors (ARNI), whereas BNP can be falsely elevated under this therapy.

The imaging method of choice in suspected heart failure and for assessing the course of existing heart failure is **echocardiography (Chap. 2.3).** It allows for the precise quantification of left ventricular volumes and ejection fraction as well as the diagnosis of other, possibly even causal structural cardiac changes (e.g. valvular heart diseases, left ventricular hypertrophy, amyloidosis, etc.). Additionally, diastolic function can be assessed using various parameters, and in the presence of typical symptoms and signs of heart failure with normal ejection fraction, the diagnosis of HFpEF can be made. ◘ Figure 13.8 summarizes a diagnostic algorithm for suspected heart failure.

13.4 Therapy

Any symptomatic heart failure, but also any left ventricular pump dysfunction with an ejection fraction < 50% (Stage NYHA I or Stage B) without symptoms, constitutes an indication for treatment.

The **goals of drug therapy** are:
- Improvement of exercise performance and quality of life,
- Slowing or inhibition of progression,
- Improvement of prognosis: reduction of mortality and hospitalizations for heart failure.

Depending on the severity and progression of the disease, various forms of therapy are used. Drug therapy forms the basis of treatment for all forms of heart failure (◘ Fig. 13.9).

■ **General Measures**

For every patient, causal therapeutic approaches to eliminate the cause of their

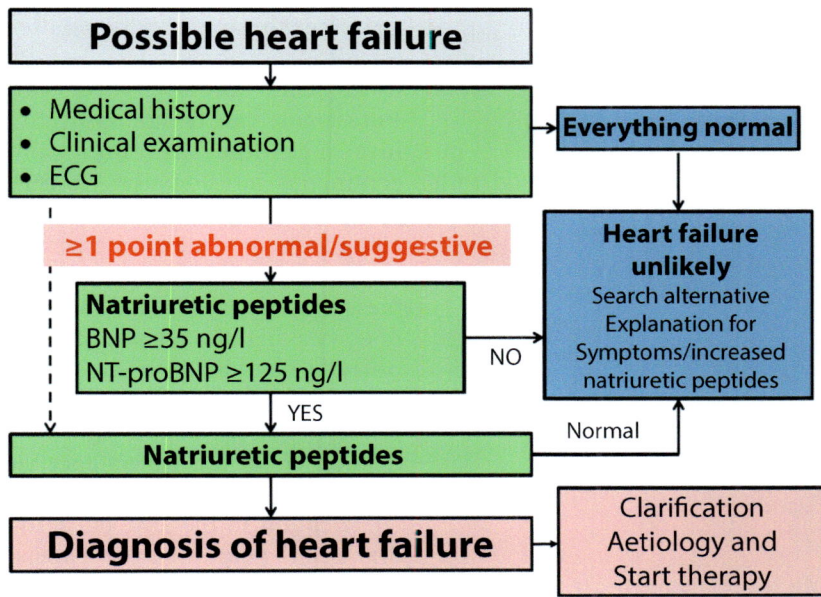

◘ **Fig. 13.8** Diagnostic algorithm for suspected heart failure. (Source: Pocketcard, Swiss Working Group for Heart Failure 2022)

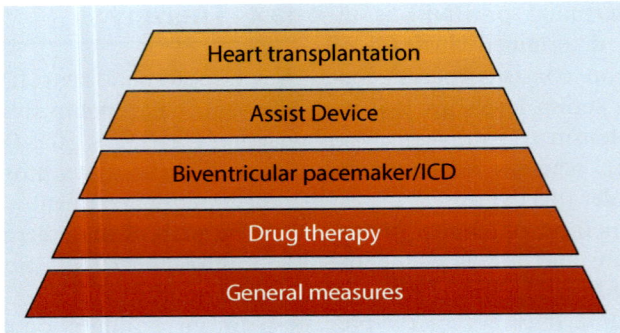

Fig. 13.9 Therapy options for heart failure

heart failure should first be exhausted, such as antihypertensive medication for hypertensive patients, stopping the use of NSAIDs among others. A change in lifestyle (including smoking cessation) is also an important factor in heart failure therapy:
- Aim for normal weight or body mass index,
- Reduce salt intake (< 6 g/day),
- Maintain constant fluid intake ($\leq$ 2 l/day)—regular weight checks (rapid weight gain is always due to fluid retention!),
- Regular exercise once the patient is well reated with stable heart failure, avoid strenuous activities,
- Assure regular medication intake (non-compliance is associated with mortality and hospitalisation).

> Although alcohol abstinence is generally prescribed in heart failure (as alcohol can cause alcohol-induced cardiomyopathy), no negative impact of moderate alcohol consumption (1–2 glasses/day) on the clinical course could be documented so far.

- **Acute Therapy**

! Acute decompensated heart failure is a clinical emergency.

In acute decompensated heart failure and especially in cardiogenic shock, it is crucial to quickly identify and address **treatable causes** (e.g., acute coronary syndrome, arrhythmias, valvular heart disease). A rapid evaluation of the clinical presentation regarding volume and perfusion status is also essential for further therapy. In most cases, **volume overload (congestion)** is predominant, which should be treated with diuretics. Specifically, in the presence of severe right heart failure, venous congestion in the liver and intestines significantly impairs the absorption of orally administered medications (diuretic pseudo-resistance). Thus, intravenous therapy with loop diuretics (furosemide) is the preferred treatment modality in acute decompensated heart failure. Furosemide can be administered as repetitive single doses, 2–3 times daily, or as a continuous infusion using a perfusor. An optimal diuretic response is achieved with 100–150 ml of urine output per hour within the first 6 hours. With stable systolic blood pressure values > 110 mmHg, intravenous vasodilators, such as nitrates or nitroprusside, can also be used. Nitrates reduce preload by increasing venous pooling. The principle of venous pooling is based on the dilation of venous capacitance vessels and small venules, which leads to increased water retention in the legs, but leads to withdrawal of fluid from the circulation and ideally from the lungs. Nitroprusside acts primarily on the venous, but also on the arterial vascular system as a vasodilator. An

Heart Failure

efficient reduction of preload and afterload increases stroke volume and reduces congestion, eventually contributing to improved end-organ perfusion.

❗ Vasodilators should be used cautiously and with adequate monitoring, as a potentially dangerous drop in blood pressure, hypokalemia and hyponatremia as well as reanl failure can occur, especially in acute decompensated heart failure.

If hypotension (sBP < 90 mmHg) with **reduced cardiac output and critical end-organ perfusion** is predominant, the use of positive inotrops (e.g., with dobutamine) may be necessary. This may also be required in volume overload with renal hypoperfusion to break the vicious cycle of volume overload → ventricular dilation → reduced pump function → decreased renal perfusion → volume retention → organ congestion dysfunction (kidney edema and dysfunction, etc.) → increased volume overload. Additionally, intravenous phosphodiesterase inhibitors or calcium sensitizers such as milrinone or levosimendan can be considered to improve cardiac output. These have both positive inotropic and vasodilatory effects. In severe hypotension and cardiogenic shock, vasopressors (e.g., norepinephrine) are often used in addition to inotropes to stabilize blood pressure and maintain adequate end-organ perfusion.

❗ Therapy with positive inotropes must be initiated cautiously under continuous hemodynamic monitoring, as numerous potentially life-threatening complications such as hypotension, hypertension, and arrhythmias up to ventricular fibrillation can occur.

However, if acute decompensation or cardiogenic shock cannot be controlled with medication, there is the option of a temporary or permanent assist device implantation (*Mechanical Cardiac Support*; MCS) as *Destination Therapy* or as a *Bridge-to-Transplant* for a highly urgent (*super urgent*) heart transplant.

▪ Long-term Medication Therapy

Long-term medication therapy has seen significant advancements in recent years with the introduction of new drug classes such

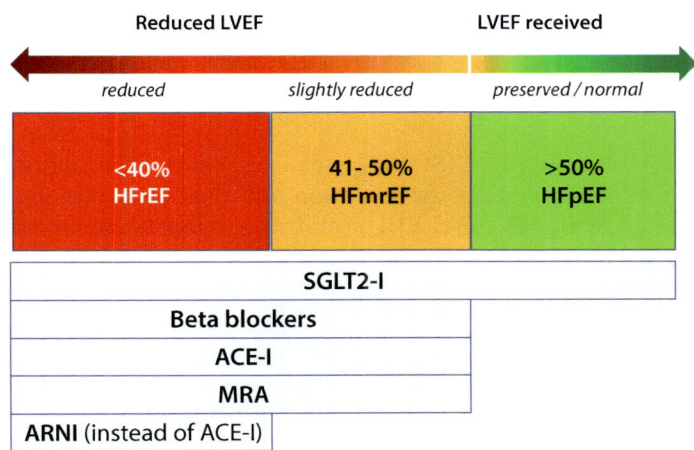

◻ **Abb. 13.10 Prognostically effective heart failure therapy according to LVEF.** *ACE-I*: Angiotensin-converting Enzyme Inhibitor, *ARNI*: Angiotensin Receptor Neprilysin Inhibitor, *MRA*: Mineralocorticoid Receptor Antagonist, *SGLT2-I*: Sodium-Glucose Co-Transporter 2 Inhibitor

Table 13.1 Pharmacological basic therapy for heart failure with reduced ejection fraction

Therapy	Indication	Advantages/Disadvantages
Loop diuretics: – Torasemide – Furosemide	Symptomatic therapy for **hypervolemia**	Effect on prognosis not proven Hypokalemia, hyponatremia (Renal failure)
ACE inhibitors (ACEI): – Enalapril – Lisinopril – Perindopril – Ramipril	Basic therapy	Prognostic +++ in HFrEF Renal protection Dry cough (Hyperkalemia) (Hypotension together with diuretics) (rarely Angioedema)
ARB (instead of ACEI): – Candesartan – Losartan – Valsartan	Alternative to ACEI, only in case of true ACEI intolerance	Prognostic ++ in HFrEF Renal protection (Hyperkalemia) (Hypotension together with diuretics)
Beta-blockers (BB): – Carvedilol (α/β-blocker) – Bisoprolol – Metoprolol – Nebivolol (also releases NO)	Basic therapy	Prognostic +++ in HFrEF Hypotension (with higher dosages) Bradycardia (with higher dosages) Contraindicated in AV block
Mineralocorticoid receptor antagonist (MRA): – Eplerenone – Spironolactone – Finerenone (non-Steroidal MRA)	Basic therapy	Prognostic +++ Hyperkalemia (Hypotension) (Gynecomastia with spironolactone)
ARNI: – Sacubitril/Valsartan	Basic therapy	Prognostic +++ in HFrEF (better than ACE inhibitors) Hypotension Renal protection (Hyperkalemia)
SGLT-2 inhibitors (SGLT2-I) – Dapagliflozin – Empagliflozin	Basic therapy	Prognostic +++ in HFrEF and HFpEF No BP effect Renal protection (lactat acidosis)

as sodium-glucose co-transporter-2 (SGLT-2) inhibitors and angiotensin receptor-neprilysin inhibitors (ARNI) (Table 13.1, Fig. 13.10). This has significantly improved the prognosis, especially in patients with HFrEF. With the exception of SGLT-2 inhibitors, which improve symptoms and clinical outcomes regardless of ejection fraction and are thus beneficial in HFrEF, HFmrEF, and HFpEF, the remaining long-term medications are mainly beneficial in HFmrEF and HFrEF and should be introduced and uptitrated as soon as possible. Since neurohormonal stimulation and thus the activation of the RAAS and the sympathetic nervous system increase with the severity of pump function impairment, RAAS inhibitors (ARNI, ACE inhibitors, MRA) and sympatholytics (beta-blockers) are particularly effective in HFrEF (Fig.13.4). In addition to improving prognosis, RAAS inhibitors counteract ventricular remodeling, which is exacerbated by the renin-angiotensin-aldosterone system. SGLT-2 inhibitors prevent the reabsorption of sodium and glucose in the proximal tubule of the kidney. This leads to increased diuresis and constriction of the efferent arteriole in the glomeruli through the activation of the tubuloglomerular feedback mechanism. As a result, intraglomerular pressure decreases. The mechanisms by which SGLT-2 inhibitors ultimately improve the prognosis of heart failure independently of left ventricular ejection fraction are still unclear but may include beneficial effects on autophagy, mitochondrial function among others. The novel Glucagon-like peptide-1 (GLP-1) with or without combination with the Glucose-dependent insulinotropic peptide (GIP) hold promise in overweight and obese patients with heart failure with improvement of quality-of-life and a reduction in heart failure hospitalisations.

In HFrEF, rapid establishment of the four therapy pillars (ARNI, BB, SGLT2-I, MRA) is crucial for prognosis. The principle here is: "First establish, then rapidly titrate up." When titrating up the beta-blocker and ARNI (or ACEI), the principle "Start low, aim high as soon as possible" applies, i.e., start with a low dose and increase the dosageas as quickly as possible (caution: hypotension, bradycardia). SGLT-2 inhibitors practically do not affect blood pressure and heart rate, while beta-blockers have a negative inotropic and bradycardic effect, which can lead to decompensation. Symptomatic hypotension can occur with too rapid titration with ARNI, beta-blockers (especially the α/β-blocker carvedilol), or ACEI in combination with diuretics.

Finally, diuretics are used in long-term therapy only in the presence of water retention and edema. The rule here is: As much as necessary, as little as possible.

> ❗ When administering mineralocorticoid receptor antagonists in parallel with other RAAS inhibitors, the risk of hyperkalemia must be considered. The concurrent administration of ARNI and ACE inhibitors is contraindicated due to overlapping mechanisms and the increased risk of angioedema.

In contrast to HFrEF, RAAS inhibitors could not improve prognosis and symptoms in HFpEF. Only SGLT-2 inhibitors show a positive effect on the rehospitalization rate and likely mortality regardless of LVEF and are therefore indicated in HFrEF, HFmrEF, and HFpEF alike. In addition to therapy with SGLT-2 inhibitors, the optimal treatment of cardiovascular risk factors and comorbidities (e.g. hypertension) is the focus in HFpEF.

The **stimulator of cyclic GMP,** vericiguat, also reduces mortality and hospitalizations in HFrEF (except in very advanced forms), but is usually only used in case of treatment resistance or intolerance to basic therapy.

In heart failure, intestinal iron absorption and mobilization of iron from the body's iron stores are reduced. This results in functional or absolute iron deficiency in up to 50% of patients. Iron deficiency should be sought in all patients with heart failure and, if present, treated with intravenous iron substitution. This can improve quality of life and physical performance and reduce rehospitalizations, but not mortality. The laboratory criteria for iron deficiency in heart failure are: ferritin < 100 ng/L (absolute iron deficiency) or ferritin 100–300 ng/L with a transferrin saturation of < 20%.

- **Device Therapy**

Implantable Cardioverter-Defibrillator (ICD)

Ventricular tachycardias and ventricular fibrillation are common causes of death in patients with heart failure, particularly in HFrEF due to infraction with scar formation. ICDs are therefore used to detect and treat such malignant ventricular arrhythmias in such patients, while in cardiomyopathies (▶ Chap. 8.1.) ICDs have not shown prognostic benefit.

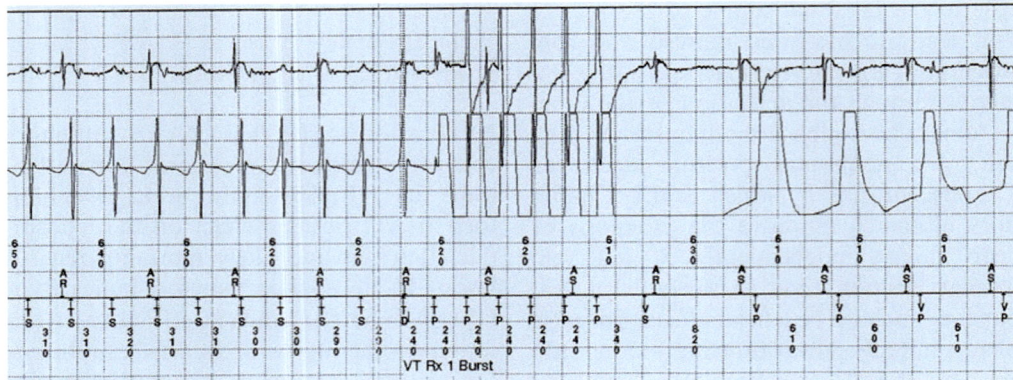

Fig. 13.11 Excerpt from an ICD interrogation in a patient with recurrent ventricular tachycardias. A ventricular tachycardia is correctly detected (*Tachycardia Sensed*, TS), which can be successfully terminated using ATP (Anti-Tachycardia Pacing, "Burst"). Subsequently, a complete AV block is shown, which is why ventricular stimulation (ventricular pacing, VP) occurs after detection of atrial excitation (atrial sensing, AS). 1st line: atrial electromyogram (EMG), 2nd line: ventricular EMG, 3rd line: marker channel with atrial (top) and ventricular (bottom) cycle lengths

▶ **Practical**

Implantable Cardioverter-Defibrillator (ICD)
ICDs are implanted in principle like pacemakers. An electrode is placed transvenously in the right ventricle, which continuously records the ventricular excitation processes. If the device diagnoses ventricular tachycardia, it attempts to terminate it using various algorithms (overstimulation, so-called *Anti-Tachycardic Pacing*, ATP, ◘ Fig. 13.11 and ▶ Chap. 12.5). If this is not successful, a shock is delivered for internal cardioversion or defibrillation. If the device detects ventricular fibrillation, it defibrillates directly, with an electrical shock as this is the only effective therapy for ventricular fibrillation.

Furthermore, every ICD can also function as a normal pacemaker, i.e., if the ventricular rate falls below a programmed threshold, stimulation in the right ventricle can occur via the defibrillator electrode just like with ordinary pacemakers. ◀

Indications for ICD Implantation
— Primary prophylactic ICD implantation
  - Ischemic cardiomyopathy (> 40 days after myocardial infarction) with LVEF < 35% in spite of optimal medical therapy
  - In non-ischemic cardiomyopathy, ICDs are overall ineffective to reduce mortality. An ICD indication must be considered individually in NYHA II/III with LVEF < 35% in spite of optimal medical therapy, ideally after genetic testing for mutations associated with a high risk of sudden death (e.g. Laminin mutations among others).
  - Hypertrophic cardiomyopathy with high arryhtmia risk (▶ Chap. 8.1)
  - Rare indications (arrhythmogenic cardiomyopathy; ▶ Chap. 8.1; Long-QT syndrome, Short-QT syndrome, Brugada syndrome with risk factors, etc.; ▶ Chap. 12.5)
— Secondary prophylactic ICD implantation
  - Patients who survived sudden cardiac death without treatable cause regardless of LVEF (Note: survived ventricular fibrillation in the con-

text of an acute myocardial infarction is not an ICD indication)
– Persistent ventricular tachycardia and LVEF < 40%

■■ Cardiac Resynchronization Therapy (*Cardiac Resynchronization Therapy*, CRT)

In symptomatic patients despite extensive medical therapy, there is also the possibility of implanting a biventricular pacemaker for the resynchronization of dyssynchronous ventricular excitation, typically in those with left bundle branch block. CRT leads in selected patients with HFrEF (see below) in addition to optimal medical therapy to an improvement in quality of life and reduction in morbidity and mortality.

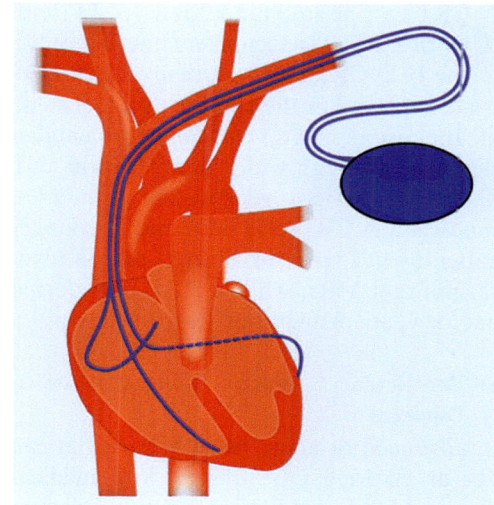

Fig. 13.12 Schematic representation of a CRT system

▶ Practical

Cardiac Resynchronization Therapy

For resynchronization, a pacemaker electrode is first anchored in the right ventricular myocardium. Additionally, another electrode is placed (also transvenously) via the coronary sinus in front of the left ventricle (Figs. 13.12 and 13.13). For optimal atrioventricular synchronization, a third electrode is anchored in the right atrium. By synchronous stimulation of the right and left ventricles, the left ventricular contraction can now be "resynchronized," leading to an increase in LVEF and reverse left ventricular remodeling.

Clinically, in the majority of cases, there is an improvement in left ventricular pump function. Additionally, a reduction in morbidity and mortality through cardiac resynchronization therapy has been demonstrated. ◀

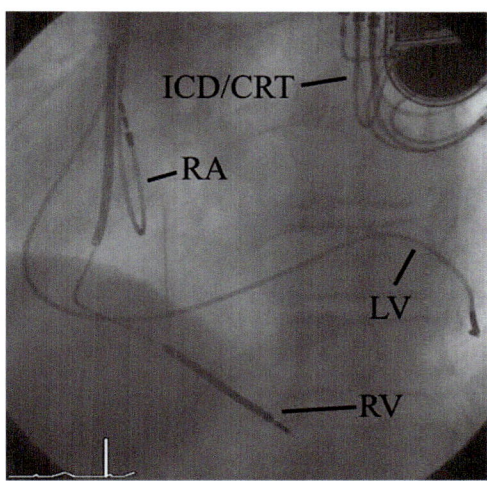

Fig. 13.13 Fluoroscopy control after successful ICD/CRT implantation. It shows a proper position of the electrodes in the right atrium (*RA*), right ventricle (*RV*), and in the coronary sinus (LV electrode)

Indications for CRT
- Symptomatic heart failure (from NYHA II) with impaired left ventricular function (LVEF < 35%) **AND**
- Widened QRS complex (> 130 ms, or even better > 150 ms) in sinus rhythm with left bundle branch block (best response to CRT)

A CRT can be implanted as CRT-D (with ICD) or CRT-P (pacemaker function only). In the ICD/CRT device, a defibrillator electrode is placed in the right ventricle instead of the usual right ventricular pacemaker electrode, through which defibrillation and, if necessary, right ventricular stimulation can occur. A CRT-D is preferred in younger patients with scars or fibrosis of the myocardium on MRI, while CRT-P is preferred in older patients without scars or fibrosis.

▪▪ Ventricular Assist Devices (Assist-Devices)

In advanced or acute heart failure that can not or no longer be treated with medication and CRT, a ventricular assist device or *Cardiac Mechanical Support* (LVAD = Left Ventricular Assist Device, BiVAD = Biventricular Assist Device), which replaces the left ventricular function or the entire heart, can be used (◘ Figs. 13.14 and 13.15)—either as a *Bridge-to-Recovery* (in cases of expected recovery of ventricular function, e.g., in severe myocarditis), as a *Bridge-to-Transplant* (bridge to heart transplantation) or more recently as a final solution (*Destination Therapy*), if no recovery is expected and the patient is not a candidate for heart transplantation. *Destination Therapy* is now prognostically comparable to heart transplantation with the new magnetic flow devices (HeartMate-3). The INTERMACS status (*Interagency Registry for Mechanically Assisted Circulatory Support*; ◘ Table 13.2) is used to assess whether a mechanically assisted system or heart transplant is necessary.

> ▶ **Practical**
>
> **Ventricular Assist Devices**
>
> The systemic venous blood is drained from the right atrium (RA, ◘ Fig. 13.13) and pumped into the pulmonary artery (PA) in case of the "right pump." Oxygen-rich blood is drained from the apex of the left ventricle

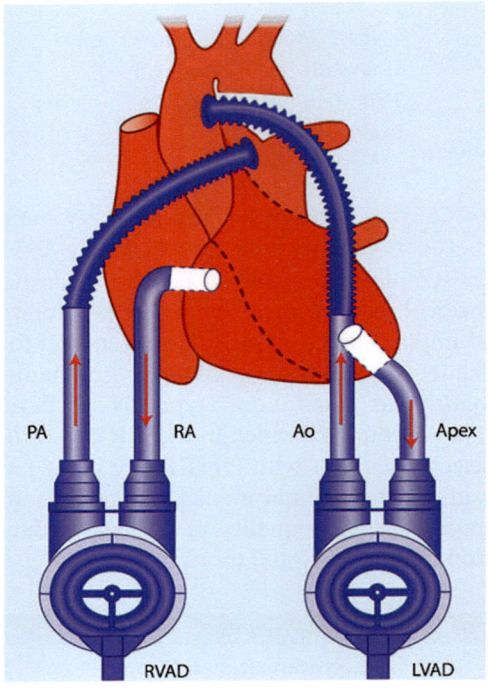

◘ **Fig. 13.14 Functional principle of a biventricular assist device.** Abbreviations see text. (With kind permission of Markus Wilhelm, University Hospital Zurich)

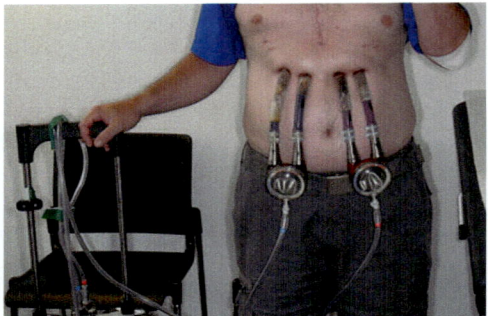

◘ **Fig. 13.15 Biventricular assist device in situ.** (With kind permission of Markus Wilhelm, University Hospital Zurich)

and pumped into the aorta (Ao) in case of the "left pump." In the case of an LVAD, the left ventricle is thus bypassed and function-

◘ **Table 13.2 INTERMACS status for assessing prognosis and indication for mechanical support systems or heart transplantation**. (With kind permission of Gummert J et al. Dtsch Arztebl Int 2019; 116: 843–8)

INTERMACS status for the classification of patients with terminal heart failure (1)
1. Cardiogenic shock ("crash and burn") NYHA class: IV System: ECLS, ECMO, percutaneous MCS One-year survival: 52.6 ± 5.6%
2. Progressive deterioration despite inotropics ("sliding on inotropes") NYHA class: IV System: ECLS, ECMO, LVAD One-year survival: 63.1 ± 3.1%
3. Stable under inotropics ("dependent stability") NYHA class: IV System: LVAD One-year survival: 78.4 ± 2.5%
4. Symptoms at rest ("frequent flyer") NYHA-Klasse: IV outpatient System: LVAD One-year survival: 78.7 ± 3.0%
5. not resilient ("housebound") NYHA class: IV outpatient System: LVAD One-year survival: 93.0 ± 3.9%*
6. limited resilience ("walking wounded") NYHA class: III System: LVAD/LVAD can be discussed as a treatment option.
7. Placeholder NYHA class: III System: LVAD can be discussed as a treatment option.

ECLS, "extracorporeal life support"; ECMO, "extracorporeal membrane oxygenation"; INTERMACS, Interagency Registry for Mechanically Assisted Circulatory Support; LVAD, "left ventricular assist device"; MCS, "mechanical circulatory support"; NYHA, New York Heart Association

*Kaplan-Meier survival probabilities ± standard error for one-year survival with LVAD therapy. Patients were censored at the time of last contact, recovery or heart transplantation. Due to small patient numbers, results for Intermacs status 5,6 and 7 were combined (1).

ally completely replaced, while in the case of a BiVAD, the entire heart is bypassed. Basically, assist devices can be implanted as external (e.g., Excor®, ◘ Fig. 13.14) or internal (e.g., Heart-Ware) systems. ◄

■■ **Heart Transplantation**

In cases of terminal heart failure that can no longer be treated by any of the described methods, there is the option of heart transplantation (HTX).

A challenge at surgery and later in the course after HTX is the management of immunosuppression, which must be precisely adjusted individually. With too **strong** immunosuppression, there is a risk of **opportunistic infections**, which are one of the greatest threats to organ transplant patients. About 30% of deaths in the first year after heart transplantation are caused by an infection. With too **weak** immunosuppression, there is a risk of **organ rejection**. For this reason, patients after HTX undergo endomyocardial biopsy at regular intervals. In this procedure, the right ventricle is probed via a sheath in the internal jugular vein (alternatively the subclavian vein or femoral vein) using a special forceps under fluoroscopic control, and several small myocardial fragments are taken from the right ventricle with a biopsy forceps. The degree of rejection (from none to hyperacute) can be determined based on the histopathological picture.

Heart transplant patients are furthermore at risk by a number of other diseases. In particular, the development of **transplant vasculopathy** (*graft vasculopathy*) is sometimes difficult to diagnose, as these patients usually do not complain of typical angina pectoris due to myocardial hypoperfusion because of the denervated heart.

Additionally, there is a risk of **malignancies** (about 15% of heart transplant patients develop a malignancy after 5 years), especially after long-term use of immunosuppressants. The most common malignancies are skin tumors.

Renal insufficiency and high blood pressure can be caused particularly by calcineurin inhibitors such as cyclosporine and tacrolimus.

Despite everything, heart transplantation in terminal heart failure has established itself as a highly effective method in well-selected patients, through which these patients with otherwise poor prognosis can continue to live for years to decades with good quality of life.

Prognosis The prognosis of heart failure is fundamentally unfavorable and comparable to the course of many carcinomas. On average, 30–40% of patients die within a year of diagnosis. The prognosis of heart failure caused by a myocardial infarction is generally worse.

Congenital Heart Defects

Helmut Baumgartner and Gerhard-Paul Diller

Contents

14.1 Introduction – 242

14.2 Congenital defects in Adulthood – 242
14.2.1 Atrial Septal Defect – 243
14.2.2 Ventricular Septal Defect – 245
14.2.3 Persistent Ductus arteriosus (PDA) – 246
14.2.4 Congenital Pulmonary Stenosis – 247
14.2.5 Coarctation of the Aorta – 248
14.2.6 Tetralogy of Fallot – 249
14.2.7 Transposition of the Great Arteries (TGA) – 251

© The Author(s), under exclusive license to Springer-Verlag GmbH, DE, part of Springer Nature 2025
T. F. Lüscher and U. Landmesser (eds.), *Cardiovascular System*,
https://doi.org/10.1007/978-3-662-70152-2_14

Congenital heart defects are the most common congenital disease in humans. About 0.8–1.1% of all newborns are born with a congenital heart defect. Thanks to advances in surgical and interventional treatment over the past 6 decades, the vast majority of children with congenital heart defects now survive into adulthood. As a result, the number of **A**dult **P**atients with **C**ongenital **H**eart defects (ACHD) is constantly increasing and currently exceeds the number of children with this condition. This trend will continue, and the median age of ACHD patients already exceeds 40 years. The vast majority of patients must be cared for in specialized centers for life. With the exception of atrial septal defects, the majority of heart defects in industrialized countries are diagnosed in infancy and childhood. Therefore, in adult cardiology, one is predominantly confronted with patients who already have a known congenital heart disease. Occasionally, however, the diagnosis must be made only in adulthood. For an adequate treatment of ACHD, a fundamental understanding of common heart defects is required. Since many patients have undergone surgical or interventional treatment, their anatomy and physiology differ from those in pediatric cardiology.

14.1 Introduction

In principle, any structure in the cardiovascular system can be affected by a malformation, and accordingly, various malformation syndromes have been described. However, the eight most common malformations together account for about 74% of all heart defects:

Congenital heart defects and their frequency in the neonatal period
- Ventricular septal defect (32%)
- Atrial septal defect (7.5%)
- Tetralogy of Fallot (7%)
- Pulmonary stenosis (7%)
- Persistent ductus arteriosus Botalli (7%)
- Aortic coarctation (5%)
- Transposition of the great arteries (4.5%)
- Aortic stenosis (4%)
- Others (26%)

Tetralogy of Fallot and complete transposition of the great arteries are examples of so-called **cyanotic heart defects**, i.e., they cause cyanosis in the newborn and are noticeable by reduced oxygen saturation and corresponding blueish skin coloration. A number of other congenital heart defects are also associated with cyanosis. In the course of correction, cyanosis is usually resolved.

Diagnostics Many heart defects cause characteristic **auscultatory findings**, and patients may also present with cyanosis, signs and symptoms of heart failure, or arrhythmias. In case of a clinical suspicion of a congenital heart defect, **echocardiography** is the method of choice to confirm the diagnosis and to evaluate any accompanying conditions. Additionally, other imaging modalities (especially MRI, CT) may be used. In case of suspected pulmonary arterial hypertension, as well as for the evaluation of the hemodynamic situation and the diagnosis of coronary stenoses, cardiac catheterization remains an important tool.

14.2 Congenital defects in Adulthood

The following discusses the most common congenital heart defects encountered in adults. In most of these patients, a "reparative" operation was performed in childhood, and the anatomy differs from the native anatomy of the heart defect.

14.2.1 Atrial Septal Defect

Atrial septal defects (ASD) are among the most common lesions in ACHD patients. Due to the lack of early symptoms and relatively discreet physical findings, ASDs are often not diagnosed in childhood. Depending on the location within the atrial septum, ASDs are classified into primum ASD (ASD I), secundum ASD (ASD II), sinus venosus defects, and unroofed coronary sinus).

Classification and Anatomy ASD II is by far the most common interatrial communication, accounting for about 80% of ASDs. It is located centrally in the region of the fossa ovalis (◘ Fig. 14.1). In case of very small defects, there is an overlap with a patent foramen ovale (PFO). ASD I is a malformation of the atrial septum in the area of the atrioventricular (AV) valves, accounting for about 15% of ASDs. It is actually a variant of the atrioventricular septal defect (AVSD), where communication exists only at the atrial level. As with all variants of AVSD, it is associated with a malformation of the mitral and tricuspid valves and varying degrees of AV valve regurgitation.

Sinus venosus defects are located near the openings of the venae cavae. The superior sinus venosus defect is much more common (~ 5% of ASDs) than the inferior type (< 1%) and is usually associated with partial or complete anomalous drainage of the right pulmonary veins.

The *unroofed coronary sinus* is a rare form of ASD characterized by a connection between the coronary sinus and the left atrium. It is almost always associated with a persistent left superior vena cava. Most ASDs occur sporadically, and the etiology is likely multifactorial. Secundum ASDs can be associated with the so-called Holt-Oram syndrome (heart-hand syndrome), which is characterized by skeletal anomalies of the upper limbs (an autosomal dominant disorder).

Pathophysiology The pathophysiology of the disease is primarily characterized by a left-to-right shunt. The shunt volume depends on the size of the defect, the relative compliance of the left and right atria, and especially the two ventricles, as well as the presence of possible AV valve regurgitation. With increasing age, left ventricular compliance decreases and the shunt volume increases. This process can be exacerbated by systemic hypertension, ischemic heart disease, cardiomyopathy, or valvular heart disease and can be accompanied by the onset of symptoms such as exercise intolerance, arrhythmias, and heart failure symptoms. In contrast, decreased right ventricular compliance due to right ventricular hypertrophy (e.g., in the context of pulmonary stenosis) or significant tricuspid regurgitation can reduce the left-to-right shunt or even lead to shunt reversal with cyanosis at rest or during exertion. Clinically, the majority of patients with ASD II present in adulthood with increasing exercise intolerance, shortness of breath, atrial arrhythmias, or right heart failure. Due to the increased pulmonary blood flow, a certain degree of pulmonary pressure elevation is to be expected, but severe pulmonary vascular disease is rare, and the Eisenmenger syndrome occurs in less than 5% of patients. In addition to supraventricular arrhythmias and right heart failure, ASDs can favor paradoxical embolisms (as do PFO's) with a risk of TIA or stroke. (► Chap. 7.7)

Echocardiography Current guidelines highlight the central role of echocardiography in determining the diagnosis and hemodynamic relevance of the defect. In cases of unexplained right ventricular dilation, an atrial communication should always be suspected. Often, the defect can only be inadequately visualized by transthoracic echocardiography (especially sinus venosus defects), and therefore transesophageal echocardiography (► Sect. 2.3) should be performed. Transesophageal echocardiog-

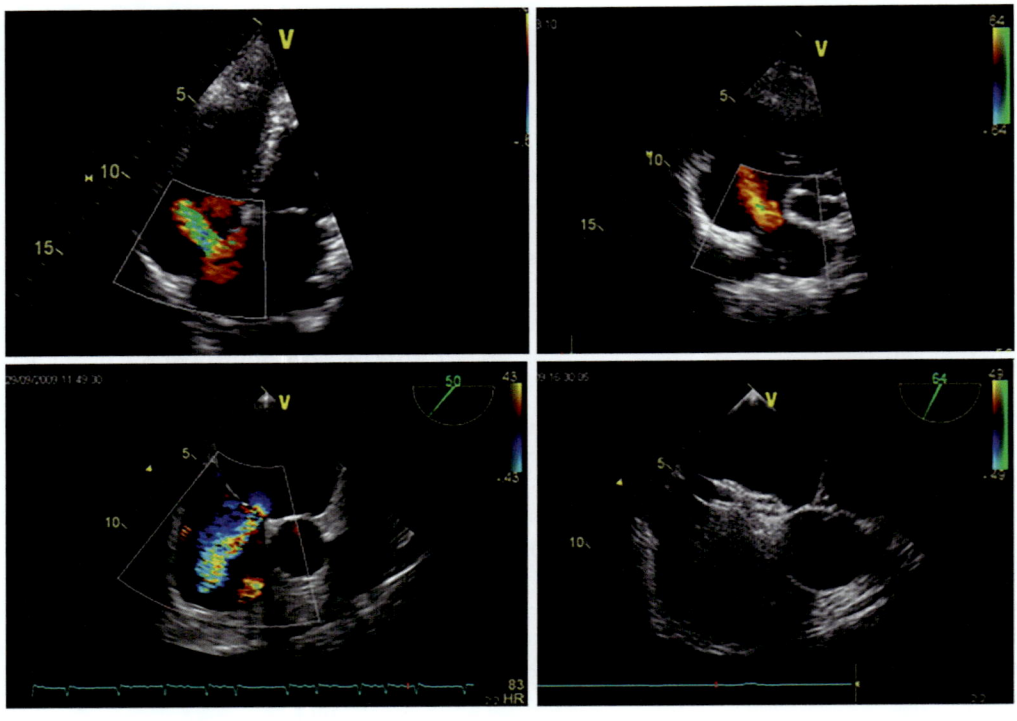

◘ Fig. 14.1 **ASD II in transthoracic view** (upper row: modified apical 4-chamber view and parasternal short axis) **as well as in transesophageal view** (lower row). Bottom left shows the view before interventional closure and bottom right after device implantation

raphy allows for better anatomical visualization of the atrial septum (especially when interventional ASD closure is being considered) and assessment of pulmonary venous return (pulmonary venous anomalies in sinus venosus defects). Transesophageal echocardiography is superior to transthoracic echocardiography, particularly in terms of measuring defect size, assessing atrial septal morphology, and rim size.

Therapy The current guidelines recommend **ASD closure** for symptomatic patients and those with a significant shunt and signs of right ventricular volume overload, regardless of symptoms. If the pulmonary vascular resistance exceeds 5 Wood units, closure should only be performed at specialized centers, if a reduction in pulmonary vascular resistance below this threshold can be demonstrated after specific therapy for pulmonary hypertension (see ▶ Chap. 5.4). In any case, only a fenestrated closure should then be considered. In cyanotic patients or those with exercise-induced cyanosis in the context of pulmonary arterial hypertension, defect closure is contraindicated. According to current guidelines, ASD closure is advisable for patients with a previous paradoxical embolism. Nowadays, secundum ASDs are usually closed interventionally using a catheter-based venous approach with septal occluders in suitable patients. Interventional closure is not an option for patients with ASD I; these patients must be referred for surgical closure. The same applies to most sinus venosus defects, although interventional closure procedures have also been successfully performed in selected patients.

14.2.2 Ventricular Septal Defect

Classification and Anatomy Ventricular septal defects (VSD) represent the most common congenital heart defect in humans. Depending on the location of the defect within the ventricular septum and its relationship to the so-called membranous septum, VSDs are classified into different forms. The most common are the so-called **perimembranous VSDs** (adjacent to the membranous septum), followed by **muscular VSDs** (which are completely located within the muscular septum).

Pathophysiology The pathophysiology of the disease depends on the size of the defect and the extent of the shunt. Small pressure-separating (so-called **restrictive**) VSDs without volume overload of the left ventricle are occasionally associated with endocarditis, but the survival rate of patients is essentially comparable to that of the general population. In contrast, large, **non-restrictive VSDs** often lead to left ventricular volume overload and eventually to heart failure and/or severe pulmonary hypertension, which ultimately results in shunt reversal and Eisenmenger syndrome. Other important complications of VSDs include: aortic regurgitation due to prolapse of semilunar valve tissue into the defect, endocarditis, subaortic stenosis, and cardiac arrhythmias.

Diagnostics In small VSDs, a thrill over the chest is often palpable, and a **pansystolic murmur** can be heard. This is often loudest in small VSDs ("*Much noise about nothing*"), while in large VSDs with pressure equalization between the ventricles, a murmur is absent. Except in patients with very limited acoustic windows, transthoracic echocardiography almost always allows for precise identification of the defect(s) and

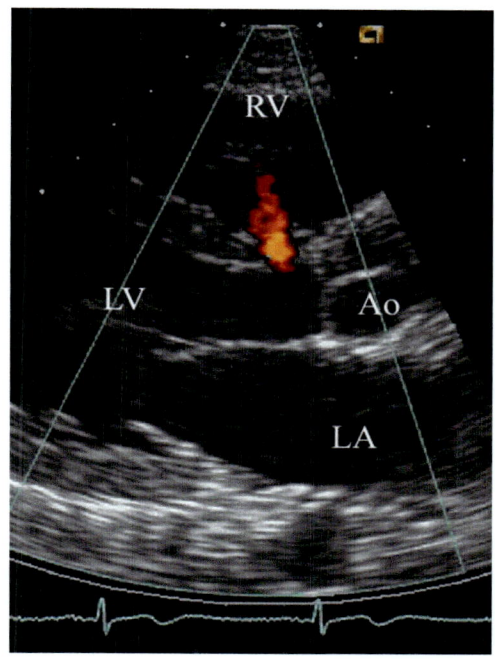

◘ **Fig. 14.2** Transthoracic Echocardiography of a typical ventricular septal defect with Doppler echocardiographic evidence of a left-to-right shunt (red)

their hemodynamic impact (◘ Fig. 14.2). Various planes should be used to visualize the defect. Special attention should be given to identifying apically located muscular VSDs, as these can be difficult to visualize. Indirect (nonspecific) signs for the presence of a hemodynamically significant VSD include unexplained left ventricular and left atrial dilation as well as increased right ventricular pressure. Therefore, in patients suspected of having a VSD, the Doppler peak velocity of tricuspid or pulmonary regurgitation should be measured. Additionally, the **Doppler velocity** over the VSD should be determined. A high velocity of turbulent flow indicates a restrictive VSD (*CW* Doppler velocity > 4 m/s). In contrast, large non-restrictive VSDs are characterized by laminar or bidirectional flow with low velocities. In cases of suspected pulmonary hypertension, invasive hemodynamic assessment is required for further therapy planning.

Therapy The current guidelines recommend the closure of a VSD in patients with a significant left-to-right shunt and signs of left ventricular volume overload (with or without symptoms), in patients with a history of infectious endocarditis, and in patients with aortic regurgitation due to a prolapse of aortic valve tissue into the defect. In patients with severe pulmonary arterial hypertension and Eisenmenger syndrome, closure is contraindicated.

Eisenmenger Physiology

Due to prolonged pressure or volume load on the pulmonary vascular bed, as occurs in congenital heart defects with a large, hemodynamically significant left-to-right shunt at the level of the ventricles or large vessels, structural changes in the pulmonary vessels with irreversible pulmonary hypertension can develop over time. If the pulmonary vascular resistance eventually exceeds the systemic vascular resistance, **shunt reversal** occurs, leading to the development of a right-to-left shunt. This results in central **cyanosis** with consequent secondary erythrocytosis.

In contrast to patients with primary pulmonary hypertension, these patients have a better long-term prognosis. A surgical or interventional shunt closure is contraindicated in these patients, as it would close the "overflow valve" and worsen the prognosis. **Therapeutically**, selective pulmonary vasodilators (especially endothelin receptor antagonists and phosphodiesterase inhibitors) are used, which can improve symptoms in these patients. A combined heart-lung transplantation or a lung transplantation with repair of the cardiac defect is a therapeutic option for some patients with severely impaired quality of life.

14.2.3 Persistent Ductus arteriosus (PDA)

The ductus arteriosus (◘ Fig. 14.3) represents an essential structure of the fetal circulation, which connects the pulmonary arteries with the descending aorta and allows the diversion of blood into the lungs. The postnatal functional closure of the ductus occurs within a few hours after birth, and the ductus is normally converted into a fibrous ligament within the first year of life.

Pathophysiology If the ductus does not close after birth, a left-to-right shunt from the aorta into the pulmonary circulation occurs. The pathophysiology varies depending on the size of the PDA. Small PDAs generally remain asymptomatic, while medium and large PDAs lead to left atrial and left ventricular **volume overload** as well as eventually **pulmonary hypertension**, which in

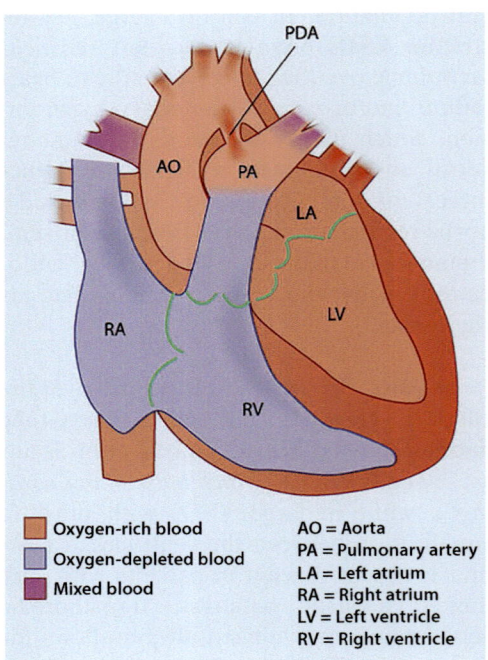

◘ Fig. 14.3 Schematic representation of the anatomical conditions in the ductus arteriosus

patients with large PDA may finally culminate in a shunt reversal and the development of Eisenmenger syndrome. Other complications include an increased risk of endarteritis and the possibility of aneurysm formation (rare).

Diagnostics The auscultatory feature of PDA is the **continuous machine-like murmur**. Diagnostically, Doppler echocardiography is the method of choice. The PDA should be visualized echocardiographically in a parasternal short-axis view. **Echocardiographically**, a characteristic diastolic flow in the pulmonary arteries can be documented (◘ Fig. 14.4). The Doppler signal usually reveals systolic-diastolic flow, but in patients with elevated pulmonary arterial pressure, the diastolic component may be absent. Diagnosing a (even large) PDA in patients with established Eisenmenger syndrome, systemic pulmonary arterial pressure, and slow bidirectional flow can be challenging. In addition to the direct assessment of the ductus, the echocardiographic examination should focus on the assessment of left ventricular dimensions and function as well as the estimated pulmonary arterial pressures (using the gradient of tricuspid regurgitation and the pulmonary acceleration time as well as the flow profile of the shunt flow itself, which reflects the pressure difference between the aorta and pulmonary arteries; see Chap. 2.3). Pulmonary hypertension and Eisenmenger syndrome can lead to right ventricular hypertrophy, dilation, and eventually failure. CT and cardiac MRI examinations can provide further anatomical information. Invasive diagnostics are required before interventional or surgical closure.

Therapy A **surgical or interventional closure** is indicated in patients with PDA and left ventricular volume overload as well as in patients with elevated pulmonary arterial pressure, but still significant left-to-right shunt. In patients with a small PDA and a continuous murmur, PDA closure can be considered to reduce the risk of endarteritis. In patients with a small silent ductus and in patients with proven Eisenmenger syndrome, closure of the ductus is not recommended. In adults with a PDA, interventional closure is nowadays the method of choice.

14.2.4 Congenital Pulmonary Stenosis

In pulmonary stenosis, there is an outflow obstruction of the right ventricle, which leads to pressure overload of the right

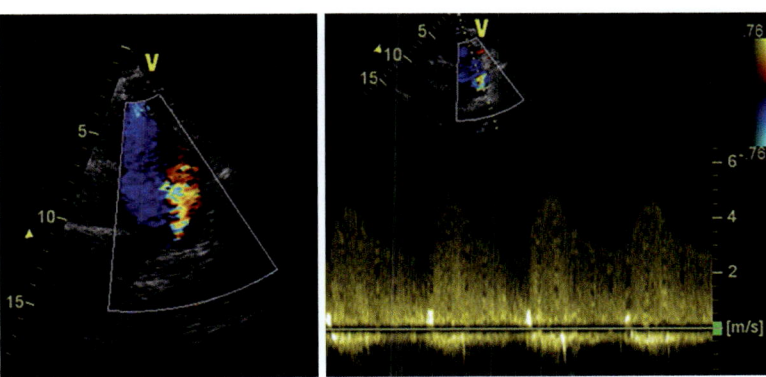

◘ Fig. 14.4 Color echocardiographic representation of the ductus arteriosus (left) as well as an example of a Doppler signal with systolic-diastolic flow over the defect (right)

ventricle and consequently to right ventricular hypertrophy. Pulmonary stenosis can occur in isolation or in the context of other defects. It can occur subvalvular, valvular, or supravalvular, or in combinations.

Diagnostics **Symptoms** of severe pulmonary stenosis include dyspnea, reduced exercise capacity, dizziness, and syncope. Additionally, signs of right heart failure may occur during the course of the disease.

In adults with operated pulmonary stenosis, pulmonary regurgitation after surgical valvulotomy (less commonly after interventional balloon valvuloplasty) is one of the most frequently encountered sequelae. The symptoms depend on the severity of the regurgitation and the right heart load and can range from nonspecific complaints (reduced performance, etc.) to manifest right heart failure. Similar symptoms can occur with residual pulmonary stenosis.

The method of choice is **echocardiography**, possibly combined with other imaging modalities (also for the evaluation of additional, corrected or uncorrected, defects). It is important in diagnostics to precisely define the level of obstruction (subvalvular, valvular, supravalvular), as this has a significant impact on the therapeutic decision.

Therapy In severe symptomatic pulmonary regurgitation, pulmonary valve replacement is often performed. In symptomatic severe valvular stenosis, interventional valvuloplasty is required, and in obstruction below or above the valve, surgical repair is necessary. The threshold for intervention is lowest when valvuloplasty is an option and highest when valve replacement is required for therapy.

14.2.5 Coarctation of the Aorta

Coarctation of the aorta (CoA) is characterized by a narrowing of the aorta near the junction of the ductus arteriosus (distal to the origin of the left subclavian artery). Morphologically, the lesion can appear either as a localized obstruction or as a hypoplastic aortic segment. Traditionally, coarctation of the aorta has been classified into pre-, para-, and post-ductal forms. However, this is of limited clinical relevance in adult patients, as the ductus is almost always closed and remodeled into a ligament. The condition is part of a generalized arteriopathy and is often associated with other lesions of the aorta (e.g., a **bicuspid aortic valve** in up to 85% of cases; ▶ Chap. 9.1 and 9.2). CoA occurs more frequently in patients with Turner (i.e. single X chromosome with webbed neck, abnormaliites of teeth, elbows and fingers) or Williams syndrome (i.e. congitive impairment, personality and facial features), congenital rubella syndrome, neurofibromatosis, and Takayasu arteritis.

Pathophysiology Severe CoA manifests in infancy, while many patients with less severe forms or those with significant collateral circulation are diagnosed only in adulthood. Signs and symptoms of CoA in these patients include **arterial hypertension** in the upper extremities (usually asymptomatic, occasionally associated with headaches, epistaxis, or dizziness), reduced blood flow to the lower extremities (**claudication of the legs**), heart failure (as a result of increased afterload, ventricular hypertrophy, and left ventricular failure), aortic dissection (due to high blood pressure and intrinsic aortic wall abnormalities such as cystic medial necrosis), endocarditis, and intracranial hemorrhages (as a result of hypertension and due to associated intracranial aneurysms). The severity of these end-organ complications depends on the degree of narrowing and in turn the height of arterial blood pressure. In the presence of significant collateral circulation, the gradient across the stenosis may be reduced. Even after surgical or interventional therapy, significant CoA can reoccur, together with the signs and symptoms of native CoA. After surgical correction, aortic aneurysms can develop, and if such an aneurysm is suspected, the aorta should be examined using CT or MRI. Upper body arterial hypertension is common even after correction without significant re- or residual CoA. It is believed that this is due to abnormal aortic compliance and intrinsic endothelial dysfunction.

Diagnostics The diagnosis of CoA is often made during a routine examination, where **high blood pressure in the upper body** with absent (or significantly weakened) femoral pulses is observed. If there is a blood pressure difference between the right arm and the legs, CoA must be sought using imaging. Upper extremity hypertension may, however, be absent depending on the degree of narrowing and the extent of collateral circulation. If there is also hypoplasia of the aortic arch, a blood pressure difference between the right and left arm is usually found. Auscultation may reveal a systolic or continuous murmur in the interscapular region.

The **echocardiographic examination** should focus on the site of the CoA as well as possible associated lesions (in particular bicuspid aortic valve with stenosis or regirgitation) and complications. Characteristic of severe CoA in transthoracic echocardiography are high Doppler velocities that persist throughout the cardiac cycle, leading to a diastolic "run-off" or "diastolic tail" phenomenon. A meaningful gradient calculation from the flow velocities is often not possible. The presence of extensive collaterals also generally makes the echocardiographic Doppler signs of coarctation of the aorta unreliable. Accurate depiction of the anatomy usually requires a CT or MRI examination.

Therapy Nowadays, interventional angioplasty is usually the treatment of choice in most centers for native or postoperative significant CoA, provided it is anatomically suitable, with **stent implantation** (Fig. 14.5). An intervention is recommended for patients with arterial hypertension and a non-invasive gradient > 20 mmHg between the upper and lower extremities. An intervention should also be considered in patients with hypertension and an aortic narrowing of > 50% relative to the aortic diameter at the level of the diaphragm in CT, MRI, or invasive angiography, even without a relevant gradient. Successful relief of significant CoA is not a guarantee for blood pressure normalization.

14.2.6 Tetralogy of Fallot

Tetralogy of Fallot is the **most common cyanotic congenital heart defect** in humans. The defect consists of a non-restrictive VSD, an overriding aorta, an obstruction of the right ventricular outflow tract, and secondary right ventricular hypertrophy (Fig. 14.6). The obstruction of the right ventricular outflow tract is usually a combination of subpulmonary and valvular obstruction. The disease is associated with a microdeletion on chromosome 22 (formerly **DiGeorge syndrome**, 22q11) in about 15–20% of cases, which generally occurs sporadically but is transmitted to offspring in 50% of cases and is often accompanied by psychiatric disorders.

Pathophysiology Patients with uncorrected tetralogy of Fallot are cyanotic. Although the non-restrictive VSD and the overriding aorta predispose to cyanosis, the severity of cyanosis mainly depends on the extent of the right ventricular outflow tract stenosis. Nowadays, patients are usually subjected to corrective surgery at diagnosis or upon the onset of symptoms in early childhood.

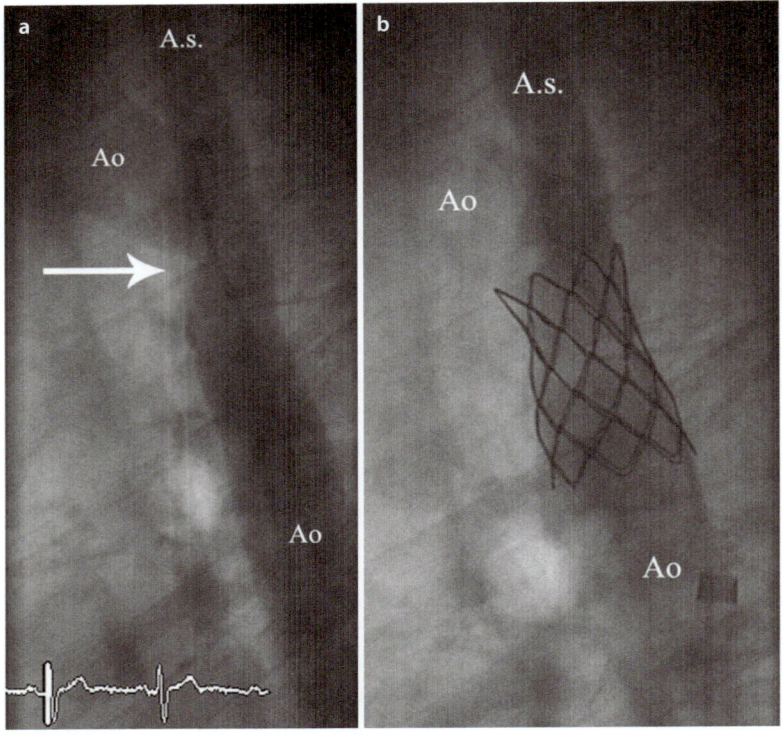

Fig. 14.5 (a, b) Coarctation of the aorta (a) before (arrow) and (b) after stent implantation. *Ao:* Aorta, *A.s.:* A subclavia sinistra

Patients with tetralogy of Fallot who were operated on several decades ago—and who are now under ACHD cardiological care—often underwent a primary palliative operation preceding a **corrective surgery**. These early palliations, aimed at increasing pulmonary blood flow, included:

- **Blalock-Taussig (BT) anastomosis**: The classic BT shunt is an end-to-side anastomosis between the subclavian artery and the ipsilateral pulmonary artery. A modified BT shunt is characterized by the insertion of a vascular graft between the subclavian artery and the pulmonary artery.
- **Waterston shunt**: Side-to-side anastomosis between the ascending aorta and the right pulmonary artery
- **Potts shunt**: Side-to-side anastomosis between the descending aorta and the left pulmonary artery

Palliative procedures can lead to a narrowing or kinking of the pulmonary arteries, pulmonary hypertension, and left ventricular volume overload. Consequently, these procedures have largely been abandoned, and a **primary correction** of Tetralogy of Fallot at the age of 6–18 months is now the treatment of choice. This is associated with a very low perioperative mortality. The corrective surgery consists of closing the VSD and eliminating the obstruction of the right ventricular outflow tract and is currently generally performed via a transatrial-transpulmonary approach. In contrast, the repair was previously performed via a right ventriculotomy, with a transannular patch typically placed to achieve "complete relief" of the right ventricular outflow tract obstruction. This approach creates an arrhythmogenic substrate in the right ventricular infundibulum and commonly lead to severe pulmonary regurgitation. The long-term results after the repair are excellent (35-year survival rate of approximately 85%). **Sequelae and complications** are, however, common and include:

- **Pulmonary regurgitation(PR)** (◘ Fig. 14.7). Previously, PR was considered a harmless sequela, but it has been shown that significant PR over time leads to right ventricular dilation and impairment of right ventricular function, constitutes a substrate for (potentially malignant) arrhythmias, and is accompanied by symptoms of heart failure. Severe PR is the norm in patients after a transannular patch repair.
- A **right ventricular dilation** and dysfunction is generally associated with severe PR.
- A **left ventricular dysfunction** can occur as a result of right ventricular dysfunction (ventriculo-ventricular interaction) and can, in itself, represent an unfavorable prognostic marker.
- An **aortic root dilation** with aortic regurgitation has been described due to intrinsic aortic wall anomalies associated with Tetralogy of Fallot.
- **Cardiac arrhythmias** and sudden cardiac death. About half of Fallot patients die suddenly. The propensity for (malignant) arrhythmias is related to hemodynamic substrates, surgical scars, and myocardial fibrosis.

Therapy Current guidelines recommend pulmonary valve replacement in symptomatic patients with severe pulmonary regurgitation and/or stenosis (defined as a right ventricular systolic pressure over 80 mmHg). Additionally, pulmonary valve replacement should be considered in asymptomatic patients with severe pulmonary regurgitation and/or stenosis, reduced objective exercise capacity, or progressive right ventricular dilation or progressive right ventricular dysfunction or progressive tricuspid regurgitation or significant right ventricular outflow tract obstruction (generally defined as right ventricular systolic pressure > 80 mmHg) or persistent arrhythmias. An aortic valve replacement should be performed in patients with severe aortic regurgitation and symptoms or signs of left ventricular dysfunction or dilation. A VSD closure is advisable in patients with residual VSD and signs of significant left ventricular volume overload. Thresholds for right ventricular volumes that warrant consideration of elective pulmonary valve replacement are based on cardiac MRI measurements and are generally 160 ml/m^2 for right ventricular end-diastolic volume and > 80 ml/m^2 for end-systolic volume.

14.2.7 Transposition of the Great Arteries (TGA)

In the transposition of the great arteries (TGA), the aorta arises from the (morphologically) right ventricle and the pulmonary artery from the (morphologically) left ventricle. In TGA, there are thus two parallel, separate circulations. For this reason, survival without a shunt (usually ASD or VSD) and corresponding blood mixing is not possible. Newborns with transposition are **severely cyanotic** and not viable without an intracardiac shunt. If such a shunt is not present, a shunt must be created postnatally as quickly as possible, usually by catheter intervention (so-called **Rashkind procedure**). In most cases, the aorta is located anterior and to the right of the pulmonary artery (~ 95% of cases), although it can sometimes be directly anterior or to the left and, in very rare cases, even posterior to the

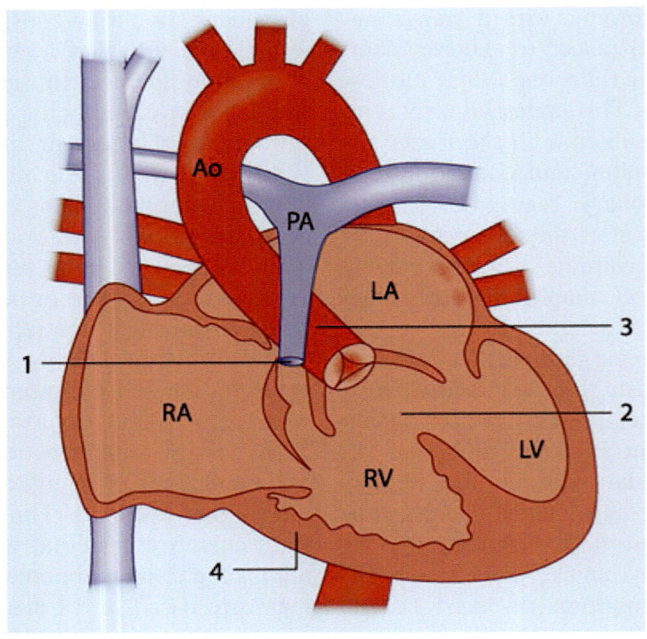

Fig. 14.6 Schematic representation of the anatomical conditions in unoperated tetralogy of Fallot. 1 = Right ventricular outflow tract obstruction; 2 = Ventricular septal defect; 3 = Overriding aorta; 4 = Right ventricular hypertrophy

pulmonary artery. Unlike the normal heart (with a crisscross arrangement of the vessels), the great vessels run parallel (side by side). The anatomy of the coronary arteries is abnormal and variable.

The primary therapy consists of **surgical repair** of the cardiac anatomy. The anatomical arterial switch correction with repositioning of the great arteries to the respective appropriate ventricle (arterial switch, **Arterial-Switch Operation**) was technically feasible only as of the late 1970s due to the required reimplantation of the coronary arteries into the neoaorta and has been routinely performed at most centers since the mid-1980s. Previously, these patients were treated with only a physiological correction, where the blood was redirected at the atrial level using so-called *baffles* (so-called **Senning** or **Mustard operation**, ◘ Fig. 14.8). Although this operation resulted in two serially connected circulations, the morphologically right ventricle still had to supply the systemic circulation (atrial switch, **Atrial-Switch Operation**, ◘ Fig. 14.4). Clinically, TGA is often classified as simple (2/3 of cases) or complex, depending on whether significant accompanying malformations are present. These typically include a VSD (~ 45% of cases), significant obstruction of the left ventricular outflow tract (~ 25%), and occasionally a CoA.

Pathophysiology in Adulthood Long-term complications after **arterial switch operation** include pulmonary artery stenoses, which sometimes require reoperation (in some series up to 10–25%), neo-aortic valve regurgitation (generally no more than moderate), and coronary artery anomalies with uncertain long-term effects.

Long-term complications after **atrial switch** (Mustard or Senning) include baffle stenoses (mostly in the upper part of the systemic venous baffle), baffle leaks, sinus node dysfunction, atrial arrhythmias, right

Congenital Heart Defects

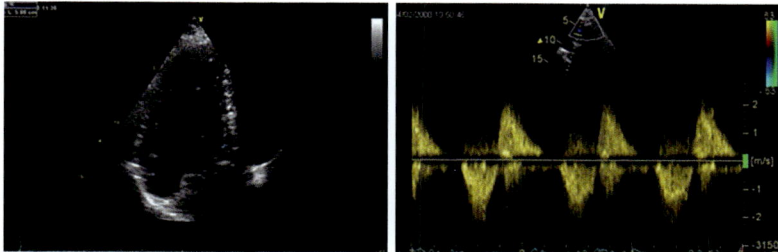

Fig. 14.7 Echocardiographic representation of right ventricular dilation (left) in an adult patient with Tetralogy of Fallot and severe pulmonary regurgitation. The Doppler echocardiographic tracing (right) shows a rapid decline in diastolic flow with the end of diastolic flow occurring before the end of diastole

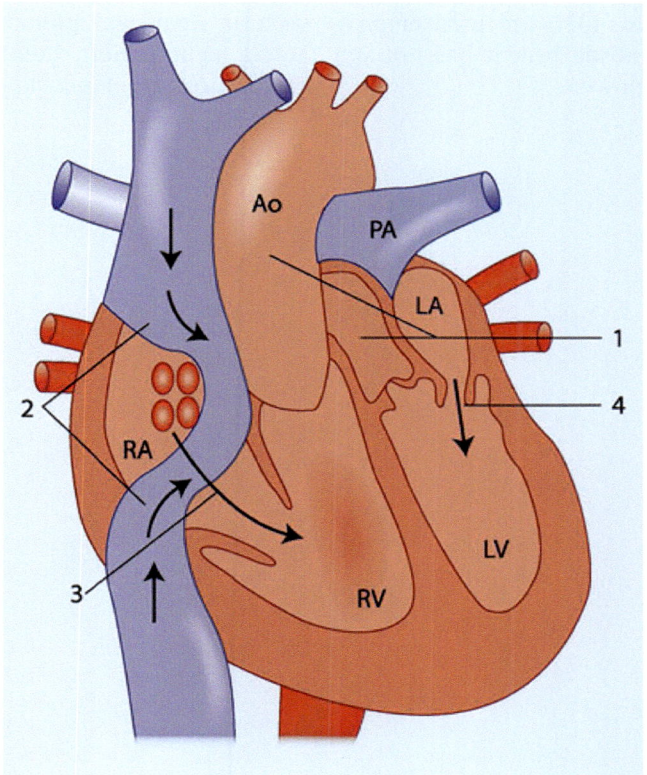

Fig. 14.8 Conditions in TGA and correction after atrial switch operation. Systemic venous blood (2) is redirected through the mitral valve (4) into the morphologically left ventricle, which pumps the blood into the pulmonary circulation (1). Pulmonary venous blood is directed into the right atrium (*RA*) and through the tricuspid valve (3) into the morphologically right ventricle (*RV*), which pumps the blood into the systemic circulation (aorta, *Ao*)

ventricular dysfunction and dilation, (functional) tricuspid regurgitation, ventricular arrhythmias, heart failure, and sudden cardiac death.

While relevant long-term complications after arterial switch are relatively rare, they are the norm after atrial switch.

Therapy Diuretics should be used for symptomatic treatment of Mustard/Senning patients with signs or symptoms of heart failure. Beta-blockers and ACE inhibitors/angiotensin II receptor antagonists and newer heart failure medications (e.g. SGLT2-I; ▶ Chap. 13.4) are used empirically. Their prognostic benefit has not yet been definitively proven.

A **surgical therapy** is recommended for severe tricuspid regurgitation in symptomatic patients with preserved systolic systemic function. Interventional procedures should be considered for patients with significant baffle obstruction. The closure of **baffle-leaks** should be performed in symptomatic patients with significant right-to-left (cyanosis) or left-to-right shunt (heart failure) and considered in asymptomatic patients. Significant obstruction of the left ventricular outflow tract must be surgically treated. In patients who had undergone an arterial switch operation, complications such as significant pulmonary stenosis or aortic regurgitation should be treated according to current guidelines.

Aortic Diseases

Martin Czerny and Christoph Nienaber

Contents

15.1 Aortic Aneurysm – 256

15.2 Aortic Dissection – 260

Earlier versions of this chapter were created by Marc Husmann, Jan Steffel, and Thomas F. Lüscher.

© The Author(s), under exclusive license to Springer-Verlag GmbH, DE, part of Springer Nature 2025
T. F. Lüscher and U. Landmesser (eds.), *Cardiovascular System*,
https://doi.org/10.1007/978-3-662-70152-2_15

An aortic aneurysm is defined as an enlargement of the aortic diameter by more than 50% of the normal value. Depending on the location, there is an indication for surgical repair at a certain size, especially with rapid size progression due to the risk of rupture, and with symptoms (associated aortic valve regurgitation, pain, compression, hoarseness etc.).

◘ Figure 15.1 shows an aneurysm of the ascending aorta with marked dilatation of the aortic diameter. In comparison, an aortic dissection is a spontaneous or traumatic splitting of the layers of the aortic wall with intramural bleeding, spreading, and accumulation of blood in the media. In the context of acute dissection, there is an acute increase in the overall vessel size (usually as a result of an acute increase in the size of the false lumen, which is only limited by the weak tunica adventitia). The dissected aorta is also commonly referred to as an aneurysm dissecans due to the increase in size, but it is a different pathology compared to the previously mentioned true aneurysm. A dissection can result from an aneurysm, but newer data increasingly suggest that the aorta is usually not enlarged prior to the dissection (thus had a normal diameter before the acute event). Rather, the elongation of the aorta seems to be a possible risk factor for the development of aortic dissection.

15.1 Aortic Aneurysm

Definition An aortic aneurysm is present when there is an increase in the aortic diameter of more than 50% of the normal value. The term "aneurysm" generally refers to the enlargement of an artery or a local enlarrgemt of a cardiac chamber (mostly due to a myiocardial infarction; ▶ Chap. 7.5).

Pathophysiology In its anatomical course, the aorta physiologically has different diameters, which decrease from proximal, i.e., from the aortic root, to distal, i.e. the iliac bifurcation. The normal value for the ascending aorta is 3–3.5 cm, for the descending thoracic aorta 2.5–3.0 cm, and for the infrarenal abdominal aorta up to 3 cm.

If there is an enlargement of all three layers of the aortic wall, a classic aortic aneurysm is present, which is also referred to as a **true aneurysm**. Morphologically, there are other special forms such as the previously mentioned aortic dissection or **aneurysm dissecans**, in which the expansion of the true and/or false lumen leads to an increase in size. Since the overall diameter of the aorta is enlarged in this case, it is also referred to as aneurysmal enlargement (▶ Sect. 15.2).

A morphologically different form is the **penetrating atherosclerotic ulcer(PAU)**, in which a local bulging of the wall occurs due to, for example, an injury or plaque

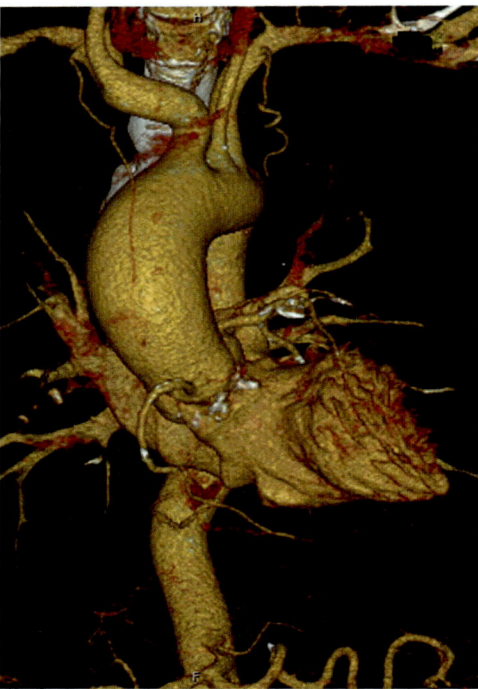

◘ Fig. 15.1 Computed tomography of an aneurysm of the ascending aorta

Aortic Diseases

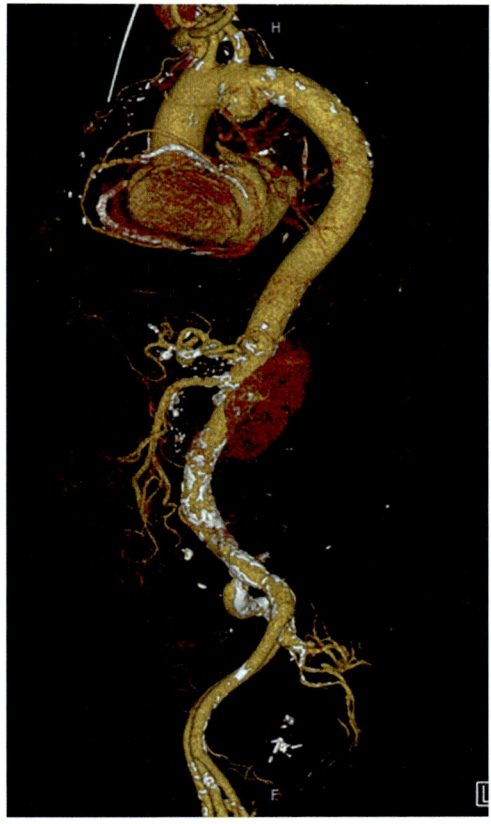

◘ **Fig. 15.2** Computed tomography of a penetrating atherosclerotic ulcer (PAU) in the aortic arch recognizable as a bulging

rupture. ◘ Figure 15.2 shows such a PAU in the aortic arch. Here, an extra- or intramural hematoma, which tamponades the leak and is covered by a connective tissue capsule over time, may develop. Thus, such a pseudoaneurysm is not a dilation of the aorta itself like in the case of a classical aneurysm, but rather a local increase in size of the vascular wall with to bulging. Classical aneurysm also develop in the distal aorta. Figure 15.3 shows a classic **infrarenal aortic aneurysm**, which is the most common sire of aneurysm formation.

❗ Degenerative aortic aneurysms should, depending on the location and size, considered for elective preventive repair to prevent an often fatal aortic rupture with massive bleeding.

Epidemiology The incidence and prevalence of aortic aneurysms is difficult to determine, as it usually remains a **clinically silent disease** for a long time. It is known that the incidence of aneurysms increases with age. In Western countries, the prevalence of **abdominal aortic aneurysm** is estimated to range between 2 and 8% with a preponderance in men compared to women and a marked increase after the age of 50 years and particulary in smokers. The incidence of **thoracic aortic aneurysms** is even harder to quantify due to their long asymptomatic clinical course. Current studies suggest an annual incidence of 5.6–10.4 cases per 100,000 patient-years. The incidence of thoracic aortic aneurysms and that of ruptured thoracic aortic aneurysms seems to be increasing, but it is unclear whether this is merely a result of better imaging diagnostics or a true change. Men are also more frequently affected by thoracic aortic aneurysms, and such patients are generally older than 60 years.

Etiology The underlying cause of aneurysm formation is usually an **arteriosclerotic remodeling** of the aortic wall. The risk factors for the development of an aortic aneurysm are therefore similar to those for arteriosclerosis (see also Chap. 7.1:
- Smoking (the most important risk factor),
- arterial hypertension,
- positive family history,
- male gender,
- age,
- dyslipidemia.

Rarer causes are **hereditary connective tissue diseases**, specifically Marfan, Ehlers-Danlos, and Loeys-Dietz syndromes, or inflammatory and mycotic aneurysms. In these cases, the patients are often younger.

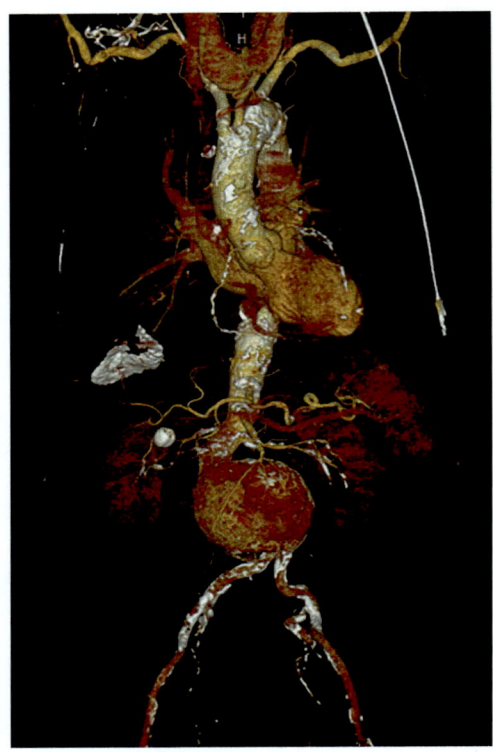

Fig. 15.3 Computed tomography of a saccular infrarenal aneurysm of the abdominal aorta

to the formation of aortic gummas. With the decline of advanced stages of syphilis in Western countries, the prevalence of syphilitic aortic aneurysm has also decreased.

Clinical Findings Aneurysms often remain clinically silent for a long time until **rupture** occurs. Alternatively, they are discovered incidentally during imaging for other causes. However, the local expansion of the aorta can lead to **compression of surrounding organs**, which, depending on the affected structure, can cause abdominal pain, back pain, dyspnea (in case of airway obstruction), dysphagia (esophageal obstruction), or hoarseness (pressure on the recurrent laryngeal nerve). Pain in the aorta itself occurs only when the adventitia is stretched or torn and is always a sign of impending rupture that should urgently be reffered to a specialized center.

> ❗ Open or covered rupture represents the main danger of any aneurysm and is associated with very high mortality. Another risk is the formation of thrombi within the aneurysm, which can lead to peripheral embolisms.

Diagnostics Physical examination rarely provides an indication of an aortic aneurysm, and if it does, it is only for large abdominal aneurysms (**pulsating tumor**). Conventional X-rays can sometimes show an enlarged, often calcified aorta and thus may only raise a suspicion for an aneurysm with low sensitivity.

> ▸ The imaging modalities of choice in the diagnosis and planning of interventions of aortic aneurysms are echocardiography or abdominal ultrasound and computed tomography angiography (CTA).

It should also be noted that although diabetes mellitus is associated with arteriosclerosis, there is a negative correlation between diabetes and thoracic and/or abdominal aortic aneurysms, and diabetes is therefore not a risk factor for the development of an aortic aneurysm.

> ▸ In Marfan syndrome, aneurysm formation typically occurs in the aortic root and ascending aorta.

The presence of a **bicuspid aortic valve** is also associated with the formation of a thoracic aneurysm, especially in the ascending aorta, with the risk of rupture being significantly increased. In the past, **syphilis** was also a major cause of aortic aneurysms, and in this case typically localized in the ascending aorta and the isthmus region, due

As regards abdominal aortic aneurysms, every **smoker > 65 years** (regardless of whether active or ex-smoker) as well as patients with a positive **family history** (men as of 55 years, women as of 65 years) should be examined once by ultrasound for the presence of an abdominal aortic aneurysm. Men aged 65 years or older should undergo a one-time examination for abdominal aortic aneurysms. Abdominal **ultrasound** or echocardiography can only visualize the ascending aorta and partially the aortic arch. The distal part of thethoracic aorta and the proximal part of the descending aorta, is a blind spot for echocardiography, as these parts can only poorly or not at all be visualized using this imaging modality. Even for the ascending aorta and the aortic arch, echocardiography is inferior to CTA and thus more suitable for screening rather than planning of further steps.

As the diagnostic tool of choice for the thoracic aorta and for planning of surgical or catheter-based interventions, **CTA** of the entire aorta and its first-order branches is the gold standard. Alternatively, magnetic resonance imaging can be considered on an individual basis (especially in young patients).

Aneurysms are consequences of advanced atherosclerosis and are often associated with coronary artery and peripheral artery disease as well as renal artery stenosis /see ▶ Chap. 4.2, 4.4 and 7.2, 7.4). Therefore, in addition to imaging the thoracoabdominal vessels, screening for vascular changes in the peripheral vessels (e.g. femoro-popliteal aneurysms, peripheral arterial occlusive disease), the cerebrovasculature , and also the coronary arteries should be considered in such patients using ultrasound or angiography, respectively.

Prognosis The rupture risk of any aneurysm depends on changes in the vascular wall as well as on the wall tension, which can be estimated using Laplace's law:

$$W = P \times r/2h$$

W: Wall tension, *P:* (blood) pressure, *r:* radius, *h:* wall thickness

The rupture risk increases accordingly with rising blood pressure and with increasing diameter of the aneurysm. The rupture riska averages up to 33% per year with a diameter of the ascending aorta of > 7 cm.

Therapy For smaller aneurysms, treatment consists of optimal management of cardiovascular risk factors. In particular, the patient should quit **smoking**, and **blood pressure** should be lowered to low-normal values using ACE inhibitors, beta-blockers, or calcium antagonists (systolic blood pressure target: < 130 mmHg). Due to the usually generalized obstructive and/or dilated atherosclerosis, patients should also be treated with a **platelet inhibitor** (e.g. Aspirin 75mg OD) and a **statin (Chap. 3.2)**. Follow-up checks using suitable imaging modalities (see above), ideally in specialized interdisciplinary aortic centers, are recommended.

The **indication for surgery** depends on the diameter and location of the aneurysm. For the ascending aorta, an elongation of > 11 cm should also be considered in the decision for elective aortic replacement. Additionally, a rapid increase in diameter (> 0.5 cm within 6 months) indicates the need for surgery. In patients with connective tissue diseases or bicuspid aortic valve, the indication for surgery sholud be considered at significantly lower aortic diameters (e.g., thoracic aneurysm diameter of 4.5 cm).

> **Surgical Indications for Aortic Aneurysm**
> - Ascending aorta: > 50–55 mm
> - Thoracic descending aorta: > 55 mm
> - Abdominal aorta: > 55 mm in men, > 45–50 mm in women

In principle, two **surgical procedures** can be considered:

Open surgical replacement involves implantation of a vascular prosthesis (tube and side-arm prosthesis as well as Y-prosthesis at the level of the aortic bifurcation). Depending on the location of the aneurysm, this may require a (hemi-)sternotomy, a laparotomy, or even a thoracoabdominal approach. Alternatively, there is the possibility of implanting an endovascular stent graft, usually via access through the common femoral artery.

Modern branched or fenestrated **stent-grafts** also allow treatment of complex aneurysms of the aortic arch or the iliac bifurcation. ◘ Figure 15.4 shows a CTA after treatment of the thoracoabdominal aorta with a fenestrated stent-graft prosthesis (*Fenestrated Endovascular Aortic Repair—EVAR*), which carries side branches for the main vessels (celiac trunk, superior mesenteric artery, and both renal arteries). However, the treatment of the ascending aorta is not possible endovascularly outside of experimental case series. An essentiel prerequisite for endovascular treatment is always the presence of a sufficiently large sealing landing zone proximal and distal to the aneurysm, which is not always present.

For aneurysms of the aortic arch, the so-called Frozen-Elephant-Trunk (FET) technique is available, a hybrid treatment method that combines the advantages of open and endovascular techniques. ◘ Figure 15.5 shows a postoperative CTA of a patient after aortic arch replacement with the FET technique, consisting of a hybrid prosthesis that has both a stent-graft and a classic vascular prosthesis component.

The **operative lethality** ranges from 1.5% in elective procedures to up to 50% in emergency procedures, whereby the perioperative mortality in emergencies could be significantly reduced by endovascular stent-grafts.

Prognosis Prognostically, short-term survival after endovascular treatment is better than after open surgical treatment due to a lower operative invasiveness of the endovascular approach and peri-operative morbidity, but in the long term, particularly due to the high rates of reinterventions after endovascular treatment, the benefit reverses to open surgical treatment. Thus, an individualized patient selection for either approach is ideally required by an interdisciplinary aortic team that offers all therapeutic options.

15.2 Aortic Dissection

Definition A dissection is characterized by a tear in the aortic wall (the so-called entry) with the formation of an intramural pseudolumen (the so-called false lumen), which extends distally and proximally.

Aortic dissection is an important manifestation of the so-called acute aortic syndrome (AAS), which also includes aortic rupture, aortitis, intramural hematoma, and penetrating aortic ulcer.

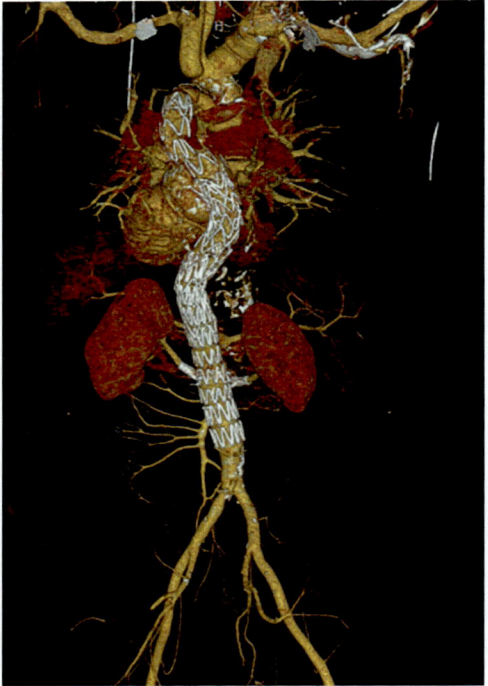

◘ **Fig. 15.4** CTA after treatment of the thoracoabdominal aorta with a fenestrated stent-graft prosthesis. (*Fenestrated Endovascular Aortic Repair—EVAR*)

Aortic Diseases

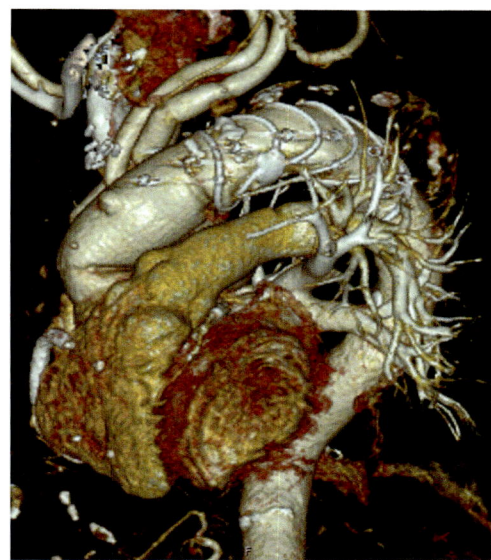

Fig. 15.5 Postoperative CTA of a patient after aortic arch replacement with the FET technique, consisting of a hybrid prosthesis that has both a stent-graft and a classic vascular prosthesis component

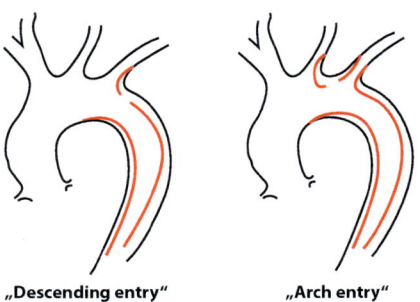

„Descending entry"   „Arch entry"

Fig. 15.6 Schematic representation of the subtypes of non-A-non-B aortic dissection

Classification The aortic dissection is classified according to Stanford definition into type A, B, and non-A-non-B aortic dissection. Furthermore, the Type-Entry-Malperfusion (TEM) classification is increasingly being adopted in clinical routine.
- In **type A dissection**, the ascending aorta is affected (with or without involvement of the aortic arch or the descending aorta).
- In **type B dissection**, only the descending aorta is affected (without involvement of the ascending aorta or the aortic arch).
- In **non-A-non-B dissection**, the aortic arch and the descending aorta are affected (without involvement of the ascending aorta), ◘ Fig. 15.6 shows the subtypes of non-A-non-B dissection— either primary entry in the descending aorta with retrograde intramural hematoma component into the aortic arch or primary entry in the aortic arch.

The **TEM classification** (◘ Fig. 15.7) conceptually follows the TNM classification from oncology. "T" stands for "type," i.e., type A, type B, and type non-A-non-B aortic dissection, "E" for the location of the primary entry—"0" if no primary entry is visible, "E1" if the primary entry is located between the aortic root and the brachiocephalic trunk, "E2" if it is located in the aortic arch, and "E3" if it is located distal to the origin of the left subclavian artery. "M" symbolically stands for "metastasis of acute aortic dissection" for the organ systems potentially involved in a "malperfusion," i.e., "M0" if no organ malperfusion is present, "M1" for coronary malperfusion, "M2" for malperfusion of the head and neck vessels, and "M3" for spinal, visceral, renal, and/or extremity malperfusion. If an organ malperfusion is associated with clinical symptoms in imaging (CTA), then a "+" is added to "M1," "M2," "M3," or the combination. This very simple classification allows an immediate assessment of the overall situation and the establishment of an initial treatment concept immediately after CTA.

Epidemiology An exact definition of the **incidence** of aortic dissection is difficult, as it is often an acutely lethal condition, and thus a high number of unreported cases labelled as sudden cardiac death is likely.

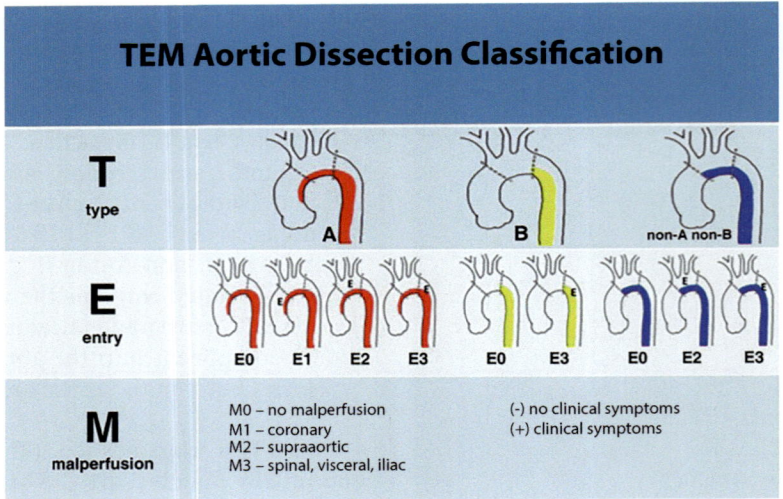

◘ Fig. 15.7 Schematic representation of the subtypes of aortic dissection according to TEM

Today, an incidence of approximately 3–6/100,000/year is assumed.

The problem of the **number of unreported cases** can be exemplified by a Japanese study: In 7% of all patients in a postmortem computed tomography study, a type A aortic dissection was actually detected contrary to the cause of death stated by the coroner.

Dissections occur more frequently in the **morning hours** (between 6 and 12 o'clock) and in **winter**. About 75% of patients suffer from arterial **hypertension**. Patients with **connective tissue diseases** (especially Marfan syndrome due to mutations in the gene for fibrillin or elastic fibers) can suffer an aortic dissection as early as adolescence or young adulthood, with the average age often being under 40 years.

Etiology Typically, the cause of a dissection is a degeneration of the media or **cystic medial necrosis**. The earlier assumption that a pre-existing aneurysm frequently leads to dissection cannot be confirmed with current data. Aortic elongation seems to be a much better predictor for type A dissection. Ultimately, however, sufficient clinical markers to prevent a dissection are lacking. 65% of all dissections begin in the ascending aorta, and 20–30% of all dissections in the area of the left subclavian artery.

Rarer etiologies include trauma, Takayasu or Horton arteritis, and iatrogenic dissections (usually after angiography or cardiac or vascular surgery).

Clinical Findings Acute aortic dissection is always a clinical emergency and requires immediate cardiac and/or vascular surgical assessment and treatment. The dissection itself causes a most severe pain (tearing, stabbing), usually between the shoulder blades. A typical feature is a migrating radiation along the anatomical course of the dissection: retrosternal, shoulder, back, abdomen.

> Through the dissection lumen, vessels that branch off in this area can be obliterated and compressed, which can lead to ischemia in the affected organs and regions and consequently functional failure.

Depending on the anatomical extent of the dissection and the degree of malperfusion, the following **additional clinical features** may thus be prominent from proximal to distal: coronary malperfusion (leading to ST-segment elevationin the ESC, angina and myocardial infarction; Chap. 7.5), supraaortic malperfusion (ischemia of the upper extremities with pain, stroke; Chap 7.7), visceral malperfusion (intestinal ischemia, acute renal failure, etc.), and iliac-femoral malperfusion (cold legs, claudication; Chap 7.6). The more organ systems are affected by malperfusion, the worse the prognosis of the patients (i.e. rule of thumb: +10% mortality per affected organ system).

In patients with type A aortic dissection, acute **aortic valve regurgitation** and/or a hemorrhagic pericardial effusion up to tamponade are also clinically prominent features in over one-third of patients. For these reasons, the huge mortality rate of acute untreated type A aortic dissection is 1–2% per hour.

> In every patient with chest pain and suspected aortic dissection, blood pressure should be measured in both arms. If there is a difference of > 15–20 mmHg, aortic dissection should be included in the differential diagnosis.

Diagnostics The diagnostic method of choice is **CTA**, which is quickly available in almost all centers and hospitals and can clearly show both the beginning of the dissection, the primary entry point, and the distal and proximal course of the dissection. Alternatively, magnetic resonance imaging (MRI) can be used (◘ Fig. 15.8), but this is more time-consuming and not readily available everywhere. In chest X-rays, thoracic aortic dissection typically shows a widening of the mediastinum, although this examination is no longer significant for diagnosis today. Echocardiographically, a proximal type A dissection can be visi-

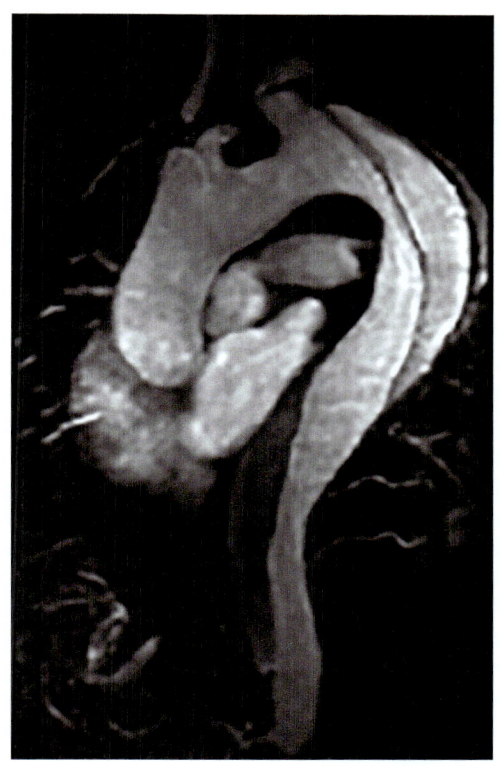

◘ **Fig. 15.8** Magnetic resonance imaging of a type A aortic dissection with a spiral dissection membrane extending into the abdominal aorta

ble, while ist further course can only be partially assessed. The ECG is almost always altered in type A dissections, but usually nonspecific except, if the take off of coronary arterees is obstructed (e.g. ST-segment elevation or depression).

Therapy Acute aortic dissection is an emergency situation. Immediate blood pressure reduction to 110 mmHg systolic with intravenous beta-blockers (possibly in combination with nitrates) and analgesia with morphine are indicated.

In the case of an acute **Type A dissection**, open surgical repair is always indicated without any alternative startegy from a prognostic point of view. The treatment consists at least of replacing the ascending aorta, usually with replacement of the small curvature of the aortic arch (so-called hemiarch replacement). In 10–20% of cases, replacement of the entire aortic arch may also be required. The goal should always be the resection of the primary entry site (the primary tear).

In contrast, acute **Type B and Type non-A-non-B aortic dissection** is initially divided into complicated and uncomplicated forms. The absence of, among other features, malperfusion, rupture/risk of rupture, and persistent pain allows the diagnosis of an **uncomplicated dissection**. In this case, conservative therapy is recommended as the initial strategy, which primarily consists of optimal blood pressure control and analgesia. If the CT findings are stable on the short-term follow-up CT, patients can be further managed in an outpatient setting. However, regular close follow-up, ideally in a specialized aortic outpatient clinic, is mandatory, as these patients have a high intervention rate (surgical or endovascular) over time.

In patients with **complicated dissection**, there is always an indication for immediate endovascular or open surgical treatment. The goal is to stabilize the dissection (prevent rupture) and/or eliminate malperfusion of affected organs. In patients with acute non-A-non-B aortic dissection, due to the poor prognosis (i.e. negative aortic remodeling of the untreated dissection with increasing risk of rupture), there is often an indication for timely intervention even in initially uncomplicated dissection.

As with classical aneurysms, interventions can be performed **open surgically, endovascularly, or through a combination** of both procedures. The procedural goal here is to close the primary entry point. If this is located in the tubular segment of the descending aorta, it can usually be achieved endovascularly with a stent graft. The closer the entry is to the aortic arch, the lower the likelihood of an adequate landing zone for a percutaneously inserted stent graft. By transposition or bypass of the supraaortic arteries (e.g., bypass from the left common carotid artery to the left subclavian artery), the subclavian artery can be overstented and a new landing zone can thereby be generated. If this is not possible, complete aortic arch replacement may also be required.

Prognosis The prognosis for **Type A dissection** depends on the extent of accompanying malperfusion or rupture and the patient's hemodynamic stability prior to surgery. Without treatment, 1–2% of patients die per hour, and about 50% of patients with Type A dissection die within the first 48 hours. The 30-day mortality rate for Type A dissection is generally more than 10% even with the best possible therapy. The 30-day mortality risk of Type A dissection can now be calculated using an online calculator at ▶ https://www.dgthg.de/de/GERAADA_Score.

For **Type B and non-A-non-B dissections**, the short-term prognosis depends on the accompanying malperfusion and the risk of rupture. The medium- to long-term prognosis is influenced by the presence of other cardiovascular diseases and the course of the aortic disease (e.g. aneurysm formation, rupture), necessitating regular check-ups at a center specialized in aortic diseases.

Tumors of the Cardiovascular System

Tatiana Manuylova and Karin Klingel

Contents

16.1 General Characteristics of Cardiac Tumors – 266

16.2 Characteristics of Selected Tumors – 267
16.2.1 Benign Tumors – 267
16.2.2 Malignant Tumors – 269

© The Author(s), under exclusive license to Springer-Verlag GmbH, DE, part of Springer Nature 2025
T. F. Lüscher and U. Landmesser (eds.), *Cardiovascular System*,
https://doi.org/10.1007/978-3-662-70152-2_16

Tumors in and on the heart are rare. Metastases are the most common. Most primary heart tumors are benign. The exceedingly rare malignant tumors are usually associated with a poor prognosis, as the therapeutic options are extremely limited.

16.1 General Characteristics of Cardiac Tumors

Epidemiology Cardiac tumours belong to a heterogeneous group that includes various primary benign and malignant as well as secondary tumors. Based on autopsy data, the frequency of cardiac tumors is 0.02%, with approximately 90% being benign and 10% malignant. Metastases from malignancies occur 20 to 30 times more frequently than primary heart tumors. In autopsies of various malignant diseases, cardiac metastases are found in 9–14%, most commonly in lung carcinoma (37%), breast carcinoma (7%), esophageal carcinoma (6%), and lymphomas (20%).

Cardiac Tumors
Primary benign cardiac tumors
- Myxoma (most common tumor in adults, rare in children)
- Fibroelastoma (most common endocardial tumor)
- Lipoma
- Rhabdomyoma (most common tumor in children)
- Fibroma
- Angioma
- Teratoma
- Cystic tumor of the atrioventricular node
- Paraganglioma

Primary malignant cardiac tumors
- Angiosarcoma (most common myocardial malignancy)
- Rhabdomyosarcoma
- Mesothelioma

Metastatic tumors
- Lung carcinoma
- Hematological neoplasms
- Breast carcinoma
- Esophageal carcinoma
- Malignant skin tumors (melanoma)
- Gastric carcinoma
- Renal cell carcinoma
- Hepatocellular carcinoma

Myxomas account for approximately 50% of all benign myocardial tumors in adults and only a few percent in children. Rhabdomyoma is the most common myocardial tumor in children (40–60%). The most common endocardial tumor is the papillary fibroelastoma. About 1% of soft tissue sarcomas are primary cardiac sarcomas, making them the most common primary myocardial malignancies. Angiosarcomas and undifferentiated pleomorphic sarcomas account for about 76% of all cardiac sarcomas. Malignant tumors of the pericardium are usually mesothelioma or pericardial carcinomatosis.

Clinical Findings The clinical manifestation of cardiac tumors is very diverse and depends on the size, location, and histological type. Some tumors, such as lipomas, are usually asymptomatic, while others, such as atrial myxomas, cause a range of symptoms primarily through obstruction of the mitral valve and outflow tract or cytokine production (including interleukin-6) with inflammation. Common nonspecific symptoms include fatigue, cough, fever, arthralgia, myalgia, and dyspnea. In cases of systemic embolization, which occurs particularly with fibroelastomas and myxomas, strokes, transient ischemic attacks (TIA), or peripheral embolisms can occur. Malignant tumors often present with bloody pericardial effusion, weight loss, and chest pain. Tumorous infiltration of the conduction pathways can lead to cardiac arrhythmias, particularly AV blockages.

> The most common severe symptoms, especially with myxoma and fibroelastoma, are transient ischemic attacks and stroke. Obstruction of the outflow tracts can cause dyspnea and exercise intolerance.

Diagnostics For diagnostics, echocardiography is particularly suitable Echocardiography (▶ Sect. 2.3), where vegetation (see Chap. 10.1), a thrombus, or a myxomatous syndrome should be excluded. Other imaging methods such as computed tomography (CT), magnetic resonance imaging (MRI), positron emission tomography (PET; ▶ Sect. 2.5) can complement the diagnosis. In the case of angiosarcomas, contrast echocardiography or angiography can visualize the vascularization to show the extent of the tumor. Essential for the therapeutic approach is the histological and cytological (e.g., obtained for associated pericardial effusion) examination to identify the exact type of tumor.

> For the clinical diagnosis of cardiac tumors, echocardiography is the method of choice.

Therapy and Prognosis The therapy of cardiac tumors is very complex and depends on the size, location, histological type, and grading. The treatment of patients must be closely coordinated by surgeons, oncologists, and radiotherapists. Surgical therapy ranges from simple tumor resections in benign tumors such as myxoma to the implantation of an artificial heart or a heart transplant if distant metastases are excluded.

> The prognosis of benign heart tumors is good, and for cardiac malignancies, it is generally poor. The prognosis of heart metastases depends on the prognosis of the primary tumors.

16.2 Characteristics of Selected Tumors

16.2.1 Benign Tumors

The **cardiac myxoma** is the most common primary tumor of the myocardium in adults and can manifest at any age, usually between 50–70 years, with women being twice as often affected than men. Ten percent of all cases are associated with the **Carney complex** (myxoma, skin nevi, and endocrinological disorders), a rare autosomal-dominant hereditary tumor syndrome. 80–90% of myxomas are found in the left atrium, near the foramen ovale. The clinical presentation is highly dependent on the location, size, and shape of the tumor. 10–20% have no symptoms, while others show symptoms of heart failure. The diagnosis is made echocardiographically (◘ Fig. 16.1) or confirmed by CT and MRI.

Macroscopically, these are yellow, white, or brown tumors of gelatinous consistency, measuring 1-10 cm. The surface is smooth or provided with very small papillae and villi, in some cases with adherent thrombotic material.

Microscopically, cardiac myxomas show relatively large Alcian blue and PAS-positive cells with eosinophilic cytoplasm and round-oval nuclei. Hemorrhages, calcifications, and hemosiderin deposits are usually also present (◘ Fig. 16.2). Myxoma cells are often immunohistochemically positive for calretinin, NSE, S100, synaptophysin, SMA, and desmin. The treatment of choice is surgical removal, with a very good prognosis in non-syndromal patients.

The **papillary fibroelastoma** is alos one of the most common cardiac tumors and the most common tumor of the valvular endocardium. Patients are on average 60–70 years old, although rare neonatal cases are also described in the literature. Fibroelastomas are often found on the mitral or aortic valves (◘ Fig. 16.3).

Etiologically, fibroelastomas belong to **hamartoma-like lesions**. Some studies show driver mutations in KRAS exon 2 or 3 in this tumor, which can lead to activation of the RAS/MAPK signaling pathway. The clinical picture is very variable and ranges from an asymptomatic course to symptoms of heart failure, syncope, systemic embolisms, and sudden cardiac death. The neoplasm can be well visualized using transesophageal echocardiography (TEE). Macroscopically, it consists of approximately 1–2 cm large, white, gelatinous structures floating in the bloodstream, resembling a sea anemone. Microscopically, the tumor consists of numerous avascular papillae with a collagen framework covered by a single layer of endothelial cells. The benign tumor has a good prognosis (◘ Fig. 16.4).

Rhabdomyomas are the most common cardiac tumors in childhood, although they are very rare after the age of 15. In up to 50% of patients, a rhabdomyoma is associated with tuberous sclerosis, so prenatal testing for mutations in the **tuberous sclerosis complex** (TSC) genes 1 and 2 is recommended. Prenatally, they can be associated with arrhythmias, fetal hydrops, and growth retardation. These tumors show a strong tendency for spontaneous regression, so a conservative approach with monitoring is generally indicated.

Rhabdomyomas occur in 90% of cases as multiple nodules in both ventricles, protruding into the heart chambers, which can

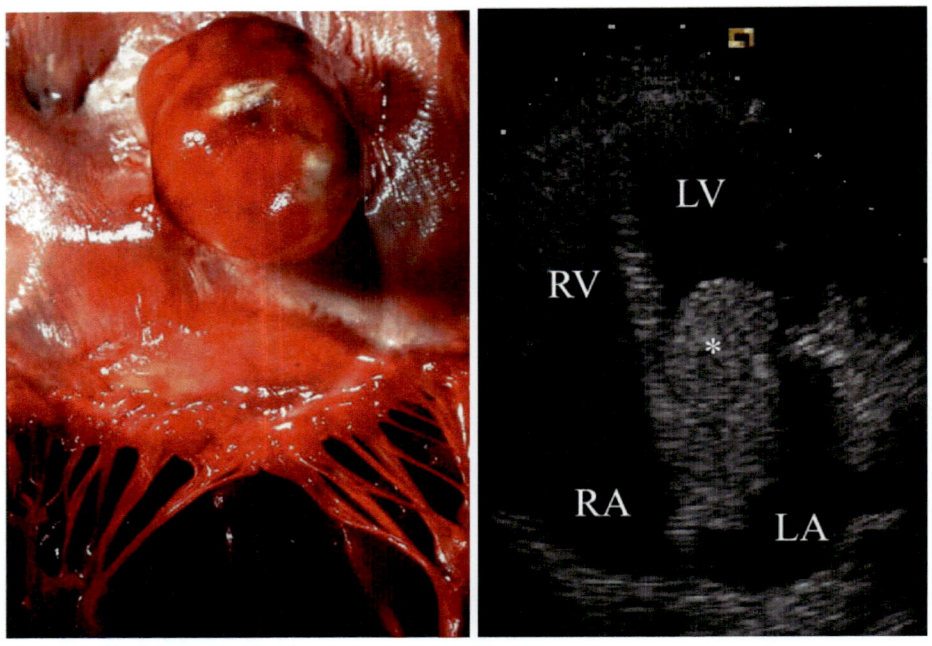

◘ **Fig. 16.1 Left atrial myxoma on the atrial septum** with anterior mitral leaflet below (left) (courtesy of Paul Vogt, Institute of Clinical Pathology, University Hospital Zurich) and echocardiographic finding (right; *LV:* left ventricle; *RV:* right ventricle; *RA:* right atrium; *LA:* left atrium; courtesy of Matthhias Greutmann).

found. The rhabdomyoma originates from myocytes that are significantly enlarged and have glycogen-rich PAS-positive inclusions in the vacuolated cytoplasm. The cardiomyocates often bleach out, leaving the cell membrane dark, making the cells appear spider-like (spider cells). Immunohistochemically, the tumor cells express typical markers for striated muscle such as myogenin, desmin, actin, and vimentin (◘ Fig. 16.5).

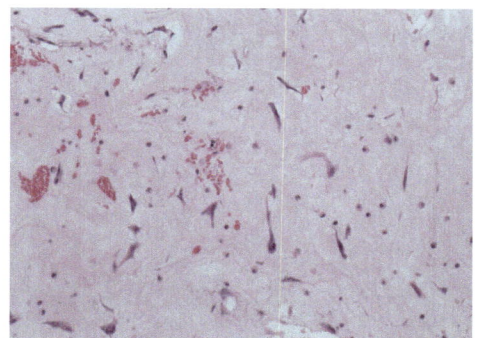

◘ Fig. 16.2 Pathological features of atrial myxoma: Hematoxylin-eosin staining of a myocardial myxoma with monomorphic histiocytoid or fibroblast-like cells in a vascular and collagen-poor myxoid stroma. Magnification 200x

16.2.2 Malignant Tumors

The **cardiac angiosarcoma** is the most common differentiated sarcoma of the myocardium. It accounts for about one-third of primary cardiac malignant tumors and predominantly affects men in the 5th and 6th decades of life. Clinically, respiratory distress, chest pain, and syncope occur, possibly also arrhythmias, hemopericardium, or right ventricular heart failure. The etiology remains mostly unclear, although rare familial cases within the framework of **Li-Fraumeni syndrome** (an autosomal dominant syndrome of children and adolescents with multiple tumors of the adrenal gland, soft tissues, bones, and breast) have been described. Angiosarcomas can occur in all areas of the heart and pericardium (◘ Fig. 16.6).

Macroscopically, there are usually broadly infiltrative growing neoplasms without clear demarcation and extensive hemorrhages and necroses. The tumor size is highly variable, ranging from 2 to 13 cm. Histologically, moderately pleomorphic, round-oval to spindle-shaped tumor cells are observed. In an epithelioid pattern, polygonal plump cells with partly strand-like, partly nest-like, or papillary growth are found. ERG is the most sensitive and specific immunohistochemical marker for detecting endothelial differentiation, with most tumors also being positive for other endothelial markers such as FLI1, CD31, and CD34 (◘ Fig. 16.7). The prognosis is

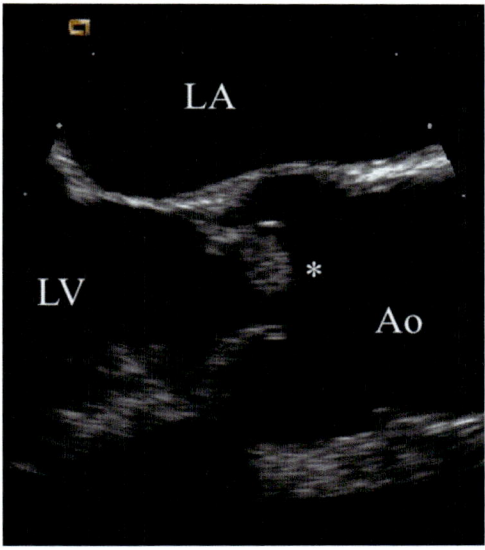

◘ Fig. 16.3 Echocardiography of an aortic fibroelastoma (*). (*LA:* Left Atrium; *LV:* Left Ventricle); *Ao:* Aorta. (Courtesy of Matthias Greutmann)

lead to obstruction of ventricular filling and outflow tract obstruction, ultimately resulting in heart failure. Occasionally, relevant cardiac arrhythmias also occur with atrial localization.

Macroscopically, whitish/yellow intramural nodules a few centimeters in size are

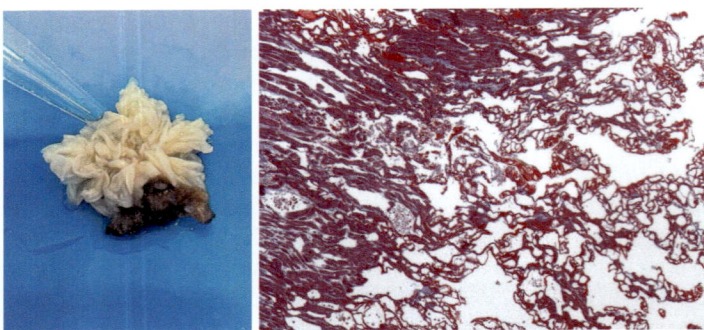

Fig. 16.4 Pathology and histology of a fibroelastoma with a typical sea anemone-like appearance (left). Histology of a papillary tumor covered with endothelium from loose connective tissue (Masson trichrome stain, 100x magnification; right)

worse than for other cardiac sarcomas and non-cardiac angiosarcomas, likely due to cardiac tamponade. The 5-year survival rate is about 10%. Unfavorable prognostic criteria include: age ≥ 45 years, tumor size > 50 mm, metastatic involvement of other organs and/or regional lymph nodes.

A **secondary cardiac involvement** in extracardiac primary tumors occurs with hematogenous myocardial metastasis of a malignancy as well as with invasion from adjacent organs. Lymphogenic metastatic involvement is typical for the pericardium. The clinical presentation is extremely variable. Diagnostics include, as with other cardiac tumors, echocardiography, CT, MRI, and PET. The therapy is directed by the primary tumor.

Cardiac metastases from a **hepatocellular carcinoma (HCC)** are very rare, with autopsy studies indicating an incidence of HCC atrial metastases of 2.7–4.1% (◘ Fig. 16.8 center). Cardiac metastases can be transcoronary hematogenous (into the myocardium), transvenous hematogenous (into the endocardium), directly invasive (into the epicardium), or retrograde lymphogenic. The prognosis remains unclear with cardiac involvement from an HCC. Besides surgical interventions, treatment options for metastases include radiation therapy and transcatheter therapy.

Melanomas frequently metastasizes to the heart, with metastases often occurring multifocally in the endocardium, myocardium (◘ Fig. 16.8 right), and/or pericardium. Tumor cells usually spread hematogenously and infiltrate the myocardium via the coronary arteries or, less commonly, via the vena cava. A disseminated melanoma affects the pericardium in > 50% of advanced cases, whereas myocardial metastases are usually diagnosed postmortem. The clinical picture is nonspecific and includes dyspnea, edema, cough, tachycardia, and chest pain.

Hematolymphatic tumors of the heart are diagnosed in about 1%. Primary cardiac lymphomas are very rare and account for only 0.5% of all extranodal lymphomas. Primary cardiac lymphomas are found in the endocardium, myocardium, and/or pericardium with or without evidence of extracardiac lesions. In contrast, secondary heart involvement in disseminated lymphomas affects 20–25% of all patients. The most common primary non-Hodgkin lymphoma is diffuse large B-cell lymphoma (≥ 80% of all cardiac lymphomas; ◘ Fig. 16.8 left). Other B- or T-cell lymphomas such as Burkitt lymphoma or primary effusion lymphoma are extremely rare.

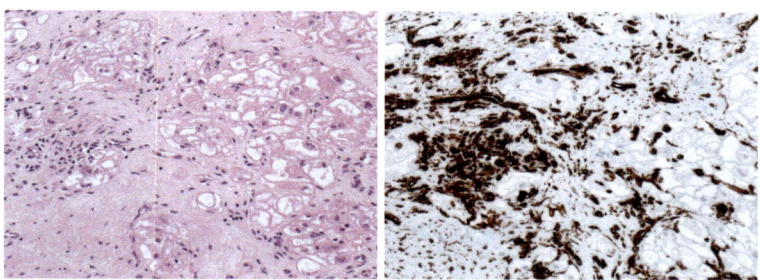

Fig. 16.5 Histology of a rhabdomyoma with vacuolated cardiomyocytes in hematoxylin-eosin staining (left) and a vimentin immunohistology (200x magnification; right)

The primary **tumors of the pericardium** include solitary fibrous tumors, sarcomas, germ cell tumors, and mesotheliomas. Tumors from mesothelial cells of the pericardium, as well as the pleura and peritoneum, are called **mesotheliomas**. Mesotheliomas of the pericardium account for about 2–4% of all cardiac tumors and about 0.3–1% of all mesotheliomas. Although the majority of pleural mesotheliomas are caused by asbestos, the etiology of pericardial mesotheliomas is still unclear. Potential risk factors include previous radiation and chemotherapy, cigarette smoking, and pre-existing cardiovascular diseases. Clinical symptoms depend on the size of the tumor in the pericardium, which can cause compression of the heart. An accompanying pericardial effusion can remain asymptomatic for a long time, often until cardiac tamponade. In imaging such as echocardiography or CT, commonly revela a thickening of the cardiac wall with nodular thickened endocardium. Cardiac mesotheliomas often show a locally aggressive growth pattern with invasion into the myocardium, pleura, large vessels, and mediastinum. Distant metastases have not yet been described. Macroscopically, a localized, nodular mesothelioma and a diffuse mesothelioma with numerous small, 2–4 mm large light nodules can be distinguished. Microscopically, according to the WHO classification 2021, an epithelioid mesothelioma, a sarcomatoid mesothelioma, a desmoplastic mesothelioma, and a biphasic mesothelioma are differentiated. Depending on the histological type, the tumor cells are of different sizes and pleomorphic. Immunohistochemically, the

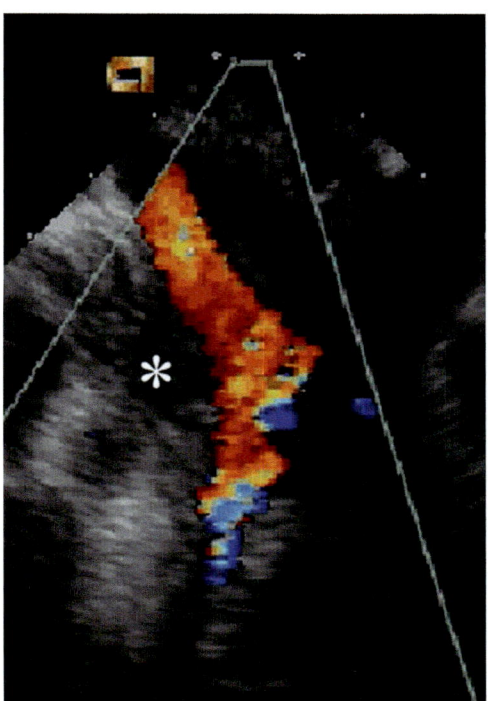

Fig. 16.6 TEE of an angiosarcoma of the pulmonary artery (*) with significant flow acceleration due to pronounced tumor-induced pulmonary obstruction. (Courtesy of Matthias Greutmann)

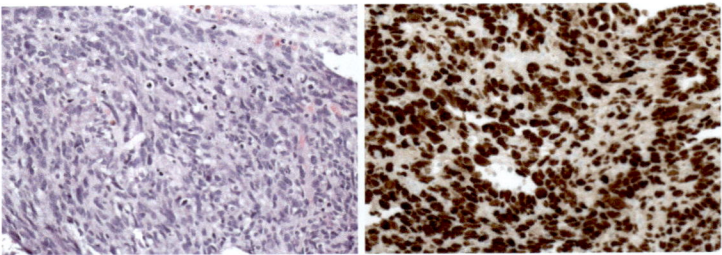

Fig. 16.7 **Histology of an angiosarcoma with spindle-shaped tumor cells** in hematoxylin-eosin staining (left) and immunohistology for detecting ERG (250x magnification; right)

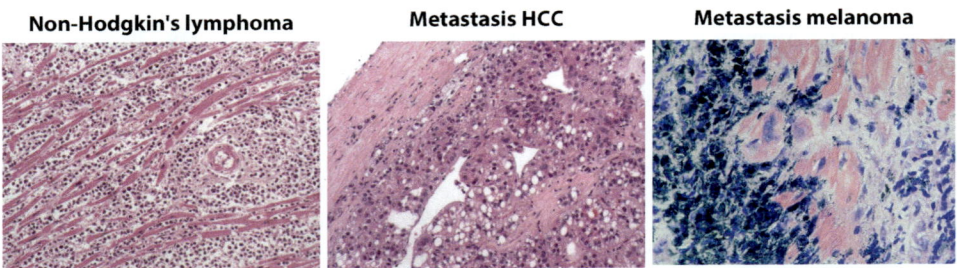

Fig. 16.8 Histology of a **non-Hodgkin lymphoma** (left; hematoxylin-eosin staining; left, 200x magnification), **a metastasis of a hepatocellular carcinoma** (middle;HCC; hematoxylin-eosin; center, 200x magnification) **and a metastasis of a melanoma** (right; Giemsa staining; right, 500x magnification)

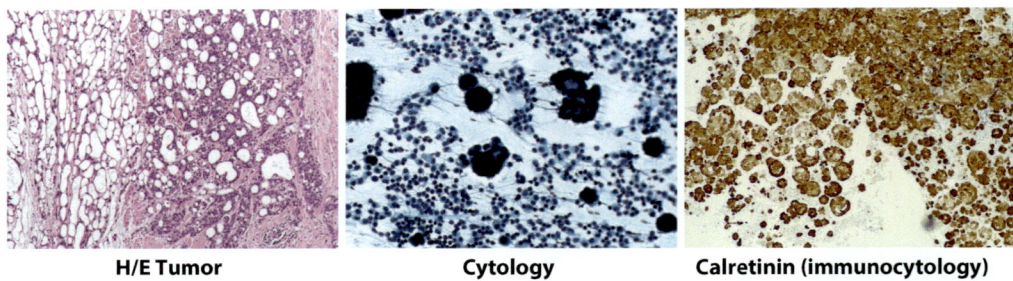

Fig. 16.9 Histology of a **cardiac mesothelioma with tumor cells of the epithelioid type** surrounded by fiber-rich stroma (hematoxylin-eosin staining; left, 200x magnification), cytology (middle), and calretinin immunocytology (right)

cells are clearly positive for AE1/3 and calretinin (Fig. 16.9). The prognosis of the disease varies and is highly dependent on the spread of the tumor.

Diseases of the Venous System

Christine Espinola-Klein and Stavros Konstantinides

Contents

17.1 Varikosis – 274

17.2 Deep Vein Thrombosis – 276

17.3 Pulmonary Embolism – 280

17.4 Pulmonary Embolism-Follow-up – 289

© The Author(s), under exclusive license to Springer-Verlag GmbH, DE, part of Springer Nature 2025
T. F. Lüscher and U. Landmesser (eds.), *Cardiovascular System*,
https://doi.org/10.1007/978-3-662-70152-2_17

17.1 Varikosis

Anatomy and Basics of Venous Flow In the extremities, there is a superficial (epifascial) and a deep (subfascial) venous system, which are separated by the fascia superficialis and connected by perforating veins. Physiologically, blood in the veins always flows from epifascial to subfascial and from bottom to top.

The flow of venous blood against gravity from bottom to top is a physiologic challlenge. To ensure flow in the direction, there are venous valves that prevent backflow in the wrong direction. Furthermore, the veins are embedded between muscle strands, so they are compressed during muscle contraction ("**muscle pump**") thereby pushing the blood flows upwards. Finally, the deep veins run alongside arteries, so they are compressedwith each pulse and emptied like a bellow.

Lastly, breathing creates a negative pressure in the thorax by moving the diaphragm distally. This causes venous blood to be sucked towards the thoracic cavity during inspiration. During expiration, the diaphragm moves upwards and the thoracic pressure is higher than the abdominal pressure, reducing venous flow. This principle is also known as the "**abdomino-thoracic two-phase pump**."

Definition, Pathophysiology, and Epidemiology Varikosis is characterized by dilatation of epifascial veins. As the diameter of the epifascial veins increases, the venous valves can no longer close tightly. This venous incompetence leads to a distal backflow of venous blood. The dilation of the epifascial veins can be localized or extensive. The term "varikosis" is derived from the Latin "varix" for knot reflecting the ballooning and turtous course of such venous segments.

In the majority of cases, there is an **idiopathic genesis**, often with a positive **family history**. In 5% of cases, varikosis is acquired, mostly due to dilation of epifascial veins that serve as collaterals after **deep vein thrombosis**.

Varikosis is common; according to current estimates, up to 20% of adults suffer from at least mild varikosis. Women are more frequently affected than men (i.e. women: men ratio = 3:1), with the first manifestation usually occurring in the 3rd decade of life, and the incidence increasing with advancing age.

Classification and Symptomatology A distinction is made between epifascial varices, which include trunk varikosis (great saphenous vein, small saphenous vein), side branch varikosis, and perforating varikosis, and cutaneous varices, which include reticular and spider vein varikosis (◘ Table 17.1).

The symptoms of varikosis vary and are commonly nonspecific. Patients complain of a feeling of tension and heaviness, itching, paresthesia, burning, evening ankle edema, pain, nocturnal foot and calf cramps, or a feeling of heat or cold. The symptoms typically increase in the evening, in warm weather, and after prolonged sitting or standing.

The **complications** of varikosis include variceal bleeding and secondary dilation of the deep veins with chronic venous insufficiency, which can even lead to leg ulcers. The risk of thrombosis is also increased,

◘ **Table 17.1** Anatomical Classification of Varikosis

Group	Subgroup
Epifascial Varikosis	Trunk varikosis – Great saphenous vein (V. saphena magna) – Small saphenous vein (V. saphena parva) Side branch varikosis Perforating varikosis
Cutaneous Varikosis	Reticular varikosis (2–4 mm) Spider vein varikosis (< 1 mm)

referred to as "thrombophlebitis."manifesting itself as painful heated skin along the thrombosed vein, which can be felt as a firm strand. It can progress to the deep venous system, resulting in deep vein thrombosis.

Diagnostics In the **medical history**, it is important to capture the symptoms, risk factors, and a familial disposition. The inspection should be performed while standing so that the varicose veins fill better and are more visible. Additionally, attention should be paid to alterations in skin structure and colour (e.g. redish colouration) indicative of chronic venous insufficiency. Finally, edema and fascial gaps in the lower leg in the case of insufficient perforating veins can be felt upon examination.

Duplex sonography is the central diagnostic tool. It allows the visualization of the epifascial and deep veins, shows post-thrombotic changes, and allows to assess the function of the venous valves and the location of backflow of the blood. In some circumstances, additional examinations such as light reflex rheography or plethysmography to assess changes in venous blood volume in the skin as a reflecting of venous blood flow in deeper veins that are connected with superficial veins via perforating veins. may be useful.

Therapy The main treatment goals are to improve congestion, to prevent the formation or healing of ulcerations, and the prophylaxis of a recurrence. Soft indications are cosmetic reasons. The decision to treat varicose veins is therefore always based on individual criteria (Fig. 17.1).

Various procedures are used for treatment. When deciding on a treatment stratgy, especially for cosmetic reasons, it should be kept in mind that epifascial veins are important bypass vessels. Therefore, any intervention should be well considered.

The onservative approach primarily involves **compression treatment**. The goal of venous compression is to reduce the epifascial blood volume and in turn backflow of blood. Usually, compression stockings of class II (approx. 30 mmHg) are used; alternatively, the legs can be wrapped with short-stretch bandages (e.g., for venous ulcers until healing). Another pillar of conservative therapy is **exercise**. The rule is: "*Better to walk and lie down than to sit and stand.*" Medications that are often used (e.g., horse chestnut) do not have sufficient

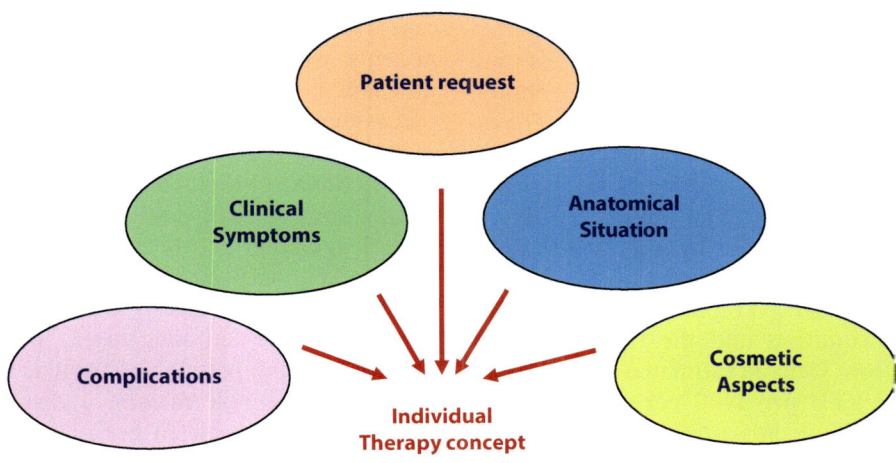

Fig. 17.1 Influencing factors on a therapy decision

evidence of effectivness and therefore cannot be recommended.

Cutaneous varicose veins can be treated using **sclerotherapy**. Here, a substance damaging the endothelium or a foamed sclerosing agent to obliterate the varicose veins is injected. For larger varicose veins, radiofrequency obliteration and endovenous **laser therapy** can be used. To that end, a catheter is inserted into the vein under ultrasound guidance. The vessel is heated and the endothelial lining destroyed, thereby obliterating the vein as the catheter is withdrawn.

Classic **varicose vein surgery** includes crossectomy, stripping, side branch extirpation, and the elimination of perforating veins. Small side branches can be eliminated through a miniphlebectomy. In *subfascial endoscopic perforator surgery* (SEPS), insufficient perforating veins are ligated using endoscopic techniques. A disadvantage of all invasive methods is a high rate of recurrences.

17.2 Deep Vein Thrombosis

Epidemiology The annual **incidence** of venous thromboembolism worldwide is 150–200 cases per 100,000 inhabitants, of which about one-third is associated with pulmonary embolisms. Since the beginning of the century, the incidence of venous thromboembolism (VTE) and particularly of pulmonary embolism (PE) has been continuously increasing in many countries. For instance, an analysis of data from the Federal Statistical Office in Germany revelead between 2005 and 2015 an increase in the annual incidence of PE by almost 30% from 85 to 109 per 100,000 persons-years. A similar trend has been reported from other European countries and the USA. A recent study from Canada estimated the incidence at 1.46 VTE per 1000 person-years, with 27% of the events presenting as PE and 73% as deep vein thrombosis. The incidence further increases with advancing age. In those over 80 years of age, the incidence was 5.3 for men and 5.2 for women per 1000 person-years. Given the demographic development, we will therefore have to expect more patients presenting with VTEs in the future.

Definition and Pathophysiology In deep vein thrombosis, there is a sudden or insidious thrombotic occlusion of at least one segment of the deep pelvic and/or leg veins. The majority of deep vein thromboses are located in the pelvic and leg veins, while thromboses of the upper extremities are much less common.

The pathophysiology of VTE was coined by Rudolf Virchow already in the 19. century as the so-called **Virchow's Triad** consisting of a combination of **reduced blood flow velocity, hypercoagulability**, and **endothelial injury** (◘ Fig. 17.2). For example, a compression of the veins, immobilization after a surgical procedure, or a previous thrombosis with an outflow obstruction can lead to reduced blood flow velocity. Increased coagulability may be due to a congenital coagulation disorder (thrombophilia), local or generalized inflammation and/or dehydration. An endothelial injury can be caused, for example, by a catheter or a local trauma. In many cases, a combination of different components are present. For instance, during pregnancy, hormonal changes lead to hypercoagulability, and the growing fetus simultaneously compresses the pelvic veins. In the context of an infection with fever, inflammation and dehydration may lead to hypercoagulability, while immobilization leads to venous stasis. A special case is the so-called May-Thurner syndrome, where crossing of the left iliac artery over the vein leads to compression of the iliac vein.

Among the **risk factors**, a distinction has to be made between persistent factors (e.g. thrombosis without a trigger factor,

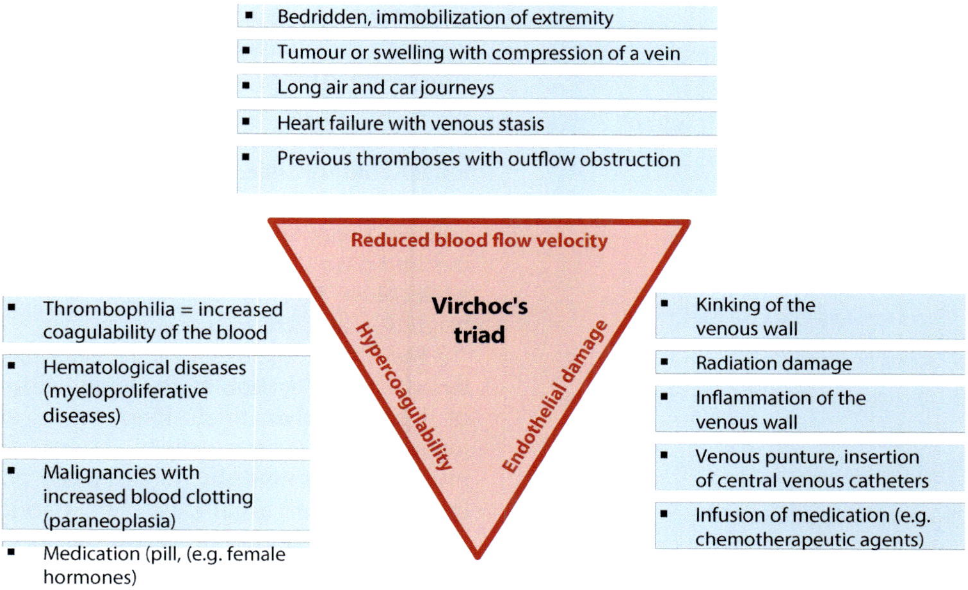

Diseases of the Venous System

- Bedridden, immobilization of extremity
- Tumour or swelling with compression of a vein
- Long air and car journeys
- Heart failure with venous stasis
- Previous thromboses with outflow obstruction

Virchoc's triad (Reduced blood flow velocity / Hypercoagulability / Endothelial damage)

- Thrombophilia = increased coagulability of the blood
- Hematological diseases (myeloproliferative diseases)
- Malignancies with increased blood clotting (paraneoplasia)
- Medication (pill, (e.g. female hormones)

- Kinking of the venous wall
- Radiation damage
- Inflammation of the venous wall
- Venous punture, insertion of central venous catheters
- Infusion of medication (e.g. chemotherapeutic agents)

Fig. 17.2 Virchow's Triad of the pathophysiology of VTE with examples

idiopathic thrombosis, often due to genetic disposition, e.g. Factor V Leiden among others) and temporary factors (e.g. triggered thrombosis). Different risk constellations are associated with different risks for a later recurrence. Therefore, the trigger of the thrombosis influences the subsequent duration of therapy.

Symptoms and Diagnosis Typical symptoms of deep vein thrombosis include unilateral swelling, pain, a feeling of tension, cyanosis, and increased venous markings through the collateral circulation via superficial veins. However, symptoms can be less typical or even absent, especially in immobilized patients. The sensitivity of the typical symptom triad of swelling, pain, and cyanosis ranges between 60% and 90% in ambulatory mobile patients, while it is below 20% in bedridden patients. However, the symptoms are not very specific, and differential diagnosis should also consider other causes of leg pain (arterial, musculoskeletal), swelling (e.g. edema due to heart failure), and cyanosis (e.g. ischemia of the extremity, acrocyanosis, chronic venous insufficiency).

The current guidelines for the diagnosis and treatment of deep vein thrombosis and PE recommend first determining the pre-test probability according to the Wells score in case of suspected deep vein thrombosis (Table 17.2). If the pre-test probability is high (at least 2 points on the **Wells score**), compression sonography is indicated as the next diagnostic step. If the pre-test probability is low, D-dimers should be determined (Fig. 17.3).

If at least 2 points are reached, the probability of thrombosis is high.

D-dimers are fibrin degradation products and are produced during any activation of the coagulation system. This means that D-dimers are released in any VTE, but also in many other conditions such as acute inflammation or arterial thromboses. D-dimers have high specificity, but low sensitivity and are therefore suitable for exclusion, but not for proof of a VTE.

◘ Table 17.2 Determination of the pre-test probability of deep vein thrombosis based on the Wells score

Criterion	Points
Active malignant disease	1
Immobilization	1
Bed rest > 3 days, major surgery < 12 weeks	1
Pain/hardening along the deep veins	1
Swelling of the entire leg	1
Calf circumference difference >3 cm	1
Pitting edema	1
Dilated superficial veins	1
Previous documented DVT	1
Alternative diagnosis at least as likely	−2

D-dimers physiologically increase with age, so age-adjusted cut-off values (age × 10 µg/L) should be used from the age of 50 onwards.

In case of a high pre-test probability or elevated D-dimers, **compression sonography** is indicated to determine whether thrombi are detectable in the deep veins. This takes advantage of the fact that a blood-filled vein can be compressed with slight pressure, with arteries serving as guide structures (◘ Fig. 17.4). In contrat, a thrombosed vein shows an internal echo and is no longer compressible. A fresh thrombus also leads to an enlargement of the venous diameter. Fresh thrombi appear homogeneous and dark ("echo-poor") on ultrasound, while older thrombi appear irregular and bright ("echo-rich").

The extent of the VTE is determined based on the **location of the levels**. A total of 4 levels (pelvis, thigh, knee region, and lower leg) have been defined. Using compression ultrasound, the femoral and popliteal veins can usually be well assessed, and in the majority of cases, the assessment of the lower leg veins o as well. The inferior vena cava and pelvic veins can only be examined using duplex sonography with color flow, which also allows to define post-thrombotic changes (e.g.residual thrombus, backflow) and is well suited for follow-up examinations.

Therapy In the case of a confirmed deep vein thrombosis, immediate and effective **anticoagulation** is required. The treat-

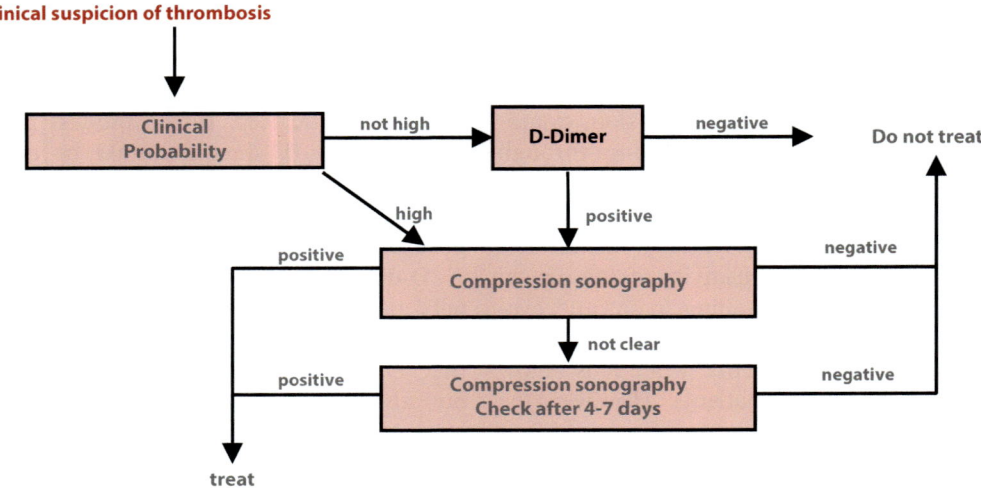

◘ Fig. 17.3 Diagnostic algorithm in case of suspected deep vein thrombosis

Diseases of the Venous System

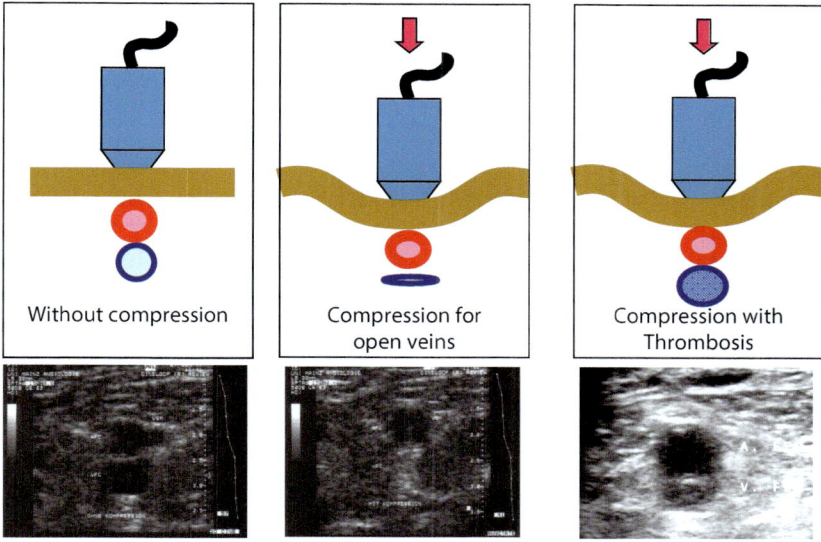

Fig. 17.4 Principle of compression sonography with ultrasound examples. (modified from Neuerburg-Heusler D. and Hennerici M., Vascular diagnostics with ultrasound, Thieme Publisher, FRG)

ment goals are to prevent thrombus growth and to support the body in breaking down evolving thrombi. The details of the initial anticoagulation are presented in ▶ Chap. 17.3, 17.4 below.

Furthermore, **compression** of the leg is recommended. After diagnosing deep VTE, mobilization is usually possible immediately, if compression has been initiated. In the case of a fresh thrombosis with a significant difference in circumference, the leg should be wrapped with short-stretch bandages or acute care stockings should be used. Once the leg is decongested, fitting a custom-made compression stocking (compression class II) is advisable. In the case of an extensive multi-level thrombosis, the entire leg should initially be compressed. Over time, a knee-high stocking is usually sufficient. The duration of compression depends on the residual findings (e.g. residual thrombi), residual valve insufficiency, and symptoms.

Usually, the extremity decongests once anticoagulation has been initiated. If there is significant initial swelling, an interventional treatment with a catheter providing local **fibrinolysis** and/or **stenting** can be considered in individual cases. Very rarely, there is massive swelling hindering a blockade arterial perfusion, i.e. phlegmasia cerulea dolens. In such cases, surgical removal of the thrombus is necessary as the the extremity may be acutely endangered.

Environmental Diagnostics and Extended Secondary Prevention The underlying cause of a thrombosis influences the likelihood of its recurrence and thus determines the subsequent duration of therapy. A venous thrombosis without a known **trigger**, is associated with an increased risk of a malignant disease within the following year. Therefore, age-adapted **tumor screening** should be performed in patients with such a VTE. An **age-adapted thrombophilia screening** should only be conducted in special cases, such in young patients with a family history of VTE. In patients with arterial and venous thromboses and/or women with a history of miscarriages, one should consider a antiphospholipid syndrome.

After completion the initial 3-6 months of anticoagulation, the question arises whether to extend or stop the therapy. A lower leg venous thrombosis is associated with a relatively low **recurrence risk** and should therefore only be anticoagulated for 3 months. Patients with a persistent risk factor (e.g. severe thrombophilia, active cancer) have a very high recurrence risk and anticoagulation should therefore be continued. In most cases, however, the decision must be made individually based on a nomber of criteria (◯ Table 17.3). If a risk factor persists, the cause remans unclear, or the VTE already is a recurrence, anticoagulation should be extented. Factors such as the type and quality of anticoagulation, the risk of bleeding, or patient's preference also play a role in decision making. If the decision is made to extend anticoagulation, there is also the option to continue at a reduced dose.

17.3 Pulmonary Embolism

Epidemiology Acute PE is the most severe clinical manifestation of VTE and the third most common cardiovascular cause of death (▶ Chap. 3.1). The mortality rate in the acute phase averages 14%, but varies depending on the severity of the PE and the presence of comorbidities. Especially in older patient, there is a high risk both for the occurrence of PE and for early death or serious complications in the acute phase.

◯ Table 17.3 Criteria favouring an extension or termination of anticoagulation after completion of the initial 3-6 months of tratment (modified according to AWMF guideline)

Criterion	Continue therapy	End therapy
Risk factor	persistent	transient
Genesis	unclear	triggered
Recurrence	yes	no
Risk of bleeding	low	high
Previous anticoagulation quality	good	bad
D-dimers (after end of therapy)	increased	normal
Residual thrombus	documented	absent
Gender	man	woman
Thrombus expansion	elongated	short-distance
Thrombus localization	proximal	distal
Severe thrombophilia	present	absent
Patient preference	if bleeding risk low	only, if safe

Diseases of the Venous System

Pathophysiology and Clinical Findings A partial or complete obstruction of one or more pulmonary arteries and their branches by embolized thrombi leads to an abrupt increase in pulmonary arterial pressure and right ventricular (RV) afterload. The "**downward spiral**" of increased myocardial oxygen demand, myocardial ischemia, and reduction of left ventricular (LV) preload results in a decrease in cardiac output and eventually a systemic blood pressure drop, hpotension and cardiogenic shock due to RV failure (◘ Fig. 17.5).

The clinical severity of acute PE encompasses a very broad clinical spectrum, from asymptomatic course to cardiogenic shock and circulatory collapse with the need for resuscitation (◘ Table 17.4).

The clinical symptoms are nonspecific. They can arise from acute RV failure, gas exchange disturbance in the lungs, or complications of PE such as infarct pneumonia

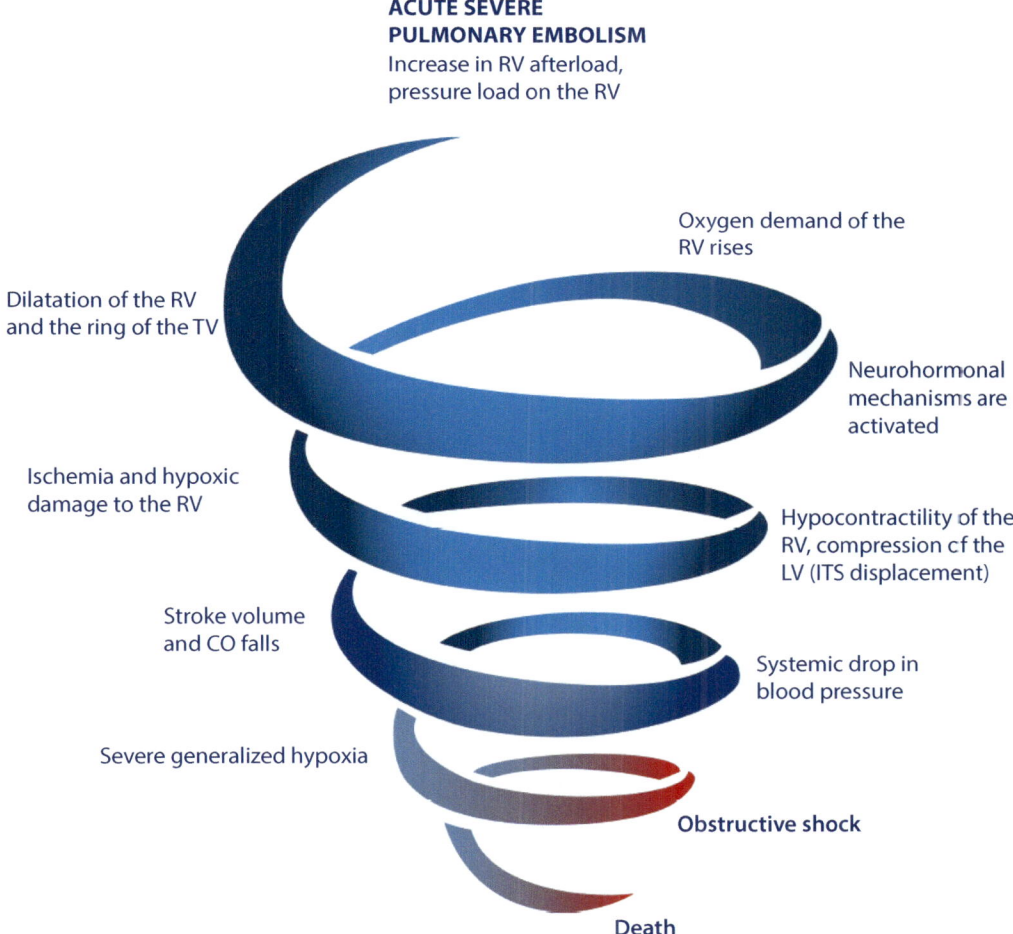

◘ **Fig. 17.5** Downward spiral of hemodynamic decompensation in acute pulmonary embolism. (*CO:* Cardiac Output, *IVS:* Interventricular Septum, *LV:* Left Ventricle, *RV:* Right Ventricle/Right Ventricular, *TV:* Tricuspid Valve)

Table 17.4 Clinical and hemodynamic instability in acute pulmonary embolism

1 Cardiac Arrest	2 Cardiogenic Shock	3 Persistent Hypotension
Need for cardiopulmonary resuscitation	SBP < 90 mmHg or vasopressors required to achieve an SBP ≥ 90 mmHg despite adequate filling pressures	SBP < 90 mmHg or SBP drop by ≥ 40 mmHg for more than 15 minutes, not due to a new arrhythmia, hypovolemia, or sepsis
	in association with	
	Organ hypoxia (altered level of consciousness, cold, clammy skin, oligo-/anuria, elevated serum lactate)	

SBP: systolic blood pressure

or pleuritis. Dyspnea is the most common symptom of PE.

Clinical Symptoms of Pulmonary Embolism
- **Orthopnea, Tachypnea** (> 20 breaths per minute)
- Reduced arterial oxygen saturation (**Hypoxemia**)
- Angina-like or pleuritic **chest pain**
- **Hemoptysis**
- Clinical signs of deep **venous thrombosis** (▶ Sect. 17.2)
- **Tachycardia** (prognostically relevant clinical sign)
- **Syncope** (also prognostically relevant, as the short-term, loss of consciousness indicates a transient drop in cardiac output)

Since no clinical symptom or sign is considered typical for a PE, an assessment of the clinical probability is recommended by applying the revised "**Geneva Score**" (● Table 17.5). These clinical decision rules include symptoms and clinical signs of a PE, but also diseases and situations that are considered risk factors for VTE and PE.

Diagnostics In hemodynamically unstable patients (● Table 17.4) with suspected

Table 17.5 Calculation of the clinical probability of a PE. (Revised Geneva Score)

Clinical Parameter	Points in the Score
Age > 65 years	1
Hemoptysis	2
Active cancer	2
Surgery or bone fracture within the previous month	2
Previous pulmonary embolism or deep vein thrombosis	3
Unilateral leg pain	3
Pain on deep palpation of the lower extremity and unilateral leg edema	4
Heart rate	
75–94 beats per minute	3
≥ 95 beats per minute	5
Clinical Probability	
Three-level probability	
Low	0–3
Intermediate	4–10
High	≥ 11
Two-level probability	
Pulmonary embolism unlikely	0–5
Pulmonary embolism likely	≥ 6

"high-risk" PE, life-saving therapy has absolute priority due to the risk of death. In this emergency situation, there is no time for specific imaging diagnostics to visualize pulmonary thrombi. Therefore, it may be sufficient to echocardiographically demonstrate acute pressure overload and RV failure without an alternative explanation (◘ Fig. 17.6) to initiate a multidisciplinary consultation for the appropriate medical, catheter-based, or surgical therapy (see below).

In initially normotensive, seemingly stable patients, the goal of diagnostics is to confirm or exclude PE with high probability through radiological or nuclear imaging modalities. The **indication for imaging** arises from the combination of clinical probability and D-dimer values to avoid misuse of these procedures (◘ Fig. 17.7).

Computed tomographic pulmonary angiography (CTPA) (◘ Fig. 17.8) is currently by far the most frequently used imaging modality in the diagnosis of pulmonary embolism.

In ◘ Table 17.6, the strengths and weaknesses or dangers of CTPA are summarized in comparison to ventilation-perfusion scintigraphy and invasive pulmonary angiography. The diagnostic sensitivity and specificity of CTPA are high. This leads to a frequently inappropriate use of CTPA without consideration of contrast agent- and radiation-related risks for patients as well as of unnecessary resource consumption. Therefore, validated diagnostic algorithms—including the estimation of clinical probability and the D-dimer test—help to restrict the use of CTPA to patients with a high risk of PE.

The **ventilation-perfusion scintigraphy (V/Q-Scan)** of the lung also remains a valid diagnostic procedure, but it is not available around the clock in all hospitals. Moreover, it is not suitable for hemodynamically unstable patients (◘ Table 17.6).

The **invasive pulmonary angiography** plays a minor role in the clinical assessment of pulmonary embolism. However, this procedure is increasingly gaining importance in certain centers, as it is used in the context of catheter-based procedures in patients with severe PE (◘ Table 17.6).

The diagnosis or exclusion of a PE in **pregnancy** is particularly challenging. Up

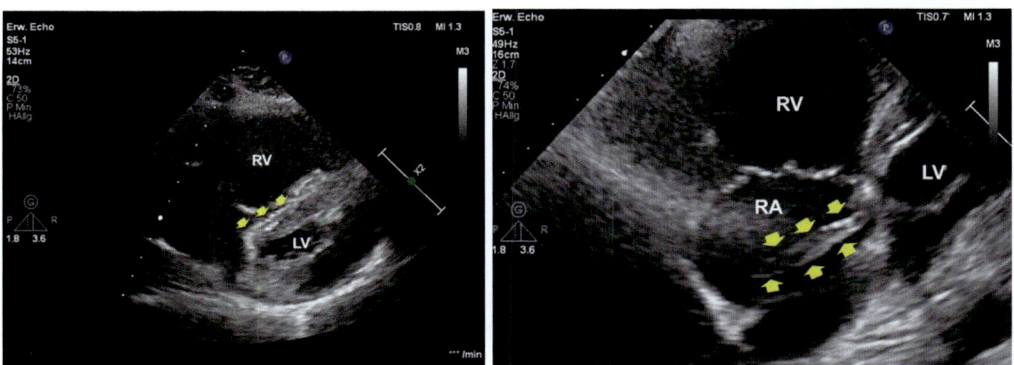

◘ **Fig. 17.6 Echocardiogram in severe pulmonary embolism.** Transthoracic echocardiogram in the emergency department of a 50-year-old patient with breast cancer, severe dyspnea, and blood pressure drop. On the left (parasternal short axis), the large RV is dilated and large compared to the compressed, small LV. The interventricular septum (arrows) is flattened due to the pressure overload of the RV (so-called D-sign of the LV). On the right (modified apical 4-chamber view), the enlargement of the RV at the expense of the LV is visible, and a large, elongated floating thrombus (arrows) is also seen in the right atrium (RA)

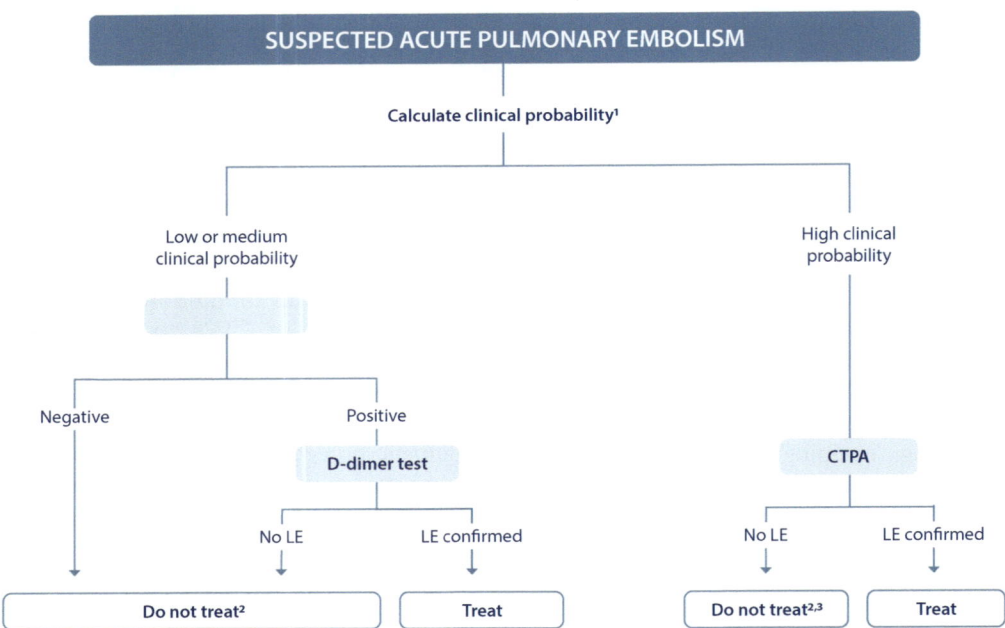

Fig. 17.7 Diagnostic steps in suspected acute pulmonary embolism. *CTPA:* computed tomographic pulmonary angiography, *PE:* pulmonary embolism.[1] Standardized assessment of clinical probability using validated scores recommended (Table 17.5).[2] "Do not treat" means: no anticoagulation after excluding pulmonary embolism. In such cases, an alternative explanation for the clinical symptoms must be searched for.[3] In case of negative CTPA despite high clinical probability, further diagnostics, e.g., ventilation-perfusion scintigraphy, can be considered.

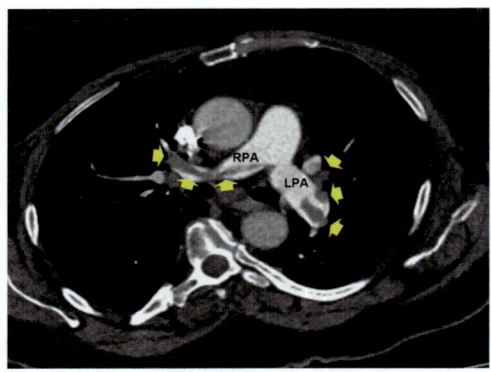

Fig. 17.8 Computer pulmonary angiogram with extensive bilateral PE. The arrows show the large thrombi as intraluminal filling defects in the right (*RPA*) and left (*LPA*) pulmonary artery

to 14% of all deaths in pregnant women are associated with PE. Therefore, a reliable diagnosis and immediate treatment once PE is confirmed are of utmost importance. Symptoms and clinical signs indicative of PE are even less specific in pregnant women. This also applies to D-dimers, as their blood levels increase during pregnancy. Structured diagnostic algorithms can reliably diagnose or exclude a PE even during pregnancy. In this context, the use of compression ultrasonography of the leg veins (e.g. detection of a VTE in case of clinical suspicion of PE → indirect PE diagnosis and indication for anticoagulation") holds a special significance. However, the following must be considered:

Diseases of the Venous System

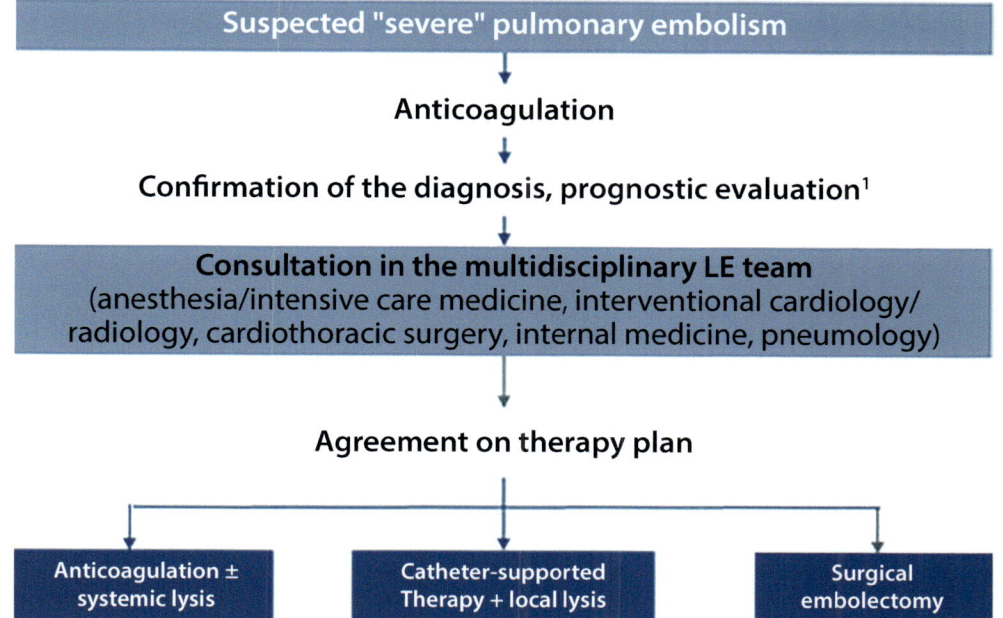

◻ **Fig. 17.9** Multidisciplinary treatment of acute pulmonary embolism with high or intermediate-high risk. *PE*: Pulmonary embolism, *RV*: right ventricular, transthoracic echocardiography
[1] Includes:
- Assessment of clinical/vital status (presence and severity of hemodynamic instability)
- Echocardiography to assess RV function and size, as well as to detect or exclude intracardiac thrombi or an open foramen ovale
- Laboratory biomarkers, particularly troponin levels

- In the case of a **positive diagnostic compression ultrasonography** of the leg veins, imaging of the pulmonary vessels is not recommended, but echocardiography should be performed for prognostic reasons to confirm or exclude pressure overload of the RV and impending RV failure.
- A negative or **unclear finding** of the compression ultrasonography does not exclude a PE and should prompt a CTPA or V/Q scan. Concerns about radiation exposure (which is relatively low for the embryo) should not lead to potentially life-threatening diagnostic uncertainty.

Severity of Acute Pulmonary Embolism While hemodynamically unstable patients in cardiogenic shock (◻ Table 17.4) are categorized as "high risk," there are predictors for an unfavorable or fatal outcome in the acute phase for the much larger group of normotensive patients at admission. **Scores for risk assessment** such as the simplified *Pulmonary Embolism Severity Index* (sPESI, ◻ Table 17.7) integrate clinical parameters
- of the severity of the acute PE event,
- the underlying disease and/or comorbidities of the patient.

Table 17.6 Comparison of imaging techniques for pulmonary embolism diagnosis

	Advantages	Disadvantages and Risks
CTPA	– Established and reliable, current "gold standard" – Provides alternative diagnoses (diseases of the heart, lungs, large thoracic vessels) – Generally available around the clock – Examination takes only a few minutes – With modern devices, relatively low effective radiation dose of 3–10 mSv[1]	– Concerns about use during pregnancy and breastfeeding due to radiation exposure to the mother's breast tissue – Contraindicated in severe renal failure due to nephrotoxicity of the contrast agent – Contraindicated in iodine allergy or hyperthyroidism – More frequent misuse in clinical routine, i.e., use without specific indication based on validated algorithms (Fig. 17.7)
V/Q-Scan	– Long-established, validated procedure – Lower radiation exposure than CTPA, no contraindication in thyroid diseases, renal failure, iodine allergy – Relatively cost-effective	– Not available in all centers and not around the clock – Interpretation of findings can be examiner-dependent – Less helpful than CTPA in searching for alternative diagnoses when excluding a PE – V/Q-SPECT promises high accuracy but still needs to be validated and standardized in prospective studies
Pulmonary Angiography	– Recently increasing use in the context of catheter-based therapies for severe pulmonary embolisms (Fig. 17.9)	– Invasive procedure – Not available in many centers or expertise not present – Effective radiation dose 10–20 mSv – Contrast agent nephrotoxic – Contraindicated in iodine allergy or hyperthyroidism

CTPA: computed tomographic pulmonary angiography, PE: pulmonary embolism, SPECT: "Single-Photon Emission Computed Tomography", V/Q-Scan: ventilation-perfusion lung scan
[1] Dose in mSv = absorbed dose in mGy × radiation weighting factor (1.0 for X-rays) × tissue weighting factor

Table 17.7 Clinical Score for Risk Assessment in the Acute Phase

Score	Parameter	Points	Risk
sPESI	Age > 80 years	1	0 points: low risk ≥ 1 point(s): increased risk
	Cancer	1	
	Chronic heart or lung disease	1	
	Heart rate ≥ 100/min	1	
	Systolic blood pressure < 100 mmHg	1	
	Arterial oxygen saturation < 90%	1	

CrCl: Creatinine Clearance, sPESI: simplified Pulmonary Embolism Severity Index

This score allows a reliable **prognostic assessment** and is particularly valuable in identifying low-risk patients who are eligible for early discharge and outpatient therapy.

In addition to determining clinical parameters, according to current guidelines, the **evaluation of RV function** is an essentiel part of risk stratification for patients with acute PE. In particular, echocardiography allows for a quick and uncomplicated assessment of cardiac morphology and hemodynamics, providing valuable information of an increased intermediate risk, such as RV dilation (i.e. ratio of diastolic RV and LV diameters). Systolic RV pressure can be reliably estimated via the velocity of the tricuspid regurgitation jet. Furthermore, TTE allows for the estimation of RV pressure load and dysfunction (TAPSE; ▶ Sect. 2.3): signs of this include hypokinesia of the free RV wall, flattened interventricular septum (D-sign), or paradoxical septal movement (Chap. 2.3). Dilation and reduced respiratory variability of the inferior vena cava indicate increased right atrial pressure and thus RV decompensation.

Initial Management **"Reperfusion therapy" for severe PE.** Systemic i.v.-thrombolysis is the first-line therapy for acute PE in hemodynaically unstable patients. If there are absolute contraindications to thrombolysis, mechanical catheter-based interventions (e.g. thrombus fragmentation, rheolytic thrombectomy, aspiration thrombectomy, rotational thrombectomy) can be used depending on local availability. Additionally, combined **pharmaco-mechanical procedures** with local, low-dose thrombolysis with or without ultrasound are available. Finally, **surgical embolectomy** is an alternative to thrombolysis or catheter intervention, but is rarely used.

To optimize the acute treatment of hemodynamically compromised PE patients, **multidisciplinary PE teams** are increasingly being established. Local treatment protocols with discussion and consideration of all therapeutic options, taking into account the available capacities and resources, enable—in consensus with the experts from the involved specialties—the selection of the best therapy (◘ Fig. 17.9).

All patients with pulmonary embolism require **therapeutic anticoagulation**. This should be initiated already upon suspicion of PE, without waiting for the results of imaging. Approved for anticoagulation are low molecular weight heparins (LMWH) and fondaparinux; alternatively, direct oral anticoagulants (**DOAC**) such as apixaban or rivaroxaban can be used (◘ Table 17.8). In this context, it is essential to note that, based on current evidence, DOACs such as edoxaban or dabigatran should only be started after at least 5 days of parenteral heparin treatment. Apixaban and rivaroxaban, on the other hand, are approved from the beginning, but must, based on recent trials, be prescribed at higher dosages initially d(apixaban; 10mg BID during the first week) or (rivaroxaban; 30mg OD for the first 3 weeks).

The initial therapy over the first 5–10 days is followed by the **chronic phase of anticoagulation** lasting at least 3 months. During this phase, the use of a DOAC is generally preferred over vitamin K antagonists (VKA), both based on guideline recommendations and experience in clinical practice. Even in patients with acute VTE on the basis of an active **cancer disease**, the DOACs Apixaban, Edoxaban, and Rivaroxaban are now validated and approved and can be used, considering the patient's bleeding risk (which is often increased in cancer patients), instead of low molecular weight heparin in the first 3–6 months.

The warnings or **contraindications** for DOACs currently apply to patients with severely impaired renal function and those

◘ Table 17.8 Anticoagulants for the treatment of acute venous thrombosis and pulmonary embolism

Heparins

Substance	Dosage	
Unfractionated heparin (i.v.)	– Start with 80 IU/kg BW bolus injection – Then continuous infusion of 18 IU/kg BW per hour, adjust infusion rate to aPTT (1.5 to 2.0 times the normal value)	
Enoxaparin (s.c.)	GFR ≥ 30 ml/min – 1 mg/kg BW twice daily	GFR < 30 ml/min – 1 mg/kg BW once daily
Dalteparin (s.c.)	– 100 IU/kg BW twice daily – Alternatively: 200 IU/kg BW (maximum dose 18,000 IU) once daily	
Tinzaparin (s.c.)	– 175 IU/kg BW (maximum dose 20,000 IU) once daily	
Fondaparinux (s.c.)	GFR ≥ 30 ml/min – BW < 50 kg: 5 mg once daily – BW 50–100 kg: 7.5 mg once daily – BW > 100 kg: 10 mg once daily	GFR < 30 ml/min – Contraindicated

Direct oral anticoagulants

Substance	Dosage
Apixaban (Xa inhibitor)	– Start with 10 mg twice daily (first week) – Then 5 mg twice daily
Edoxaban (Xa inhibitor)	– Start with heparin (first 5–10 days) – Then 60 mg once daily – Reduced dose: 30 mg once daily (GFR 15–50 ml/min or BW ≤ 60 kg)
Rivaroxaban	– Start with 15 mg twice/day (for 3 weeks) – Then 20 mg once daily – Reduced dose: 15 mg once daily (in case of increased bleeding risk)
Dabigatran (thrombin inhibitor)	– Start with heparin (first 5–10 days) – Then 150 mg twice daily – Reduced dose: 110 mg twice daily (age ≥ 80 years, concurrent verapamil intake)

aPTT: activated partial thromboplastin time, DTI: direct thrombin inhibitor, GFR: glomerular filtration rate, IU: international units, i.v.: intravenous, BW: body weight, s.c.: subcutaneous, Xa: activated factor X

being treated with strong P-glycoprotein inhibitors (e.g. amiodarone, clarithromycin, ciclosporin, verapamil, and certain protease inhibitors). Carriers of mechanical valve prostheses are also not candidates for DOAC therapy and should be further treated with Vitamin-K-Antagonists (VKA). Furthermore, DOACs are contraindicated in **pregnant patients** and during **lactation**. During pregnancy, a body weight-adjusted dosage of low molecular weight heparin is recommended for the treatment of VTE or PE. Reliable data on Fondaparinux in this context are not yet available.

In patients with PE and evidence of **antiphospholipid antibodies**, DOACs are contraindicated, if there is triple positivity and/or an arterial thrombotic event. Testing for antiphospholipid antibodies is not routinely

17.4 Pulmonary Embolism-Follow-up

- **Duration of Anticoagulation**

Patients who have survived an acute PE are generally at considerable risk for VTE recurrences and the associated morbidity and mortality. In a meta-analysis of 7'515 patients after proximal deep vein VTE or PE—without an identified thrombosis risk factor—the incidence rate of VTE recurrences was 10.3% in the 1st year after discontinuation of anticoagulation, 6.3% in the 2nd year, 3.8% annually in years 3–5, and 3.1% annually in years 5–10 leading to a cumulative incidence of 36% after 10 years. However, if a thrombosis risk factor associated with the initial or "index" event is present, the annual recurrence risk varies greatly depending on whether the triggering or contributing risk factor was strong or weak, temporary or persistent. A classification of the **VTE recurrence risk** according to the **pathogenesis of the initial event** is presented in ◘ Table 17.9.

◘ **Table 17.9** Long-term recurrence risk after pulmonary embolism

Thrombosis risk factor that led to/contributed to the acute event	Clinical examples	Estimated long-term VTE recurrence risk
Strong temporary (reversible) thrombosis risk factor	– Severe trauma with bone fractures – Major surgery, anesthesia duration > 30 min – Bed rest in hospital for at least 3 days due to acute illness or acute exacerbation of a chronic illness	– Low (< 3% annually)
Weak temporary or weak persistent thrombosis risk factor	– Minor surgery, anesthesia duration < 30 min – Hospital admission for < 3 days due to acute illness – Bed rest outside the hospital for ≥ 3 days due to acute illness or acute exacerbation of a chronic illness – Leg injury (without fracture) associated with limited mobility for ≥ 3 days – Estrogen therapy/contraception – Pregnancy or postpartum period – Long-distance flight (or car trip without breaks) – Inflammatory bowel disease – Active autoimmune disease	– Medium (3–8% annually)
No risk factor identified	–	
Strong persistent thrombosis risk factor	– Active cancer – One or more VTE episodes in history – Antiphospholipid syndrome	– High (> 8% annually)

PE: pulmonary embolism, DVT: deep vein thrombosis, VTE: venous thromboembolism

After the initial event of an acute PE, all patients should initially be anticoagulated for at least 3 months. Subsequently, anticoagulation can be discontinued, if the PE was triggered by a strong temporary, reversible thrombosis risk factor. In contrast, for patients with a history of VTE recurrences, known antiphospholipid syndrome, or active cancer, continuation of anticoagulation for an indefinite period is recommended. In all other clinical situations, the decision to continue versus discontinue anticoagulation should be based on a personalized assessment of the recurrence risk without therapy and the bleeding risk on anticoagulation. The improved safety profile (i.e. lower risk of severe bleeding) of DOACs compared to VKAs should be taken into account. In this context, existing recurrence and bleeding scores can also be helpful. These allow semi-quantification of the respective risk and can help identify

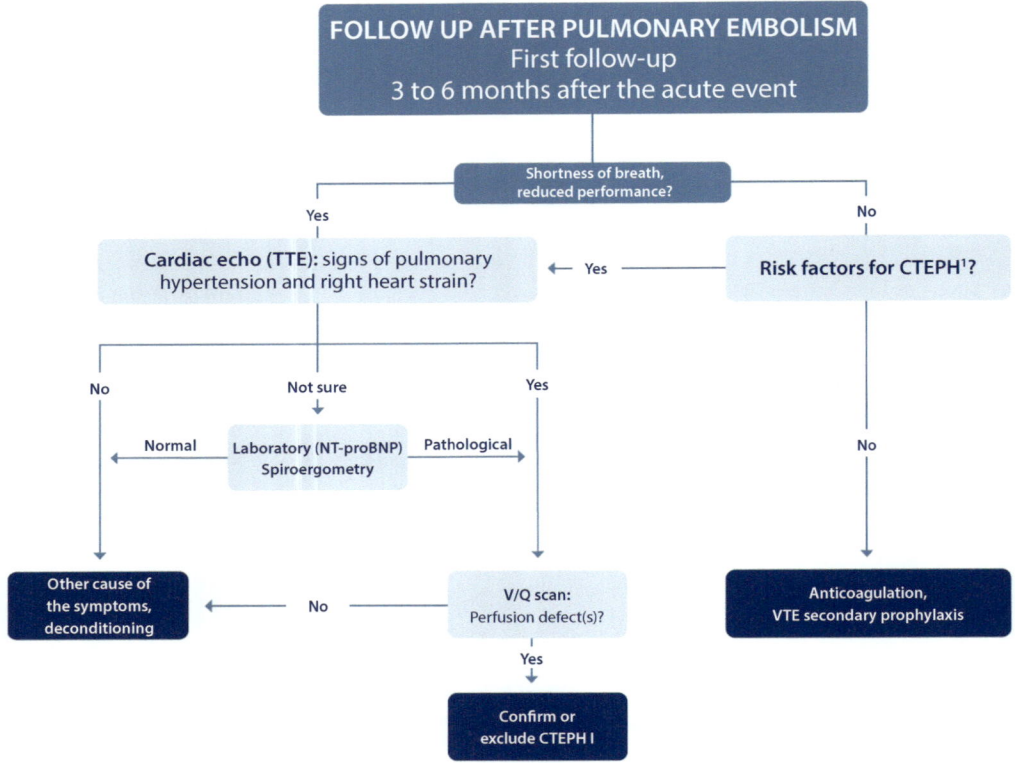

Fig. 17.10 Follow-up of pulmonary embolism. (*CTEPH:* chronic thromboembolic pulmonary hypertension, *NT-proBNP:* N-terminal *pro-brain* natriuretic peptide, *TTE:* transthoracic echocardiography, *V/Q Scan:* ventilation-perfusion lung scan, VTE: venous thromboembolism)
[1]This includes:
- Acute findings: large pulmonary arterial thrombi in the computed tomography pulmonary angiogram, echocardiographic signs of RV strain, signs of chronic, organized thrombi
- Chronic diseases and conditions: history of PE(s) or deep vein VTE(ss), ventriculo-atrial shunts for the treatment of hydrocephalus, infected permanent i.v. accesses or pacemakers, post-splenectomy, thrombophilic conditions (e.g. antiphospholipid syndrome), blood group A or B (not 0), hypothyroidism treated with thyroid hormones, cancer or myeloproliferative diseases, inflammatory bowel diseases, chronic osteomyelitis

potentially reversible and treatable bleeding risk factors.

The recommendation for or against extended anticoagulation should be explicitly explained to the patient, discussed with him or her, and the joint decision documented in the patient's record. The criteria listed in ◘ Table 17.3 provide a decision aid for everyday practice. In case of extended anticoagulation with apixaban or rivaroxaban, the dose should generally be halved (to 2.5 mg BID of apixaban or 10 mg OD rivaroxabany) 6 months after PE. Regular follow-up checks (at least once a year) are recommended for all patients.

- **Early Detection and Treatment of Late Effects**

Apart from assessing the duration and dosage of anticoagulation as well as its monitoring, patient follow-up afteran acute PE has the following goals: **a)** rehabilitation, treatment of comorbidities, modification of cardiovascular risk factors, if necessary, behavioral therapy for patients with persistent symptoms, **b)** early detection of signs of possible chronic thromboembolic pulmonary hypertension (CTEPH) and timely referral to a CTEPH expert center.

The recommended **pulmonary embolism follow-up** is illustrated in ◘ Fig. 17.10 in the form of an algorithm.

GPSR Compliance

The European Union's (EU) General Product Safety Regulation (GPSR) is a set of rules that requires consumer products to be safe and our obligations to ensure this.

If you have any concerns about our products, you can contact us on ProductSafety@springernature.com

In case Publisher is established outside the EU, the EU authorized representative is:

Springer Nature Customer Service Center GmbH
Europaplatz 3
69115 Heidelberg, Germany

Batch number: 08795092

Printed by Printforce, the Netherlands